"Dr. Neal Barnard is a brilliant visionary, one of the leading pioneers in educating the public about the healing power of diet and nutrition. In *Foods That Fight Pain* he offers scientifically based rationales for nutritional therapies to help alleviate the everyday pains for which conventional medicine often has so little to offer. This may be one of the most practical and useful books you will ever read. I highly recommend it."
　—Dean Ornish, M.D., author of *Dr. Dean Ornish's Program for Reversing Heart Disease*

"Neal Barnard's book separates the wheat from the chaff in nutritional literature."
　—Benjamin Spock, M.D.

"If we all were more careful in our choices of food and drink, our health would improve enormously. Dr. Barnard has been advocating healthful nutrition for many years. His message is beginning to be heard."
　—William C. Roberts, editor-in-chief, *American Journal of Cardiology*, and director, Baylor Cardiovascular Institute

"Once again Dr. Barnard is pushing the frontiers of therapeutic nutrition. The science is clearly on his side, and it will be further vindicated by those who follow his altogether sensible and intelligent dietary lifestyle."
　—Hans Diehl, DrHSc, MPH, Lifestyle Medicine Institute

"Dr. Barnard's *Foods that Fight Pain* is an incredibly valuable resource."
　—Ron Cridland, M.D., Health Promotion Clinic

"Dr. Neal Barnard is the only person who has both the scientific background and the knowledge of nutrition to write this book. It will, in a natural way, free many people from pain and eliminate their need for drugs that cause dangerous side effects."
　—Henry J. Heimlich, M.D., president, The Heimlich Institute

Also by Neal Barnard, M.D.

Food for Life
Eat Right, Live Longer

Foods That Fight Pain

Revolutionary New Strategies for Maximum Pain Relief

Neal Barnard, M.D.

with menus and recipes by Jennifer Raymond

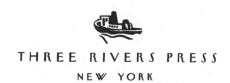

THREE RIVERS PRESS

NEW YORK

Published by Three Rivers Press, New York, New York.
Member of the Crown Publishing Group.

Random House, Inc. New York, Toronto, London, Sydney,
Auckland
www.randomhouse.com

THREE RIVERS PRESS is a registered trademark and
the Three Rivers Press colophon is a trademark of Random
House, Inc.

Originally published in hardcover by Harmony Books in 1998.

Printed in the United States of America

Design by Barbara Balch

Library of Congress Cataloging-in-Publication Data

Barnard, Neal D., 1953–
    Foods that fight pain : Revolutionary new strategies for
maximum pain relief / Neal Barnard, with menus and recipes
by Jennifer Raymond. — 1st ed.
    Includes index.
    1. Pain—Diet therapy. I. Raymond, Jennifer. II. Title.
RB127.B355   1998
616'.0472—dc21   97-43242

ISBN 0-609-80436-7

20 19 18 17 16 15

A Note to the Reader

My goal is to provide you with information on the power of foods for health. However, neither this book nor any other can take the place of individualized medical care or advice. If you have any medical condition, are overweight, or are on medication, please talk with your doctor about how dietary changes, exercise, and other medical treatments can affect your health.

The science of nutrition grows gradually as time goes on, so I encourage you to consult other sources of information, including the references listed in this volume.

With any dietary change, it is important to insure complete nutrition. Be sure to include a source of vitamin B_{12} in your routine, which could include any common multivitamin, fortified soymilk or cereals, or a vitamin B_{12} supplement of five micrograms or more per day.

I wish you the very best of health.

Contents

Acknowledgments   ix

Preface   xi

Introduction: How Foods Fight Pain   1

PART I: CONDITIONS RELATED TO POOR CIRCULATION   5

1 Oh, My Aching Back!   7

2 Dissolving Chest Pain, Cleaning
   Your Arteries   23

PART II: FOOD SENSITIVITIES AND INFLAMMATORY PAIN   39

3 Migraine Knockouts   41

4 Foods for Other Kinds of Headaches   64

5 Cooling Your Joints   72

6 Curing Stomachaches and Digestive
   Problems   97

7 Fibromyalgia   116

PART III: HORMONE-RELATED CONDITIONS   123

8 Using Foods Against Menstrual Pain   125

9 Breast Pain   142

10 Cancer Pain   146

PART IV: METABOLIC AND IMMUNE PROBLEMS 165

11 Carpal Tunnel Syndrome 167

12 Diabetes 173

13 Herpes and Shingles 182

14 Sickle-Cell Anemia 188

15 Kidney Stones and Urinary Infections 192

PART V: ACTIVITY, REST, AND FOOD 201

16 Exercise and Endorphins 203

17 Rest and Sleep 206

18 Yogurt and Corn Dogs: Why Our Bodies Rebel
    Against Certain Foods 211

19 From Laboratory to Kitchen 219

PART VI: MENUS AND RECIPES BY JENNIFER RAYMOND 223

The Elimination Diet 228

Recipes Suitable for the Elimination Diet 234

Low-Fat Recipes Without Cholesterol or Animal
    Protein 254

About Baking Powder 299

Ingredients That May Be New to You 301

Notes 305

Resources 335

Recommended Reading 336

Index 338

Acknowledgments

I owe a debt of gratitude to the many people who made this book possible:

Patti Breitman's clarity of vision, unflagging support, and enormous skill as a literary agent nurtured this project from concept to fruition.

Peter Guzzardi's editorial skill and his rare combination of enthusiasm and objectivity made the writer's task a pleasure.

Jennifer Raymond provided wonderful menus and recipes and also lent her skills as a cooking instructor to our research participants, changing many lives forever.

Andrew Nicholson, M.D., took the lead in the Physicians Committee for Responsible Medicine's research that yielded a new and much improved dietary treatment of diabetes.

Anthony Scialli, M.D., of the Department of Obstetrics and Gynecology at the Georgetown University School of Medicine, shared his expertise in designing and implementing our research on menstrual pain.

Gabe Mirkin, M.D., Diana Rich, and Pat Mill generously allowed us to use their outstanding nutrition-teaching facility for our research.

Donna Hurlock, M.D., Lisa Talev, Miyun Park, Neva Davis, Kathy Savory, Steven Ragland, and Cathy DeLuca devoted many late nights to keeping our research on track, while Tony Perfetto and Quest Diagnostics helped us over many scientific hurdles.

Our research participants put in enormous amounts of time and effort and submitted to examinations, questionnaires, and laboratory tests in order to contribute to our research studies.

David Perlmutter, M.D., a wise and skilled physician, provided many helpful insights on the nutritional approach to migraines.

Richard Wurtman, M.D., of the Massachusetts Institute of Technology; Robert Zurier, M.D., of the Division of Rheumatology at the University of Massachusetts Medical Center; David Eisenberg of Health from the Sun supplement manufacturers of Sunapee, New Hampshire; C. Peter N. Watson, M.D.; and Eduardo Siguel, M.D., Ph.D., generously responded to my numerous questions about research details.

Ellen Moore, Bruce Burdick, and Claire Musickant kindly allowed me to share their experiences to encourage others to look to the power of foods for health.

Dean Buchanan of the Apothecary in Bethesda, Maryland, shared his invaluable knowledge of the power of botanical treatments.

Preface

We all suffer pain from time to time, and for some of us that pain has become a recurring, and sometimes constant, presence in our lives. In this book I would like to offer you an approach to pain that is different—and perhaps more powerful—than anything else you have ever tried. It is based on the premise that foods have medicinal value, a notion that has long been accepted in the medical traditions of China, India, Native America, and other cultures around the world and is now being confirmed by the latest Western medical research.

Foods can fight pain. In the pages ahead, we'll discuss how this works, and specifically which foods or supplements will be most effective for your pain, along with recipes for turning those foods into delicious meals. But for the moment I want to establish something important: There is nothing speculative or far-out about the premise that foods can fight pain. On the contrary. The ideas presented in this book are drawn from a wealth of new research from prestigious medical centers around the world.

Years ago, findings showing that foods work against pain, even pain in its most severe forms, led to tentative and sometimes controversial theories. Physicians and scientists then rigorously investigated these concepts in human research volunteers. Today, after years of testing, discarding, and refining, we have arrived at a revolutionary way of thinking about pain. Research studies have given us the scientific basis not only for why foods work this magic but also how to put it to use. This book translates these powerful new laboratory findings into simple steps that you can use.

Nutrients work against pain in four ways. They can reduce damage at the site of injury, cool your body's inflammatory response, provide analgesia on pain nerves themselves, and even work within the brain to reduce pain sensitivity.

The most important approach for you depends on the kind of pain you have. If you have arthritis, your goal is to stop the joint damage along with the pain. If you have cancer pain or chest pain, you can choose foods to affect the disease process itself. If you have shingles, diabetic nerve pains, or carpal tunnel syndrome, you need to fix a problem within the nerves. If you have a chronic backache, headaches, abdominal pain, or cramps, you just want the pain to disappear. Specific foods can help with all of these.

NEVER TOO LATE

Among the most striking breakthroughs in recent years is the discovery of contributors to back pain. Certainly, back pain is the last thing one would ever associate with foods. It is usually caused by pinched nerves, muscle strains, injuries, and osteoporosis, and so far as most of us are concerned, that has been the end of the story.

Treatment has consisted of anti-inflammatory drugs, heating pads, bed rest, physical therapy, and—all too often—surgery. And virtually every scientific review of back pain treatments found that they simply did not work well for most people.

In 1995, doctors at the University of Washington and the Seattle Veterans Affairs Medical Center reported in *Medical Clinics of North America* that the annual medical costs for low back pain had reached $24 billion, and that the majority of patients seen in back clinics for chronic pain had already had at least two operations. In spite of this enormous expense and the terrible burden to the patient, doctors lamented the poor success rate of surgery in alleviating pain.[1]

In 1996, neurosurgeons from the Johns Hopkins University School of Medicine wrote in the *Journal of Spinal Disorders*, "Despite its high prevalence and the multiple burdens associated with it, low back pain remains poorly understood, inadequately diagnosed, and ineffectively treated."[2]

A whole new perspective came from a close look at the spine itself. Researchers have examined the spines of people with back pain, performing detailed autopsy studies of those who had been treated for back pain and later died from accidents or other causes. They have found that the leathery disks that are supposed to act as cushions between the bony vertebrae have often degenerated. When the disk's tough outer layer disintegrates, its soft interior tissues can squeeze out and pinch a nerve. Sometimes whole disks are destroyed and vertebrae end up crushing against each other.

This was not a surprise; we have long known that degenerated disks can lead to pinched nerves. The news came when researchers looked at why the disks and vertebrae degenerated.

A pair of lumbar arteries carries blood to each vertebra. When these arteries are wide open, they carry oxygen and nutrients to the hardworking backbone. Like every other part of your body—your heart, your brain, your joints, and every other organ and tissue—your back needs a good blood supply in order to heal from the traumas of day-to-day life.

But surprisingly often, these arteries were clogged with plaque. In fact, they had exactly the same kind of blockages that clog the arteries to the heart, causing heart attacks, or to the brain, causing strokes.

When the lumbar arteries are blocked, the oxygen and nutrients that are essential for helping the spine recover from wear and tear are cut off, and the waste products that cells produce begin to build up, irritating sensitive nerves. The autopsy studies clearly showed that the greater the artery blockage, the worse the degeneration of the disks, making it more likely that vertebrae would shift, disks would rupture, and nerves would get pinched, causing chronic pain.

It turns out that one in ten people in Western countries has an advanced blockage in one or more of these arteries *by age twenty.*

If this is all new to you, do not be surprised. No one—not even orthopedic surgeons—knew much about what was causing disks to degenerate until quite recently. But this discovery opened up a fascinating possibility: perhaps improved circulation could prevent back pain. After all, we have learned a lot about how to stop arteries from becoming blocked elsewhere in the body, and there is no reason that we cannot do so in the back.

But it also forced us to ask another question that might be even more important: Can we reopen blocked arteries and restore blood flow to an aching spine?

By the mid-1990s, we already knew that artery blockages could be reversed, at least in other parts of the body. Dr. Dean Ornish, a young Harvard-trained physician, now on the faculty of the University of California at San Francisco, proved beyond any reasonable doubt that if we change our diets enough, and avoid smoking, excessive stress, and sedentary habits, the arteries start to *clean themselves out*. These steps reversed coronary artery blockages in 82 percent of Ornish's research subjects. It also works in the arteries to the legs. The next question— one that researchers are just beginning to tackle—is, will it work in the back, too?

Imagine what that could mean to the millions of people suffering with chronic back pain, and the millions more for whom it is just around the corner. Most people with back pain, however, do not realize what is going on in their lumbar arteries, nor do they know how foods and lifestyle changes might be able to affect them.

We will take a detailed look at this work in progress in chapter 1. I raise it here simply to illustrate a critical point: the old idea that chronic pain is a one-way street is undergoing a dramatic change, and the key comes from understanding how nutrients can help the body's natural restorative processes.

DIFFERENT FOODS FOR DIFFERENT KINDS OF PAIN

Research studies have revealed special effects of certain foods and nutrients, as we will see in detail in the chapters that follow. Rice or peppermint oil, for example, can soothe your digestive tract. Ginger and the herb feverfew can prevent migraines, and coffee sometimes cures them. Natural plant oils can reduce arthritis pain. Cranberry juice can fight the pain of bladder infections. Vitamin B_6 can even increase your pain resistance, to name just a few.

Whether we are talking about back pain, migraines, cancer pain, or anything else, there are three basic principles to using foods to fight pain.

I will spell them out briefly here and, in the chapters that follow, will show you how to apply them.

1. Choose pain-safe foods. In headaches, joint pains, and digestive pains, for example, the key is not so much in adding new foods as in finding out which foods have caused your pain and avoiding them, while building your meals from foods that virtually never cause symptoms for anyone.

In the *Lancet* of October 12, 1991, arthritis researchers announced the results of a carefully controlled study that tested how avoiding certain foods could reduce inflammation. Often the culprits were as seemingly innocent as a glass of milk, a tomato, wheat bread, or eggs. By avoiding specific foods, many patients improved dramatically: pain diminished or went away, and joint stiffness was no longer the routine morning misery. The same benefit has been seen for migraines. While there are also benefits to be gained from certain supplements, particularly natural anti-inflammatory plant oils, identifying your own sensitivities is an enormously important first step.

Sugar may affect pain, at least in certain circumstances. As we will see in chapter 12, researchers at the Veterans Administration Medical Center in Minneapolis tested its effects on a group of young men. They attached a clip to the web of skin between their fingers and wired the clip to an electrical stimulator. They gradually increased the voltage and asked the men to say when they felt any pain and at what point they found it intolerable. As the researchers then infused a dose of sugar, the volunteers found that they could feel the pain sooner and more intensely. The researchers then tested diabetics, who tend to have more sugar in their blood than other people, and found that they too were more sensitive to pain than other people.

What would it mean if some part of your diet, whether it was sugar or anything else, caused pain to hurt just a bit extra, without your realizing what was causing this problem? In fact, many foods trigger pain and aggravate inflammation. Choosing pain-safe foods is as important as bringing the special healing foods in.

2. Add soothing foods that ease your pain. Foods that improve blood flow are of obvious importance in angina, back pain, and leg pains. Foods that relieve inflammation help your joints to cool down. Other foods balance hormones and will come to your rescue if you have men-

strual pain, endometriosis, fibroids, or breast pain. Hormone-adjusting foods have also been the subject of considerable research in cancer, as we will see.

3. Use supplements if you need them. I encourage you to explore the benefits of herbs, extracts, and vitamins that can treat painful conditions. Some have been in use for a long time and have been tested in good research studies, as we will see. Do this under your doctor's care, so that a nutritional approach can be integrated with other medical measures as needed, and so that you have a solid diagnosis.

WHY DIDN'T MY DOCTOR TELL ME?

In presenting the information in this book, I have given particular emphasis to dietary approaches that have been tested in reputable research studies. Science usually begins with anecdotal observations, followed by small research studies that establish the foundation for more controlled studies. I will not avoid these two lines of evidence if that is the best we can do in certain areas, but the better the test, the more confidence we can have that a new approach will actually do what it is supposed to. I have included references to scientific journals for those who would like to refer to them, as well as information about treatments that are just now emerging.

Unfortunately, your doctor is not likely to tell you—and may well not know—most of what you will read in this book. In treating pain, many doctors rely on a restricted range of treatments, while vital research showing what is actually causing the problem and how to correct it often gathers dust in medical libraries.

The fact is, when a shiny nugget of potentially lifesaving information appears in a medical journal, few doctors will ever see it. For even the most conscientious doctors, it is a challenge to keep up with more than a few of the thousands of journals that appear every month, even though the very answers we are seeking might be found there. Only a handful of these journals ever publicize their findings in the popular press. The vital information they hold is simply buried in medical archives.

Of course, it is a very different story when a research study favors the use of a new drug. Then the drug company will hire a public relations firm, pay for massive mailings to physicians, and advertise in medical journals. The company will sponsor medical conferences that highlight the role of the drug and pay speakers to discuss it. Drug companies, motivated by potentially millions of dollars in profits, are skilled at getting a busy doctor's attention. But no industry makes money if you *stop* eating a food that causes your migraines. No surgical supply company makes a cent if you open your arteries naturally through diet and lifestyle. A pharmaceutical company's bottom line does not improve if you use natural anti-inflammatory foods instead of expensive drugs. And without the PR machinery paid for by industry, some of the most important findings never make their way onto a doctor's desk. Patients with arthritis, migraines, menstrual cramps, or even cancer who ask their doctors what they should be eating to regain their health get no answers, simply because no one has brought new information to the doctor's attention.

In spite of the economic forces that often slow progress, we have every reason to be optimistic about the future of medicine. More and more doctors are integrating nutrition into their practices, and scientific journals are responding with reports on its efficacy. Studies in leading allergy journals are showing the links between migraines and food sensitivities, the *Journal of Rheumatology* has published a series of reports on how foods affect the joints, the *Lancet* is reporting the new approaches to back pain and heart disease, and the *Journal of the American Medical Association* confirms the value of something as simple as cranberry juice for bladder infections.

USE WHAT WORKS

When it comes to our health, we simply want what works. Often that means a change in diet, since every hormone, neurotransmitter, and blood cell in your body needs nutrients to do its job. On the other hand, sometimes the best choice is a prescription. Most ulcers, for example, are caused by a bacterial infection, and all the "ulcer diets" in the world are not nearly as effective as two weeks of antibiotics. In fact, I have included information on treating ulcers with drugs just so you can get back to the foods you may have been missing.

Please use the information in this book in consultation with your doctor. If you have pain, you need a diagnosis. No matter what treatment you are choosing, your doctor can clarify your other treatment options, monitor your progress, look out for any adverse effects, and can be educated by you as your symptoms improve.

However, this does not mean surrendering your good judgment. It always pays to get a second opinion—or a third, if necessary—if there is any doubt about the right treatment for your condition.

NO BIG COMMITMENT

As you use the approaches in this book, let me encourage you to focus on the short term. There is no need to make a lifetime commitment to change your diet or anything else. All I ask is that you be willing to explore the power of a dietary approach. In most cases it only takes a couple of weeks to see the beginnings of the wonders it can work for you. Everyone is unique, and what works for one person may not work for someone else. That is as true of nutritional treatments as it is of surgery and medications. But if you focus on the short term, you can give it a really good try. If it works for you, then you'll be motivated to stick with it. Try it; that's all I ask.

Along with doctors from Georgetown University Medical Center and the Physicians Committee for Responsible Medicine, I recently completed a study using very-low-fat diets to balance hormones in women with debilitating menstrual pain. Most of the research subjects were a bit daunted by the idea of making major changes in their diets. However, the fact that they only had to do so for eight weeks (two menstrual cycles) made it much more approachable. For the first two weeks, they tried different recipes, figuring out what to eat at work or at restaurants, gradually adapting to new tastes. As they adjusted to the new diet, they discovered that it helped them lose weight, boosted their energy, and for many, reduced their pain.

After eight weeks, the study required them to return to their previous way of eating to compare the effects of the new diet versus the old. By that time, many of the research subjects did not want to change back. They asked, "Do I really have to return to my old way of eating? Can I keep at least some of the new diet?" The foods they had once loved were quickly forgotten when they found a healthier way to eat. Focusing on the short term makes change easier.

The chapters in this book have been separated into six major sections. We begin with conditions related to poor circulation, including back pain and chest pain. We focus on how to use foods and other factors to restore blood flow and also look at some surprising benefits that certain foods have, apart from their effect on circulation.

In the second section, we see how food sensitivities can trigger migraines and other headaches, arthritis, digestive problems, and fibromyalgia. Again, food sensitivities are not the whole story, and we will also look at how certain foods can help reduce inflammation and other aspects of relieving pain. We will then see how hormones influence menstrual pain, breast pain, and cancer pain, and how foods can affect them. Finally, we will look at metabolic and immune problems, including carpal tunnel syndrome, diabetic pains, herpes sores, shingles, sickle-cell anemia, and kidney stones.

As you will see, these sections overlap considerably. Improving circulation is not only important for your back and your heart; it also helps alleviate diabetic nerve pain. Likewise, information on balancing your hormones that is central to menstrual pain is also important for migraines, arthritis, and carpal tunnel syndrome. You can start anywhere in this book, and each chapter can be read separately. If something from another chapter is important for you to know, I will refer you to it.

We will finish off with sections on exercise, rest, and sleep, and recipes that put the principles of this book to work. Along the way, we will take a look at why it is that certain foods that should be perfectly healthy can cause problems for so many of us.

Let me encourage you to look at all the chapters in this book, beyond whatever symptoms may be of concern right now. The principles for restoring blood flow and using foods to balance hormones, in particular, are critically important for many aspects of how we feel, not to mention how long we live. Also, you may have friends or loved ones who could benefit from the information presented here.

For maximal benefit, please follow the instructions in each chapter as carefully as you would a doctor's prescription. It does not take long to feel the wonderful effects that foods can provide. I hope you enjoy your exploration of the power of foods and wish you the very best of health.

How Foods Fight Pain

Biologically speaking, pain is not a localized event. It is a series of reactions, starting at the site of injury. When someone steps on your toe, your joints flare up, or a migraine kicks in, the injured area then sends a signal through the nervous system to your brain. Only when your brain receives and interprets the signal do you feel any pain. If the injured area or the nerves become inflamed, the damage and pain can intensify.

We can tackle pain at any one of four major links in the chain: the initial injury, the inflammatory response, the pain message traveling through the nerves, and even the brain's perception of pain. In the chapters that follow, we will use each of these strategies, depending on the type of pain you have.

USING FOODS AGAINST INJURY AND IRRITATION

Pain, of course, is an essential part of life. If you could not feel a burn when you touched a hot stove or a bee sting when a swarm surrounded you, a small injury could become a much bigger one. Pain is a danger signal that lets you take quick action. But when pain does not stop, we need to find a way to shut it off.

For many kinds of pain, we aim to stop the local injury. If you have chest pain, for example, your priority is not to keep the nerves from carrying a pain message or to prevent your brain from receiving it. Your goal is to avoid a heart attack or at least limit the damage. Sometimes this requires emergency care, and doctors have many high-tech ways to dissolve clots and crush plaques. As we will see in chapter 2, food and lifestyle changes can, over the long run, rival the power of drugs or surgery in restoring circulation and preventing heart damage.

The same holds true for migraines, sore joints, kidney stones, pains in the digestive tract, and herpes sores, among many other kinds of pain. In each case, diet changes or supplements can help protect against the assault on your tissues. Researchers have also tested how diet affects cancer, with the aim of reducing the risk of painful recurrences.

Foods can not only help prevent these injuries; they can also help shape your body's response. When your joints ache, for example, the pain, stiffness, and even the joint damage itself are caused by an inflammatory response that has gotten out of control. As we will see in chapter 5, inflammation is controlled by natural compounds called prostaglandins, and their chemical relatives, all of which are made from traces of fat that have been stored inside your cells. Some fats tend to fan the flames of inflammation, while others cool them down, and you can tip the balance one way or the other every time you put food on your plate.

Likewise, migraines and menstrual cramps are not caused by trauma. Rather, the chemicals in your body that control pain and inflammation are acting up and need to be brought into better balance. As we will see, sex hormones play a role in these conditions, and possibly in some forms of arthritis, too. Foods have a major influence over the concentration of these hormones in your blood and how active they are.

The goal in each of these situations is not to influence your brain's ability to feel pain, but to stop the damage itself.

FOODS AND NERVE FUNCTION

No matter how much irritation or injury there may be to any part of your body, you feel nothing until the pain message reaches your brain. Pain is carried in fine nerve fibers that lead to the spinal cord, where they connect to other nerve cells leading straight to the brain.

Some strategies for reducing pain focus on the nerves themselves. One example comes from diabetes. Sometimes people who have had this illness for several years develop pains in their legs and feet. This is due either to a toxic effect in the nerves that occurs when blood sugar builds up, or to poor circulation in the tiny blood vessels that nourish the nerves. For most patients, these nerve problems and poor circulation worsen gradually over time. However, recent research shows that a combination of foods and exercises lowers blood sugar, improves circulation, and relieves pain decisively and quickly in most patients.

Likewise, the nerve symptoms of carpal tunnel syndrome have been treated successfully with vitamin B_6, which probably works both on the nerves themselves and in the brain.

Hot chili peppers contain a remarkable substance called *capsaicin,* which is what gives peppers their zing. But more importantly, in the right dose, it blocks the nerves' ability to transmit pain messages. Specifically, it depletes a chemical called substance P, which is the chemical messenger that lets one pain nerve carry its message to another nerve. Capsaicin is the active ingredient in pain ointments that are used for arthritis, shingles, and postmastectomy pain.

By the way, although pain nerves are very fine and rather slow to conduct messages—the country roads of the nervous system—sensory messages of touch and pressure travel in large nerves that carry messages much faster, which is why you know you stubbed your toe or bumped your knee a fraction of a second before the pain actually kicks in.

BOOSTING PAIN RESISTANCE

Your body makes natural painkillers, called *enkephalins* (meaning literally "in the head") and *endorphins* (as in "endogenous morphine"). Enkephalins are made in the adrenals, small glands that sit on top of your kidneys. Endorphins are made in the pituitary gland at the base of your brain. They really do act like morphine. Their principal site of action is within the brain and nerves themselves, and they also travel in your bloodstream.

The active hallucinations that are sometimes reported after near-death experiences have been attributed to endorphins and enkephalins released after trauma and shock.

To manipulate these natural painkillers, we turn to exercise. As we will see in chapter 16, researchers have tested pain tolerance in athletes.

A six-mile run stimulates endorphin release that is roughly equivalent to ten milligrams of morphine, and you can take advantage of endorphins well before you can go this distance.

The amino acid *tryptophan* has been used to reduce pain. In the brain, it produces *serotonin,* a brain chemical that influences pain sensitivity, moods, and sleep. Tryptophan was popular in the United States until a manufacturing contaminant in some batches caused a rare blood disorder, and it was pulled off the market. However, high-carbohydrate foods increase tryptophan concentration in the blood safely and reliably, and they do the same in your brain. For some people, high-carbohydrate foods have a mild antidepressant effect. They can also induce sleep and sometimes reduce pain.

Painkilling drugs, heat, and massage have been around for a long time, and they are helpful in many applications. Acupuncture, long used in Asia, has shaken off the initial skepticism with which it was greeted by Western medicine and has proven its worth. Chiropractic had a harder battle, but has likewise established its role in certain aspects of pain management.

Foods and judiciously chosen nutrient supplements also give us new ways to stop local tissue injury, reduce pain impulses within nerves, and even limit the brain's perception of pain. The remainder of this book details the application of these principles to specific kinds of pain.

PART I

CONDITIONS RELATED TO

POOR CIRCULATION

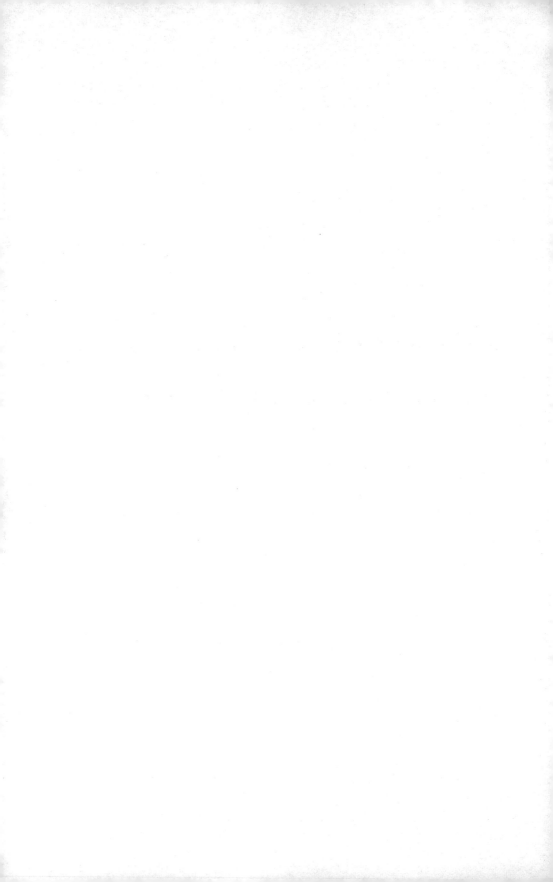

CHAPTER 1

Oh, My Aching Back!

O f all the symptoms that are related to foods, perhaps the most surprising is back pain. After all, we have long assumed that it is caused by heavy lifting, twisting or turning, injuries, sleeping on a soft mattress, osteoporosis, or a disk that has gone bad on its own, but not by anything in our diet. However, surprising new evidence shows that foods may well play a critical role in determining whether your back rebounds from the traumas of day-to-day life or succumbs to them.

Back pain is common. Between 60 and 80 percent of people in Western countries develop significant back pain at some point in their lives, and 20 to 30 percent have it at any given time.[1]

When low back pain lasts only a day or two, it is usually attributed to muscle strain, although there is rarely any identifiable injury or finding on a physical examination that would nail down a diagnosis.[2]

When back pain persists, it can often be traced to a problem in one of the disks, the leathery cushions that separate one vertebra from another. Each disk has a tough outer sheath that covers a soft inner core. If the sheath deteriorates, the interior tissues can herniate outward, pushing on a nerve root or even on the spinal cord itself. The result is pain, numbness, or other nerve symptoms. A break in the disk can also stimulate inflammation, irritating the nerves and causing the back muscles to tighten up in response.[3] About two-thirds of people with persistent back pain have pinched or irritated nerves.

Disk degeneration can also let the vertebrae crush against each other or shift out of line. In a condition called *spinal stenosis*, a degenerated disk lets the vertebrae collapse toward each other, turning and twisting

7

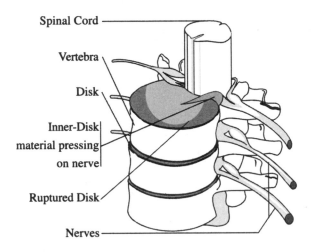

Spinal Cord

Vertebra

Disk

Inner-Disk
material pressing
on nerve

Ruptured Disk

Nerves

The disk's leathery outer shell covers a soft core. If the outer shell breaks, the inner core can squeeze out and press against the nerves as they emerge from the spine. The disk's inner tissues can also spark an inflammatory reaction that irritates the nerves.

in such a way that they narrow the already small bony passageway for the nerves at the bottom of the spinal cord.[4,5]

Sometimes people have pain without any signs of nerve compression or irritation. The pain may come from nerves that have grown into the damaged disks like roots into soil. Normally, pain nerves do not enter past the outer surface of the disk. But researchers examining specimens removed at surgery found that pain nerves sometimes grow into degenerated disks, following blood vessels that grow as part of the repair process.[6]

The changes of rheumatoid arthritis can occur in the spine, a condition called *ankylosing spondylitis*. (*Ankylosing* means stiffening; *spondylitis* means inflammation of the vertebrae.) See chapter 5 for the principles of how foods affect arthritis, including that in the spine. Some cases of back pain are caused by fibromyalgia (see chapter 7) or by complications from previous surgery.

CHILDREN AND BACKACHES

Back pain in children can result from muscle trauma, fractures, infections, tumors, or other conditions. Because some of these conditions require rapid treatment, children with back pain always need to be promptly evaluated by a physician.[7]

Kids can sometimes cause backaches for their parents. Backaches are a frequent symptom in pregnancy and postpartum, especially in mothers who are young, overweight, or who have had back problems in the past. Parenting often leads to sore backs in both men and women, for reasons that are not mysterious.[8] A 1995 study of firefighters and police officers showed that, as hazardous as those professions are, those who also have children are nearly twice as likely to suffer from back problems.[9]

AVOID SURGERY IF YOU CAN

When I was in medical school, I cringed every time I had do a preoperative exam on a patient headed for back surgery. My concern was not just that the surgery—removing a disk, for example—was very invasive. The problem was that many patients seemed to have as much pain after surgery as before, sometimes even more. Some patients came back weeks or months afterward with various complications and had to be operated on again. I am not the only one to have noticed the problem. Although operating on bulging disks may seem sensible and sometimes inevitable, research studies have shown three things:

For many patients, surgery does not reduce their pain. Numerous articles have appeared in medical journals noting that, while sometimes surgery is necessary to prevent nerve damage, in the vast majority of cases it is not and can often make things worse.

Second, researchers who have done X rays, CT scans, and MRIs on perfectly healthy people with no back symptoms at all have found protruding disks and other "abnormalities" in at least 20 percent of them.[10]

Third, damaged disks often improve spontaneously. Even when tissue from the interior of the disk has herniated out, it is often resorbed on its own.[11]

A recent review of eleven countries showed that surgery rates are not determined by how badly operations are needed. The determining factor was the per capita supply of orthopedic surgeons and neurosurgeons, with the United States at the top of the list. The sole exception to this finding was Sweden, where there are plenty of surgeons, but they are paid for a forty- to forty-eight-hour week, not by the operation.

In America, the number of operations for low back pain increased 55 percent from 1979 to 1990, and surgery for spinal stenosis increased by 400 percent during the same period. Surgeons have begun to call for greater use of more conservative measures, reserving surgery for those with persistent or progressive nerve symptoms.[2,10]

STAY ACTIVE, DON'T REST IN BED

Research has visited a similar change of heart on the most traditional and seemingly innocuous recommendation for back pain—a day or two of bed rest. In a 1995 English study, doctors asked twenty patients with acute back pain—pain that had been present for a week or less—to rest in bed for forty-eight hours. They asked a second group to *avoid* any bed rest between 9 A.M. and 9 P.M. Most patients in both groups improved significantly within a week, which is typical in acute back pain episodes. But more patients in the active group had fully recovered in seven days than in the bed-rest group.[12] Other studies have shown the same thing. For most people, bed rest actually slows recovery. By staying active, patients keep the back flexible and improve blood flow.

A research team in Oslo, Norway, decided to prescribe the opposite of bed rest for a group of 463 people whose back problems were serious enough that they needed to take at least eight weeks' absence from work. They were encouraged not to rest, but to stay active and flexible to enhance blood flow to the back and speed up repair. They had to resist the urge to guard their backs too much with inactivity and were told that "the worst thing they could do to their backs was to be too careful." To put this study in perspective, people who have already missed eight weeks of work have a 60 percent chance of still being out after six months. The researchers found, however, that keeping patients active cut that figure to 30 percent.[3] Aerobic exercise has also proven useful for spinal stenosis, replacing the immobilization that was once routine.[5]

Just as many doctors were becoming resigned to the uselessness of their treatments for chronic back pain, we came to find that the body has ways to heal itself. They are not perfect, but when doctors resist the urge to immobilize patients or to operate when it can be avoided, the body can gradually recover in many cases. Indeed, a new, more optimistic view of back problems is emerging, and it comes from a look at the underlying cause.

A NEW UNDERSTANDING OF BACK PAIN

Disks and vertebrae are subjected to minor stresses every time you walk, stand up, sit down, pick something up, or twist suddenly—hundreds of times each day. To recover from this wear and tear, the spine needs a good blood supply to bring in vital oxygen and nutrients and carry away the cells' waste products. This blood supply comes from the lumbar arteries, which branch off of the aorta, the body's main pipeline, as it passes from the heart downward along the spine toward the legs. Arteries bring in oxygen and nutrients, and veins carry away cellular wastes.

Unfortunately, of all the arteries in the human body, the abdominal aorta is among the first to develop *atherosclerotic plaques*, bumps that slowly grow and end up blocking the flow of blood.

A team of researchers in Helsinki, Finland, conducted autopsies on people who had died of various causes unrelated to back pain. They carefully examined the condition of their spines and the arteries that lead to the spine. With surprising frequency, these arteries were blocked. The average person with a history of back pain was found to have two arteries to the lower back completely blocked, and at least one more that was narrowed but not yet blocked. People who had not reported back pain had fewer blockages.[13]

Earlier studies had shown that children already have the beginnings of atherosclerosis in their abdominal arteries by age ten, and that advanced blockages are present in some people—perhaps as many as 10 percent—*by age twenty*. A favorite place for plaques to form is right at the opening of one of the lumbar arteries.[14]

You can predict the results. Vertebrae and disks that would normally be nourished with every heartbeat become increasingly cut off from their normal supply line. They resort to getting whatever oxygen and nutrients they can from smaller blood vessels passing by. The result, researchers believe, is that the disks start to degenerate. At that point, if you pick up a box of books or move too vigorously, without a sturdy, resilient disk in place, vertebrae could begin to shift from their normal position. Or a disk can rupture, spilling its inner core material. Nerves passing by could get pinched. Reduced blood flow also means that waste products accumulate in tissues and irritate sensitive nerve endings.

Could it be that back pain begins not in the back muscles or the spine but in the arteries? Could the same kind of artery blockages that slow blood flow to the heart, leading to a heart attack, or to the brain, causing a stroke, actually encourage the degeneration of the disks and the back pain that results?

Indeed, the Finnish researchers found that people who suffered from chronic back pain had clogged lumbar arteries much more often than people without back pain, and *the greater the blockage, the worse the degeneration in the disk it supplied.*[13,15]

These findings helped explain something that had puzzled spine researchers for a long time: people with back pain tend to have characteristics that point to artery problems, similar to those in heart patients. They are more likely to smoke, to be under stress, and to have other signs of poor circulation, such as pains in the chest and calves.[16–18] Smoking and stress, of course, contribute to clogged arteries, and chest and leg pains are signs that the blockages have already formed.

Here is where foods come in. *Artery blockages are not inevitable. Healthful foods and other lifestyle factors can prevent artery blockages from forming,* and this is as true in the abdominal aorta as it is in the arteries to the heart.

Artery blockages in one part of the body often indicate the same problem elsewhere. A person with blocked arteries in the heart is likely to have them in the arteries to the legs, too. A man who develops impotence in midlife, which is a sign of disrupted blood flow, has a one in four risk of a heart attack or stroke within two years. Impotence is simply a sign that the arterial system is accumulating blockages.

If back pain is the result of clogged lumbar arteries, then preventing these blockages should be a priority. This calls for the same steps that prevent artery blockages in the heart: a low-fat, zero-cholesterol diet, regular physical activity, avoiding tobacco, and keeping stress in bounds. These steps are covered in detail in chapter 2, on chest pain.

A difference in menu partly explains why elderly Japanese-American women have less risk of back pain than their Caucasian counterparts. Those who retain some of the traditional Japanese diet have a menu that is much lower in fat and cholesterol than the typical American diet, because the Japanese diet is much richer in grains (particularly rice), vegetables, and bean products, and much lower in animal products. A study of 645 women living in Hawaii, whose average age was seventy-four, showed that Japanese-Americans have only half the risk of back pain of Caucasian women.[19] Of course, an optimal diet does more than help keep arteries open. It also helps prevent weight problems, arthritis, and osteoporosis, as we will see below, all of which are linked to back problems.

CAN BACK PAIN BE REVERSED?

It makes sense that we could use foods to keep our arteries open and that this might help prevent the degeneration of disks and vertebrae. But this line of research opened up another fascinating possibility. We know that it is possible to *reverse* artery blockages and *improve* blood flow in the vast majority of cases. Dr. Dean Ornish and other researchers have demonstrated this reversal process in the heart, and it has also been shown in the arteries to the legs. So far, researchers have not looked to see whether the same thing happens in the arteries to the back, but there is every reason to believe it does.

If reduced blood flow has caused a buildup of waste products in the tissues, irritating nerve endings and causing pain, then opening these arteries again through diet and lifestyle changes may actually alleviate pain.

Once disks and vertebrae have degenerated, simply reopening the arteries is not likely to restore them (although restoring bones weakened by osteoporosis is possible, as we will shortly see), but it may well prevent further harm. However, further research should examine the possibility that an artery-opening lifestyle, along with the body's natural ability to clean up herniated disk material, can return the spine to better health than might otherwise be possible.

The foods that work in artery-opening research do not include chicken, fish, and "lean" beef. Even at their best, they all have enough cholesterol and fat to keep blockages growing. Grains, vegetables, fruits, and beans, on the other hand, have no cholesterol at all and, in their natural state, almost no fat. As a result, they allow something to happen in your body that never happened before. A low-fat, vegetarian diet, along with mild exercise, avoiding tobacco, and reducing stress, lowers most people's blood cholesterol dramatically, helps prevent artery blockages from growing, and actually allows the arteries' natural healing processes to start cleaning out the accumulated plaque to open them up again. An artery-opening program is presented in chapter 2. It is elegantly simple and very effective.

There is another advantage to an artery-opening menu. It is among the most powerful means of losing weight and of keeping it off over the long run, which provides a tremendous help for an aching back.[17]

By the way, it is not just the foods you bring home from the grocery store that contribute to back pain. The car you carry them in might play a role, too. Certain vibration frequencies aggravate disk problems. While your auto dealer will not give you the figures on vibration, researchers do test them from time to time. The most recent reports, dating from the 1980s, favored Volvo, Subaru, and Peugeot, whose drivers had less risk of disk damage, while drivers of other cars, including all American makes, had a higher risk.[20] Tractors and trucks are in a league of their own, often subjecting the driver to serious vibration.

Dietary factors are not everything when it comes to back problems. Trauma is a frequent contributor to back pain, particularly for those whose jobs demand lifting heavy loads in a warehouse, helping patients in a hospital, participating in sports, or engaging in other rugged activities. However, a good diet and reasonable precautions can help you weather the wear and tear of everyday life.

VITAMIN B₆, TRYPTOPHAN, AND GINGER

Researchers are testing certain nutritional supplements to see if they can help back pain. While these findings are still emerging, they are well worth a closer look.

Vitamin B$_6$, which has long been used to treat carpal tunnel syndrome, has also been used for back pain, and evidence suggests that it helps. It does not relax muscles that are tied up in spasms or restore a damaged disk, but it apparently does increase your pain resistance. When patients who are taking anti-inflammatory drugs add vitamin B$_6$ to their regimen, they get better pain control with less medication.[21]

It may also be useful in preventing a relapse. Researchers using B$_6$, along with other B vitamins, in patients with acute back pain found that it cut the relapse rate in half over the following six months.[22] Large-scale clinical trials have not yet been conducted.

A safe dose of B$_6$ is 50–150 mg per day. Daily doses of 200 mg or higher should be avoided, however, as they are associated with nerve damage.

The amino acid tryptophan may also help. It works by increasing the amount of serotonin in the brain. Serotonin is a natural brain chemical that is important in pain control, sleep, and moods. Researchers at the Veterans Administration Hospital in San Diego, California, gave supplements of a related compound, 5-hydroxytryptophan, to a group of men with chronic back pain due to disk disease. They found a modest but consistent reduction in pain.[23] The same effect was found in healthy subjects given two grams of tryptophan and tested for their perception of experimentally induced pain.[24]

However, tryptophan is not currently available in the United States. It was removed from the market after several cases of an unusual blood disorder and other symptoms were linked with its use. While it appears that the problem was caused not by tryptophan itself but by a manufacturing contaminant, it still cannot be legally sold. The compound 5-hydroxytryptophan is still available. However, it is not a naturally occurring amino acid, so it is more like a drug than a nutritional supplement.

The safest way to boost tryptophan naturally is to eat carbohydrate-rich foods, such as potatoes, rice, pasta, and bread. They naturally stimulate the passage of tryptophan into the brain, where it turns to serotonin automatically. See chapter 7 for more details.

Ginger, the common spice, also appears to help block inflammation in musculoskeletal disorders. It has been found to be useful in arthritis and many other conditions, but controlled trials have not yet been conducted.

The amount used is one-half to one teaspoon (one to two grams) of powdered ginger each day, allowing four to twelve weeks for benefits to appear.[25]

PREVENTING AND REVERSING OSTEOPOROSIS

Bone-thinning osteoporosis can lead to small and not-so-small fractures in the vertebrae. As these breaks progress, the spine can become severely bent forward. Although doctors often turn to calcium supplements or hormone treatments to slow bone loss, another approach addresses the real causes much more directly.

Most cases of osteoporosis have nothing to do with inadequate calcium intake. They are caused by overly rapid calcium loss, which, in turn, is caused by five factors:

1. Animal protein. The protein in fish, poultry, red meat, and eggs tends to leach calcium from the bones. This calcium passes into the bloodstream, then filters through the kidneys into the urine. Plant protein does not appear to have this effect. As a 1994 report in the *American Journal of Clinical Nutrition* showed, when volunteers switched from a typical American diet to a vegetarian diet, their calcium losses were reduced to less than half what they had been.[26] Plant-based diets provide adequate protein without the excesses and help your calcium stay in your bones where it belongs.

2. Sodium. Sodium also tends to encourage calcium to pass through the kidneys. People who reduce their sodium intake to one to two grams per day cut their calcium requirement by an average of 160 mg per day. To do that, avoid salty snack foods and canned goods with added sodium, and keep salt use low on the stove and at the table.[27]

3. Caffeine's diuretic effect causes water to be lost via the kidneys, and calcium goes along with it. If you have more than two cups of coffee per day, have decaf.[28]

4. Tobacco. Smokers lose calcium. A study of identical twins showed that if one twin had been a long-term smoker and the other had not, the smoker had more than a 40 percent higher risk of a fracture.[29]

5. Inactivity. Active people keep calcium in their bones, while sedentary people tend to lose calcium.

Sugar encourages calcium losses as well, although it has not been as extensively studied as the other five factors. As we will see in chapter 15, sugar's effect on calcium is sufficient to increase the risk of calcium oxalate stones in the urinary tract.[30]

Vitamin D is also important, as it controls how efficiently your body absorbs and retains calcium. A few minutes of sunlight on your skin each day normally produces all the vitamin D you need. If you get little or no sun exposure, you can get vitamin D from any multiple vitamin. The recommended dietary allowance is 200 IU (5 mcg) per day.

By controlling these basic factors, you can have an enormous influence on whether calcium stays in your bones or drains out of your body.

BETTER CALCIUM SOURCES

Companies that produce dairy products and calcium supplements would like you to believe that extra calcium is the answer for strong bones. Certainly, your bones need calcium, but adding calcium to your diet does little, if any, good if you are not controlling your calcium losses by avoiding animal protein and paying attention to the other factors noted above.

A landmark research report from the Harvard Nurses' Health Study showed the futility of relying on dairy products to protect the bones. The study followed 77,761 women, aged thirty-four to fifty-nine, over a twelve-year period and found that those who drank three or more glasses of milk per day had no reduction at all in the risk of hip or arm fractures, compared to those who drank little or no milk. In fact, the milk drinkers' fracture rates were slightly *higher.*[31]

Other studies support these findings. Statistics show, ironically enough, that the countries with the highest calcium intakes actually have higher, not lower, risk of osteoporosis, compared to countries with low calcium intakes.

The reason for this apparent contradiction is not so complex. Countries with high calcium intakes are also those with large dairy industries. After about four years of age, dairy cattle are less able to produce the quantities of milk they made when they were younger, and they soon end up as hamburger. Since all countries with dairy industries also have large meat industries, it is the meat consumption that is so common in these

CALCIUM AND MAGNESIUM IN FOODS

	CALCIUM (MG)	MAGNESIUM (MG)
Apricots, raw (3 medium)	15	8
Barley (1 cup)	57	158
Black turtle beans (1 cup, boiled)	103	91
Broccoli (1 cup, boiled)	94	38
Brown rice (1 cup, cooked)	20	86
Brussels sprouts (8 sprouts)	56	32
Butternut squash (1 cup, boiled)	84	60
Chickpeas (1 cup, canned)	80	78
Collards (1 cup, boiled)	358	52
Corn bread (1 2-ounce piece)	133	—
Dates, dried (10 medium)	27	29
English muffin	92	11
Figs, dried (10 medium)	269	111
Great northern beans (1 cup, boiled)	121	88
Green beans (1 cup, boiled)	58	32
Kale (1 cup, boiled)	94	24
Lentils (1 cup, boiled)	37	71
Lima beans (1 cup, boiled)	32	82
Mustard greens (1 cup, boiled)	150	20
Navel orange (1 medium)	56	15
Navy beans (1 cup, boiled)	128	107
Oatmeal, instant (2 packets)	326	70
Orange juice, calcium-fortified (1 cup)	270	—
Peas (1 cup, boiled)	44	62
Pinto beans (1 cup, boiled)	82	95
Raisins (⅔ cup)	53	35
Soybeans (1 cup, boiled)	175	148
Spinach (1 cup, boiled)	244	158
Sweet potato (1 cup, boiled)	70	32
Swiss chard (1 cup, boiled)	102	152
Tofu (½ cup)	258	118
Vegetarian baked beans (1 cup)	128	82
White beans (1 cup, boiled)	161	113

SOURCE: J. A. T. Pennington, *Bowes and Church's Food Values of Portions Commonly Used*, 16th ed. (Philadelphia: J. B. Lippincott, 1994).

countries that gets the blame for their high rates of osteoporosis. Dairy products also contain animal protein, which may encourage the loss of some of the calcium they supply.

It is easy to get plenty of healthful calcium without animal protein. The most healthful sources are green leafy vegetables and legumes, "greens and beans" for short.

Broccoli, brussels sprouts, collards, kale, mustard greens, Swiss chard, and other greens are loaded with highly absorbable calcium. The exception is spinach, which contains a large amount of calcium but tends to hold on to it tenaciously, so you will absorb less of it.

Beans are humble foods, and you might not know that they are loaded with calcium. Actually, more than 100 mg of calcium are in a plate of baked beans. If you prefer chickpeas, tofu, or other beans or bean products, you will find plenty of calcium there, as well. These foods also contain magnesium, which your body uses along with calcium to build bones.

If you are looking for a concentrated calcium source, calcium-fortified orange juice contains roughly 300 mg of calcium per cup in a highly absorbable form. Dairy products do contain calcium, but it is accompanied by animal proteins, lactose sugar, animal growth factors, various drugs and contaminants, and a substantial amount of fat and cholesterol in all but the defatted versions.

When you control your calcium losses, you need much less calcium in your diet. Even so, you do need some. According to the World Health Organization, you should get 400–500 mg of calcium per day. American standards are higher, at 800 mg per day or even more, partly because the meat, salt, caffeine, tobacco, and physical inactivity of American life leads to unnaturally rapid loss of calcium through the kidneys, and also because America's dairy industry has had a major and thoroughly unhelpful influence on health recommendations.

PROTECTING BONES WITHOUT THE RISKS OF HORMONES

If you are a woman, your doctor is likely to recommend estrogen supplements after menopause as a way to slow osteoporosis, although the effect is not much over the long run and is rarely able to stop or reverse it.

Many women find these hormones distasteful because the most commonly prescribed brand, Premarin, is actually made from pregnant mares' urine, from whence comes its name. The well-publicized pictures of tens of thousands of horses chained by the neck on urine production farms are disquieting to say the least. (Other brands are synthetic or plant-derived, but have not been marketed as aggressively as Premarin.)

What has many physicians worried is that estrogens increase the risk of breast cancer. The Harvard Nurses' Health Study found that women taking estrogens have 30 to 80 percent more breast cancer, compared to other women.[32] Adding progesterone derivatives, such as Provera, does not offset this increased risk. Given that the lifetime risk of breast cancer in North American women is already one in eight, anything that increases that risk even further is of obvious concern.

Controlling calcium losses is a much safer strategy. If you already have osteoporosis, there is an additional step that you might consider to reverse it.

REVERSING OSTEOPOROSIS

One of the most exciting breakthroughs in recent research is the discovery that a natural, nonprescription preparation, called natural progesterone, actually helps build healthy new bone where it has been lost.

By a fluke of nature, an exact copy of human progesterone exists in wild yams, soybeans, and certain other plants. The amount in cooked foods is not enough to help, but it is easy for manufacturers to isolate the progesterone and put it into a transdermal skin cream. The progesterone passes through the skin into the bloodstream. It reaches the bone, where it stimulates bone-building cells, called osteoblasts, to build healthy new bone. In one three-year study of postmenopausal women treated with natural progesterone, bone density increased by about 15 percent, which is more than enough to have a major effect on fracture risk.[33]

Many products with "wild yam extract" on their labels do not contain enough progesterone to be of any benefit. However, the most popular brand, called Pro-Gest, does have adequate and effective natural progesterone. It is available from Transitions for Health (800-648-8211).

OSTEOPOROSIS IN MEN

Osteoporosis is less common in men than in women, and its causes are somewhat different. In about half the cases, a specific cause can be identified and addressed:[34]

• Steroid medications, such as prednisone, are a common cause of bone loss and fractures. If you are receiving steroids, you will want to work with your doctor to minimize the dose and to explore other treatments.

• Alcohol can weaken your bones, apparently by reducing the body's ability to make new bone to replace normal losses. The effect is probably only significant if you have more than two drinks per day of spirits, beer, or wine.

• A lower than normal amount of testosterone can encourage osteoporosis. About 40 percent of men over seventy years of age have decreased levels of testosterone.[34]

In many of the remaining cases, the causes are excessive calcium losses and inadequate vitamin D. The first part of the solution is to avoid animal protein, excess salt and caffeine, and tobacco, and to stay physically active. Second, take vitamin D supplements as prescribed by your physician. The usual amount is 200 IU (5 mcg) per day, but may be doubled if you get no sun exposure at all. If you have trouble absorbing calcium due to reduced stomach acid, your doctor can recommend hydrochloric acid supplements.

WHAT TO DO ABOUT COMMON BACK PAIN

1. See your doctor. A good diagnosis is important. Most back pain resolves on its own, but sometimes it can be a sign of infection, cancer, or other serious illness that needs prompt treatment. Seek help immediately if you have new, severe, or acute nerve symptoms, nerve symptoms that progress or involve both sides, or incontinence or difficulty urinating. Back pain in children should always be evaluated promptly.

2. Follow an artery-opening menu and lifestyle, including a low-fat, vegetarian diet, regular exercise, keeping stress within manageable limits, and no smoking, as described in chapter 2. This is important advice for everyone, but especially for those with back pain. Drawing your nutri-

tion from plant sources not only helps you clear away artery blockages, it also helps keep calcium in your bones.

3. Keep salt use to a minimum in food preparation and at the table, consuming only one to two grams daily. If you have more than two cups of coffee per day, use decaffeinated brands. These steps also help keep calcium where it belongs.

4. Follow a regular exercise program, with the guidance of your physician. Exercise reduces pain, strengthens back muscles, helps open arteries, and protects your bones. Bed rest usually does more harm than good for a sore back.

5. Vitamin B_6 (50–150 mg per day) and powdered ginger (one-half to one teaspoon per day or one to two grams) may prove useful adjuncts for back pain. If you wish to try 5-hydroxytryptophan, I recommend doing so under your doctor's supervision, as it remains experimental at this point.

6. Be cautious about surgery, and always get a second opinion. However, in some cases surgery is essential, particularly when your nerves are damaged, and your doctor will evaluate your symptoms with this in mind.

7. Chiropractic treatments can help. While once dismissed by mainstream medicine, controlled studies have supported the use of chiropractic treatments in selected patients with lower back pain.[35,36]

8. Simple painkillers, such as acetaminophen or ibuprofen, can be helpful. In general, it is wise to avoid narcotic painkillers in treating back pain. Narcotics have an important place in treating cancer pain, where they are prescribed on an ongoing basis, so withdrawal is not an issue. They are also useful in sickle-cell crises, where they are used briefly. Back pain, however, can be persistent and recurrent, setting the stage for narcotic addiction.

9. Natural progesterone can be used to reverse osteoporosis in women. Transdermal creams, such as Pro-Gest, are most convenient. The normal dose is to use up a two-ounce jar over two to three weeks each month, spreading it on areas of thin skin, then stop until the beginning of the next month.

CHAPTER 2

Dissolving Chest Pain, Cleaning Your Arteries

We used to think of chest pain as a chronic condition requiring endless prescription medicines, ending too often with a trip to the operating room. As arteries that supply blood to the heart muscle gradually become blocked by plaques of cholesterol, fat, cells, and debris, the heart muscle starves for oxygen. Drugs might reduce the pain temporarily, but sooner or later a bypass operation or a plaque-busting angioplasty is necessary to restore blood flow to the heart. The alternative is a heart attack.

Heart bypass surgery is now routine in Western countries, even at the risk that some will not survive the procedure. In about 6 percent of cases, it causes brain damage.[1] And it is only temporary. Within six to eight years, repeat surgery is needed to clean out the arteries again.

From this dismal scenario much more attractive choices have emerged. In this chapter, we will see how foods can cut your cholesterol dramatically. Garlic, oats, soy products, and oddly enough, beans and walnuts are some of the foods that have shown this effect in research studies.

But the most important advance, by far, is research showing that a four-step program of simple diet and lifestyle changes actually lets the arteries begin to *clean themselves out*, without medication or surgery. Chest pain melts away, and blockages in the arteries actually shrink noticeably within the first year.

Researchers first showed that blockages can be reversed in the arteries to the legs. This was important because blockages in these arteries

23

lead to muscle pains after even a short walk, a condition called *claudication*. But more importantly, if it is possible to reverse blockages in the leg arteries, that means it can be done in other arteries, too, even in the heart itself.

Dr. Dean Ornish, a young, Harvard-trained physician, showed that, indeed, heart disease can be reversed. His research papers in the *Lancet* in 1990 and the *Journal of the American Medical Association* in 1995 are now milestones of modern medicine.[2,3] Dr. Ornish's research subjects were heart patients in the San Francisco Bay area. The control group was asked to follow the instructions of their regular doctors. In most cases, that meant favoring fish and chicken over red meat, taking the skin off the chicken before cooking it, quitting smoking, and trying to stay active.

A second group of patients got a completely different program. They were asked to follow a vegetarian diet, which meant spaghetti marinara, minestrone, bean burritos, vegetable chili, rice pilaf, etc., but no red meat, poultry, or fish. The goal was to essentially eliminate animal fat and cholesterol. This was new for them, but they were given classes in how to prepare meals and some prepared foods to take home. They were also asked not to smoke, to take a half-hour walk each day (or an hour three times a week), and to practice stress management exercises, such as yoga or meditation.

A year later, each patient had an angiogram, a special X ray that measures artery blockages. The results were then compared to the same test done at the beginning of the study. The findings made medical history. The patients in the first group, who had been eating skinless chicken breast and fish day after day, were not getting better. In fact, the average patient was actually worse off after a year than at the beginning of the study. Their artery blockages were continuing to grow, even though they had followed their doctors' advice. Regrettably, these results confirmed that the old-fashioned "heart diet" is simply too weak to stop artery blockages from progressing.

The second group, however, had a completely different experience. When their angiograms were put on the viewing screen and their blockages were measured, it was clear that something new was happening in their arteries. They were actually starting to *clean themselves out*, so much so that *the difference was clearly visible in 82 percent of patients in the first year.*

This wonderful result was achieved without medications or surgery. Their artery blockages shrank simply by using vegetarian foods, along with mild regular exercise, stress management, and no smoking.

Their chest pain went away long before the year was up. Within a matter of weeks, in fact, the pain diminished and eventually disappeared. They also lost weight—more than twenty pounds, on average—and felt more energetic than they had in years.

AND THE PATIENTS LOVE IT

When these results first appeared, some questioned how easy it was to follow this kind of diet, saying it really didn't matter how well it worked if it was too arduous. I examined that question in a study with Dr. Ornish and his colleague Dr. Larry Scherwitz. We interviewed all the subjects in both original groups, using quantitative measures of how well the subjects liked the food, how much effort was required to prepare it, how their families reacted, whether they would prefer the diet or prescription drugs, and whether they planned to stick with the new foods in the future.

The results were revealing. At first, the vegetarian group did grumble a bit about their diet. They had to learn new ways of thinking about food and new cooking techniques, and it took about six weeks for them to feel really comfortable with them. However, they also found that their tastes changed. They came to appreciate subtle flavors and began to really enjoy the new foods.

Their experience was rather like people who switch from whole milk to skim. At first, most people find that skim milk seems watery and unpalatable, but in a few weeks they adjust. At that point, whole milk seems much too thick, a bit like paint. This is not to say that skim milk should be part of a heart diet, since all dairy products have disadvantages,* but I raise this common experience simply to illustrate how quickly we can adapt to lower-fat foods and new tastes.

What surprised me was the reaction of the control group that had been eating chicken, fish, and "lean" meats. They grumbled about their

---

*Although skim milk eliminates dairy fat, it does not eliminate dairy proteins, lactose sugar, or contaminants. Dairy proteins tend to raise cholesterol levels, compared to plant proteins. Related health effects are summarized on pages 103 and 213.

diet, too. Several reported that the pleasures of life were gone, that they were eating nothing but chicken and fish night after night. Most importantly, they were getting little reward for all their effort. They still needed medication and still had pain.[4]

The moral of the story is that people grumble about *any* change in their routine, but after a few weeks they adapt to it. And if the change brings major rewards, people want to stick with it. So doctors might as well prescribe the more powerful diet—the vegetarian diet—rather than the old "heart diet" that is little more than a placebo.

During the interviews, several patients wanted me to know how much the new diet meant to them. One, whose cholesterol dropped from 250 to around 100 with the diet, emphasized that doctors should never assume that patients are unwilling to try something new. "Too many doctors have projected their own values onto other people who don't share them," he said. Another said, "I'm amazed at what it's done for me. I'd recommend it to anyone."

In this chapter, I will show you how these powerful, artery-opening steps work, and how easy it is to get started. If you are even the slightest bit hesitant, let me encourage you to try this approach for just three weeks. That is not enough time to see the full effect, but it is enough for the benefits to begin. You may well be surprised at how powerful they can be.

USING YOUR NATURAL HEALING PROCESSES

Your arteries are ready to clean out the accumulated plaques, at least to a degree. But this will never happen if your blood is loaded with particles of cholesterol and fat that stop your natural healing mechanisms from working. Simple changes in food choices can stop that constant irritation and let the healing begin.

To see the importance of this, let's take a closer look at what cholesterol and fat do in the body and why the diet change works so well.

NO-CHOLESTEROL FOODS

A small amount of cholesterol is normally made by your liver for use as a kind of cement that holds cell membranes together. It is also a raw material for building hormones, such as estrogen and testosterone. However, even a small increase in the number of cholesterol particles in your blood encourages the growth of plaques in the arteries. Cholesterol enters the artery wall, stimulating the overgrowth of the muscle cells that are there to strengthen it, like steel bands on a tire. In meat-eating cultures, this process begins during childhood and progresses slowly but surely until artery blockages bring the patient into the emergency room.

Certain foods actually contain cholesterol, and others stimulate the liver to make extra cholesterol. The result is that you will have too much of this "cement" in your bloodstream. It ends up where it does not belong—in plaques that look like raised bumps on the walls of your arteries, which gradually block the flow of blood.[5-7]

The cholesterol in foods comes from animal products. Chickens, cows, fish, and all other animals have livers, just as you do, and they have been busily making cholesterol and packing it into their cells. So any animal product on your plate—meat, milk, eggs, or any other animal tissue— adds some of the animal's cholesterol to your own.

Here is how the cholesterol you eat affects the cholesterol in your blood: Four ounces of beef contains roughly 100 mg of cholesterol. And every 100 mg of cholesterol in your daily routine adds about 5 points to your blood cholesterol level (that is 5 mg per deciliter, or 0.1 millimoles per liter for those using the new international system). Most people consume 500–600 mg of cholesterol every day, which is good for roughly 25–30 extra points (0.5–0.6 millimoles per liter) on their blood cholesterol level. This is the effect of the cholesterol alone. The fat in foods adds to this problem, and we'll see what it does shortly.

Four ounces of beef is a small serving, about the size of a pack of cigarettes. But what may be more surprising is that *chicken contains about the same amount of cholesterol as beef.* Chicken can be slightly lower in fat, depending on how it is prepared, but every four-ounce serving of chicken holds close to 100 mg of cholesterol. You will also find 100 mg of cholesterol in three cups of whole milk, or in just half an egg.

On the other hand, since plants have no liver to make cholesterol, there is no cholesterol at all in any foods from plants. There is no cholesterol in spaghetti noodles, tomatoes, baked beans, bananas, broccoli, cantaloupes, or any other plant food. This is the first reason why you want plant foods to replace animal products on your plate. The second, and more important, reason relates to fat.

KEEPING FATS TO A MINIMUM

When I was growing up in North Dakota, my mother used to fry strips of bacon to serve with eggs and toast. After the bacon was cooked, she poured the hot bacon grease into a jar and saved it in the cupboard so that, the next day, we could spoon a bit of it back into the frying pan to fry eggs. As bacon grease cools, it turns into a waxy solid, which is a sign that it is loaded with *saturated fat.* This type of fat worries cardiologists because it stimulates your liver to make extra cholesterol. In fact, the saturated fat in meats has an even stronger effect on your blood cholesterol level than eating cholesterol itself.

Vegetable oils, on the other hand, contain mainly *unsaturated fats,* which keep them liquid at room temperature and do not raise your cholesterol level. Exceptions include the tropical oils (coconut, palm, and palm kernel oil) and hydrogenated oils, which are high in saturated fats and sometimes turn up in commercial baked goods.

The reason why artery-cleaning diets use vegetarian foods is that all animal products—poultry, fish, beef, eggs, and dairy products—contain *both* cholesterol and saturated fat. Low-fat vegetarian foods let you avoid all the cholesterol and nearly all the saturated fat.

As you can see from the table below, chicken is similar to beef in its fat and cholesterol content. Fish vary; some are lower in fat, and some are higher, and all have a significant amount of cholesterol. But plant foods are in a league of their own. Vegetables, fruits, grains, and legumes have *no cholesterol at all,* and nearly all are well below 10 percent fat.

As you might guess, a switch from beef to chicken does not lower your cholesterol level much. In fact, in a careful study conducted jointly by five different clinics, researchers found typical "heart diets" that include moderate amounts of chicken and fish only reduce cholesterol levels by about 5 percent. That is not enough to prevent a heart attack or save you from cholesterol-lowering drugs, let alone reverse heart disease.[8]

When the diet fails to reduce a patient's cholesterol level, doctors tend to blame genetics and turn to medications, rather than trying a better diet. But all heart patients deserve to try a vegetarian diet. For most patients, even a few weeks will begin to show how well it works. Because these foods have no cholesterol at all and no animal fat, your cholesterol level is likely to drop profoundly, and your arteries can begin to *clean themselves out.*

ANIMAL PRODUCTS VS. PLANT FOODS: NO CONTEST

	FAT (% OF CALORIES)	CHOLESTEROL (MG)
Beef top round, lean, 4 oz.	25	103
Pork tenderloin, lean, 4 oz.	26	106
Chicken breast, skinless, 4 oz.	23	97
Turkey breast, skinless, 4 oz.	18	79
Halibut, 4 oz.	19	47
Chinook salmon, 4 oz.	52	96
Baked beans	4	0
Cauliflower	6	0
Lentils	3	0
Potato	1	0
Rice	2	0
Spaghetti noodles	4	0
Spinach	9	0
Sweet potato	1	0

SOURCE: J. A. T. Pennington, *Bowes and Church's Food Values of Portions Commonly Used,* 16th ed. (Philadelphia: J. B. Lippincott, 1994).

Try the simple guidelines below for three weeks. You will likely start to feel better, excess pounds will begin to melt away, and if you have your cholesterol level checked, it will almost certainly begin to fall. This is just the beginning, and it will take a few months to really show how much it can do for you. The recipes in the back of this book will make the transition easy. They come from Jennifer Raymond, with whom I have collaborated on several other books and who is a cooking instructor in Dr. Ornish's remarkable program.

HOW TO PLAN YOUR ARTERY-OPENING MEALS

Planning a heart-healthy menu is easy, and your arteries will do the rest.

1. Base your meals on these four food groups:

grains: rice, pasta, bread, oatmeal, cereal, etc.

legumes: beans, peas, chickpeas, and lentils

vegetables: asparagus, broccoli, carrots, cauliflower, potatoes, spinach, sweet potatoes, Swiss chard, etc.

fruits: apples, bananas, oranges, pears, strawberries, etc.

2. Avoid all animal products. Meats, poultry, fish, eggs, and dairy products all contain cholesterol and nearly all are high in fat. It is important to avoid them *completely.* Including even small amounts can have a surprising effect on your cholesterol, not to mention their tendency to seduce your taste buds toward fattier tastes.

3. Keep vegetable oils to a minimum. Cooking oils, shortening, and salad oils sneak into foods and can contribute fats that raise your cholesterol level. Even though vegetable oils are better than animal fat, they do contain some saturated fat, because all fats and oils are mixtures.

While we tend to think of olive oil and other oils as pure (and even "virgin"), keep in mind that they are highly concentrated and biologically unnatural. Olive oil is made by extracting the oil from thousands of olives and discarding the pulp. Corn oil is, likewise, extracted from many ears of corn, leaving behind their complex carbohydrates, fiber, and protein. They can affect your cholesterol level if used in more than modest amounts.

4. To insure complete nutrition, it is important to have a source of vitamin B_{12}, which could include any common multivitamin, fortified soymilk or cereals, or a vitamin B_{12} supplement of 5 mcg or more per day.

To turn these guidelines into meals, some people like to keep things basic and familiar: salads, baked beans, mashed potatoes, green beans, broccoli, or lentil, vegetable, or split pea soup. Some like to take advantage of the meat substitutes that have appeared in grocery stores in recent years: burgers, hot dogs, and sandwich "meats," all made from various soy and wheat derivatives. Others prefer "ethnic" cuisine: minestrone, spaghetti marinara, pasta *e fagioli,* Mexican bean burritos with Spanish rice, curries, Middle Eastern hummus, vegetable sushi, etc.

If fatty toppings are your nemesis, you'll find no shortage of healthier choices. Have jam or cinnamon on toast instead of butter or margarine. Try Dijon mustard on a baked potato. Look at the range of fat-free salad dressings on supermarket shelves. Be sure to read labels on commercially prepared foods. Hydrogenated and partially hydrogenated oils in snack foods, baked goods, and margarines behave like animal fats and will increase your cholesterol level.

HOW MUCH IS SATURATED FAT?

Figures show how much of the fat in each product is saturated:

ANIMAL FATS		VEGETABLE OILS		TROPICAL OILS	
Beef tallow	50%	Canola oil	7%	Coconut oil	87%
Chicken fat	30	Corn oil	13	Palm kernel oil	82
Pork fat (lard)	39	Cottonseed oil	26	Palm oil	49
Turkey fat	30	Olive oil	13		
		Peanut oil	17		
		Safflower oil	9		
		Sesame oil	14		
		Soybean oil	15		
		Sunflower oil	10		

SOURCE: J. A. T. Pennington, *Bowes and Church's Food Values of Portions Commonly Used*, 16th Ed. (Philadelphia: J. B. Lippincott, 1994).

FOODS WITH SPECIAL EFFECTS

Certain foods have special effects, lowering your cholesterol even further and protecting against the damage that cholesterol can cause. They are not a substitute for the low-fat, vegetarian diet that is essential for cleaning away artery blockages, but they can add to its benefits.

• Oat products contain *soluble fiber* that lowers cholesterol levels. Soluble fiber is also found in beans, barley, vegetables, and fruits. A four-ounce serving of beans every day cuts cholesterol levels significantly.[9]

• Soy products have a special cholesterol-lowering effect, apart from the fact that they have no cholesterol or animal fat. If your burger is made of soybeans instead of beef, you'll skip all the animal fat and cholesterol and get soy's extra cholesterol-lowering benefit in the bargain.[10]

• Garlic lowers cholesterol, and a little bit goes a long way. The effect amount is one-half to one clove per day.[11]

• Walnuts have a special cholesterol-lowering effect. They are as high in fat as any other nut, but somehow they have redeemed themselves with an ability to reduce cholesterol levels that has not been fully explained. The amount shown to work in research studies is three ounces a day for four weeks.[12]

• Foods that are rich in beta-carotene, vitamin E, and vitamin C can reduce the damaging effects of cholesterol in your blood.[13] They do this, believe it or not, by protecting cholesterol particles from being damaged as they travel in the blood. Damaged cholesterol particles end up being absorbed into the artery wall, which is actually how plaques start in the first place. If cholesterol is allowed to go to where it belongs without being damaged in transit, as it were, the risk of blockage formation is less. Orange vegetables, such as carrots, sweet potatoes, and pumpkins, are rich in beta-carotene, as are green, leafy vegetables. Grains, vegetables, and beans are rich in vitamin E. Citrus fruits, like many other fruits and vegetables, are rich in vitamin C.

• Be careful about iron. Iron accelerates heart disease, apparently by acting as a catalyst for the production of free radicals that can damage cholesterol and increase the risk of plaque formation.[14,15] Your red blood cells do need some iron to carry oxygen, but excesses can be risky.

There are advantages to getting your iron from plant sources— green, leafy vegetables and legumes—rather than from meat. The iron in plant products is in a form that your body can absorb more of when it is low in iron, and less of when it already has plenty. Meat, on the other hand, contains a form of iron called *heme iron*, which defies the body's attempts to regulate it. It passes into the bloodstream even when you already have more than enough, as most men and postmenopausal women do. A recent Harvard study showed that the iron in meat increases the risk of heart problems, while iron from plant sources does not.[15] See page 91 for guidelines on how to check your iron level and what to do about it.

• Certain B vitamins can help prevent heart attacks. Vitamins B_6, B_{12}, and folic acid help break down an amino acid called *homocysteine*, which tends to build up in the blood in some people and encourages artery blockages. A study of American physicians found that those in the top 5 percent of homocysteine levels had triple the risk of a heart attack, compared to those with lower levels. Researchers are still defining what is a dangerous homocysteine level, but numbers above 12 micromoles per liter are likely to be considered high.[16,17]

Beans, vegetables, and fruits are rich in folic acid and vitamin B_6. Typical daily multiple vitamins provide an adequate amount of these vitamins, along with vitamin B_{12}. Animal products are very low in folic acid and are actually high in an amino acid called methionine, which produces the dangerous homocysteine.

UNDERSTANDING THE MEDICAL TERMS

Angina means chest pain caused by an inadequate blood supply to the heart.

Atherosclerosis, sometimes called hardening of the arteries, is when small bumps, or *plaques,* made of cholesterol, fat, and overgrowing cells, form inside your arteries, slowing the flow of blood.

Claudication means leg pains that come when the arteries to the legs are blocked by plaques. It comes when you walk or climb the stairs, and it usually goes away when you rest. Blockages in the leg arteries have been shown to be reversible, just as blockages in the coronary arteries are.

Coronary arteries nourish the heart muscle. Their name comes from the fact that they ring the heart like a crown.

A *myocardial infarction* is a heart attack. The coronary arteries become blocked and a portion of the heart muscle dies from lack of oxygen.

A *stroke* is when a part of the brain dies due to a blockage or break in the arteries.

CHECKING YOUR CHOLESTEROL LEVEL

A cholesterol test can help predict your risk of heart problems. Keep in mind, however:

• A cholesterol test is not perfect. It is a general indicator of risk, not an infallible measure.

• Cholesterol tests do not predict anything other than heart disease. A low cholesterol level is not a reason to dig into chicken wings and fish sandwiches. Colon, breast, and prostate cancer, diabetes, gallstones, weight problems, and many other conditions are linked to the same fatty foods that cause heart problems, and a low cholesterol level indicates nothing about your risk for these conditions.

• Cholesterol in the foods you eat increases your risk of artery blockages, apart from its effect on the amount of cholesterol in your blood. A long-term study examined men working at the Western Electric Company near Chicago, starting in 1957 and 1958 and running for the next twenty-five years. Researchers found that those whose meals contained more cholesterol were much more likely to die of heart disease—as much as twice as likely—*regardless of their blood cholesterol level.*[7] The take-home message is that it is always good to avoid eating foods that contain cholesterol—that is, animal products—whatever your blood cholesterol level may be.

• In addition to checking your total cholesterol, your doctor will also check how much of your cholesterol is in the form of high-density lipoprotein (HDL). HDL particles are the form of cholesterol your body uses to transport it for elimination. It is sometimes called good cholesterol, because it is leaving your body. If your HDL level is low, this means that the cholesterol in your blood is staying around for a while. Happily, you can change that. Exercise and vitamin C–rich foods can increase the amount that is in the "good" HDL form. Smoking and being overweight tend to reduce HDL.[18,19]

Do not be alarmed if a healthy, vegetarian diet reduces your HDL along with the other forms of cholesterol. It simply means that you have less cholesterol in your body, so there is less cholesterol leaving. The fraction of your total cholesterol that is in the HDL form is likely to improve.

• There is no "good" cholesterol in foods. Cholesterol in foods is always a disadvantage. The HDL in your blood is considered "good" only because it is leaving your body.

• Triglycerides are special fat molecules that are built in your liver and travel in your bloodstream. At high levels, they increase the risk of heart problems. Foods can help you lower them. Low-fat diets generally reduce triglycerides along with cholesterol levels, and beans, other legumes, and garlic have a special triglyceride-lowering effect.[9] Exercise and losing weight also lower triglycerides.[19] Sugars, including natural fruit sugars, can raise triglycerides.

HOW TO READ YOUR CHOLESTEROL TEST

Doctors will first check your total cholesterol level—that is, the combined amount of all the different types of cholesterol in your blood. Here is a thumbnail guide to interpreting the results. U.S. authorities measure cholesterol levels in milligrams per deciliter. Most other countries use a different unit, millimoles per liter, which is listed in parentheses.

> Above 240 mg/dl (6.2 mmol/l): High risk
> 200–240 mg/dl (5.2–6.2 mmol/l): Above-average risk
> 205 mg/dl (5.3 mmol/l): Average for U.S. adults
> 150 mg/dl (3.9 mmol/l) or less: Very low risk

If your total cholesterol level is 150 mg per deciliter (3.9 mmol per liter) or below, your risk of heart problems is extremely low. Your goal should be to have your blood cholesterol level in this range, not at the arbitrary levels set by government authorities (e.g., 200 mg/dl or 5.2 mmol/l), which offer no protection at all.

If your total cholesterol is higher than 150, your doctor will check how much of your cholesterol is in the form of high-density lipoprotein (HDL). Ideally the HDL level should be about one-third of the total. For most North Americans, only about 20 percent of their total cholesterol is HDL. This means that not enough of the cholesterol in your body is leaving.

Triglyceride levels above 150 mg/dl (1.7 mmol/l) are considered high and add to your risk of heart problems.

HOW MUCH OF YOUR CHOLESTEROL IS "GOOD" CHOLESTEROL?

The following figures, from the Framingham Heart Study, show for various groups how much of the total cholesterol is in the HDL form.[20] HDL is the "good" form of cholesterol that is leaving the body.

Average male with heart disease	17%
Average female with heart disease	19
Average male without heart disease	20
Average female without heart disease	23
Average Boston Marathon runner	29
Ideal	near 33
Average vegetarian	34

NIACIN WHEN YOU NEED IT

If you have followed a perfect vegetarian diet, have been generous with beans, vegetables, and grains, have been vigilant about hidden fats in pastries and snack foods, and still have a high cholesterol level, you are no doubt wondering if you should take additional steps. Between 5 and 10 percent of people with high cholesterol levels can blame the problem on genetics. If you are in this group, the best diet in the world will not overpower your liver's tendency to make cholesterol.

Do not assume that your problem is genetic, however, until you have tested yourself by following a diet that avoids animal products completely and keeps vegetable oils to a bare minimum. After six to eight weeks, a cholesterol test will show whether you are improving. Even small deviations from a vegetarian diet can cause cholesterol levels to climb in many people.

If your problem *is* genetic, avoiding cholesterol and fat in your diet is still a good idea. Evidence shows that consuming less cholesterol reduces your risk of heart problems, *even if your blood cholesterol level does not decrease.*[7] It also reduces your risk of many other health problems.

If you are considering medications, at the top of the list is vitamin B_3, or niacin. Its benefits are now well established. It reduces total cholesterol levels by 15–20 percent, cuts triglycerides by 20–50 percent, and increases HDL (the good cholesterol) by 15–20 percent.[21]

Niacin treatment usually begins at doses of 100–250 mg one to three times a day with meals and is gradually increased. Most people need one to three grams per day, split between two to three doses.

Its major side effect is an uncomfortable flushing or itching that occurs in almost everyone who takes it. These effects gradually diminish over time and can be further reduced by taking niacin with meals, using aspirin, and avoiding alcohol and hot liquids at the time you take it.

Less commonly, niacin can cause liver problems, gastritis, and gout and can aggravate diabetes. These effects are much more common at doses higher than three grams per day, and particularly when sustained-release varieties are used.[21,22]

Niacin should be used as an addition to a low-fat, vegetarian diet, never as a replacement for it.

PUTTING IT ALL TOGETHER

While changing your diet is the cornerstone of opening your arteries, here are the other parts of the program:

• Physical activity: Heart disease reversal programs prescribe a brisk walk for a half hour each day or an hour three times per week. You can substitute any equivalent activity. If you have chest pain or any history of heart problems, or if you are over forty, check with your doctor before increasing your activity level. Exercise puts added strain on your heart.

As you begin, you are likely to feel more energetic and to want to push yourself a bit. Resist this urge until your doctor gives you the okay. One of the great dangers for recovering heart patients is doing too much too soon.

• Smoking cessation: Smoking poisons your arteries. When you quit, your heart risk drops back to normal quickly, within one year.[20] Whether you use nicotine gum or patches or simply quit on your own, keep trying until you succeed. I myself smoked cigarettes for a few years and soon learned how difficult it is to stop. Keep trying. Once you get a week or two as a nonsmoker under your belt, it will get easier, and ultimately you will succeed.

• Stress reduction: Emotional stress causes the fight-or-flight hormones to be released into your blood. They can increase your cholesterol level and your risk of heart disease.[20] Stress-reducing exercises are described in chapter 17.

• Controlling your blood pressure: High blood pressure increases the tendency for blockages to form in the arteries, and bringing it down is essential. Cutting down on salt helps a little, but the basic artery-opening diet presented above is actually even more powerful for lowering your blood pressure. Many people on medications for high blood pressure in research studies no longer require them when they switch to a low-fat, vegetarian diet.[23,24] No one knows exactly why it works so well, but it is probably because cutting out meat, dairy products, and added fats reduces the viscosity (or "thickness") of the blood, which in turn brings down blood pressure.[25]

If you are on medications for high blood pressure, you will likely need less—or perhaps none at all—if you follow this artery-opening program. Do not stop them on your own, however. Let your doctor monitor your blood pressure and guide you in your use of medicines.

FREE OF PAIN

If chest pain has you on a tether, it is time to free yourself. By making the right kind of diet and lifestyle changes, even long-standing artery blockages can be reversed. It does not matter how old you are. Whether you are in your forties or your nineties, you can reverse your heart disease, dissolve your pain, and begin to enjoy a full life again.

PART II

FOOD SENSITIVITIES AND

INFLAMMATORY PAIN

CHAPTER 3

Migraine Knockouts

W hen I was an intern at George Washington University Hospital in Washington, D.C., I first saw the misery of migraines. A young woman had suddenly begun seeing flashing lights the previous day, and then her head started to pound with throbbing pain. This had never happened to her before. As the pain intensified, she feared she might be having a stroke. But she calmed herself down and tried to sleep. After a restless night, the pain was as bad as ever.

Unfortunately, the emergency room was characteristically busy that day, so she had to spend most of the morning in the waiting room with an out-of-focus television blaring out commercials that were loud enough for the deafest patient to hear. She was then grilled by a skeptical medical student who had been taught that drug addicts sometimes feign headaches to get narcotic painkillers.

After several necessary but fruitless tests to check for more dangerous causes of headache, we were finally able to give her pain relievers. In her case, they were about as helpful as the ancient Egyptian treatment for migraine, which required sufferers to put grain in the mouth of a clay crocodile and bind it to their heads with a strip of linen bearing the names of the gods.[1] (Sometimes medications do a world of good, but too often they are clay crocodiles.)

That was in 1980. Not for another three years did the first of a series of controlled research studies reveal something that I wish I could have passed along to the young woman in the emergency room: migraines are often triggered by foods. About a dozen common foods can cause headaches, which is often not appreciated until the migraine sufferer happens to avoid them for whatever reason and finds that the headaches become rare or even disappear completely.

Later research showed that not only do certain foods seem to cause migraines, but some nutrients can be used to prevent or even treat them. Coffee can sometimes knock out a migraine. Foods that are rich in magnesium, calcium, complex carbohydrates, and fiber have been used to cure migraines by restoring the natural balance of brain chemistry. Clinical reports began to show that ginger—the ordinary kitchen spice—can help prevent and treat migraines with none of the side effects of drugs. Controlled studies showed that the leaves of a wild plant called feverfew effectively reduce migraine frequency for many people. Not every headache sufferer benefits from diet changes or supplements, but many do.

WHAT KIND OF HEADACHE DO YOU HAVE?

Let's start by identifying the kind of headache you have. This is important, because some types need urgent medical treatment. Also, diet changes work for some headaches, but not others, as is true for some painkillers. Most migraine treatments, for example, are useless for tension headaches.

A *migraine* is not just a bad headache. It has a characteristic pattern. It usually involves just one side of your head and is a throbbing pain rather than a dull, constant ache. Along with it, you are likely to have nausea, vomiting, and sensitivity to light and sounds. A migraine is not fleeting. It lasts for anywhere from four hours to three days. You may get a brief warning aura of flashing lights, blind spots, or blurred vision, although most migraines arrive unannounced. Migraines can start up at any age and tend to run in families.

The prevailing theory about their cause is that, in response to some trigger—foods, perfume, cigarette smoke, stress, sunlight, too much or little sleep, or changing weather—blood vessels inside the brain constrict, sometimes leading to the peculiar visual auras and other sensations. The blood vessels then expand, causing nerve endings to send a painful signal to the brain centers that perceive pain.[2]

A *cluster headache* lasts only an hour or so, but it is excruciating. It centers around one eye, which turns red and begins to water. Its name comes from the fact that it occurs in clusters, arriving day after day on the same side of your head, and then vanishes for months. It does not bring the light sensitivity or visual aura that are characteristic of migraines. And while sleep will often make a migraine go away, it will not do a thing for cluster headaches.

A *tension headache* is a diffuse, constant ache, rather than a throbbing or stabbing pain. As its name implies, it will hit when you are stressed and go away when you relax.

A *sinus headache* is a constant ache in the forehead or under your eyes. It is often caused by environmental allergies. Foods can be the culprit or can aggravate the effects of other allergens. Cluster, tension, and sinus headaches are covered in chapter 4.

Caffeine withdrawal causes a dull headache. It is no great trick to diagnose it. If you are a coffee drinker, it kicks in when you miss your daily dose, and a cup of coffee quickly relieves it.

LESS COMMON CAUSES

Doctors are also on the lookout for headaches resulting from injuries, fever, medical illnesses, dental problems, and other less common causes.

Temporal arteritis is a one-sided, throbbing headache caused by an inflamed artery on the side of your head, which is firm to the touch but sensitive. You will also notice that you have been feeling run-down and tired for some time and have pains in your muscles and joints. Your doctor will do a blood test, called a sedimentation rate, and will appear disconcerted by the result, which in temporal arteritis is often high. The doctor will then insist on prescribing steroids to prevent serious complications, such as blindness, and that is good advice.

Glaucoma sometimes presents as a headache with eye pain and vomiting.

Blood vessel abnormalities can cause headaches that arrive repeatedly on the same side of the head. By contrast, migraines will at least occasionally affect either side of your head, and cluster headaches will often switch sides when a new cluster begins. Neither of these generally has the nerve symptoms that blood vessel abnormalities can bring.

If you have a headache without having had them before, and it has slowly increased in intensity and frequency and does not fit the typical pattern of a migraine, cluster, or tension headache, your doctor will run tests looking for increased pressure inside the skull or other causes.

SEE YOUR DOCTOR

Your doctor should evaluate your headache, especially if headaches are new for you, are unusually severe or persistent, or are accompanied by any of these characteristics:
- fever
- a change in your strength, coordination, or senses
- neck or back pain
- a chronic run-down feeling with pain in your muscles or joints
- drowsiness
- difficulty thinking or concentrating
- progressive worsening over time
- the headache awakens you from sleep
- the headache follows head trauma

FIGHTING MIGRAINES WITH FOOD

While the proof of food's role in migraines is recent, it was as long ago as 1778 that John Fothergill wrote in his text on the "sick headache," "My opinion of this disease is that for the most part it proceeds from inattention to diet, either in respect to kind or quantity or both." He laid the blame at "milk and butter, fat meats and spices, especially common black pepper and meat pies and rich baked puddings."[3]

Research studies have allowed us to be much more specific, both in identifying problem foods and also in finding foods that work as treatments. Let's first take a look at those that can cause migraines because the easiest solution may be simply to avoid them.

FIND YOUR MIGRAINE TRIGGERS

Clinicians have systematically eliminated various foods from migraine sufferers' diets and have found that, in many cases, the headaches diminish or even go away completely. They then return the suspect foods to the diet in a disguised form to see if the headaches come back.

In 1983, researchers at the Hospital for Sick Children in London reported their results for eighty-eight children with severe, frequent migraines who began an elimination diet. Of this group, seventy-eight recovered completely, and four improved greatly. In addition, some children who also had seizures found that their seizures stopped. The researchers then reintroduced various foods and found that they sparked migraine recurrences in all but eight. In subsequent tests using disguised foods, the vast majority of children again became symptom-free when trigger foods were avoided. Migraines returned when trigger foods were added to the diet.[4]

In adults, anywhere between 20 and 50 percent have a reduction or elimination of their headaches when common trigger foods are avoided.[5,6]

By compiling the results from hundreds of patients, we are now able to separate migraine triggers from safe foods. Sometimes a single food is to blame, but you are more likely to be sensitive to several triggers, often foods you would least suspect.[4,5,7]

Did you ever see the play *Arsenic and Old Lace*, which was also made into a Cary Grant movie? Two elderly ladies decide to help people escape the troubles of everyday life by poisoning them with arsenic. A large dose could kill you quickly, but a small dose given daily builds up slowly, causing weakness and aches and pains that seem to come out of nowhere. A headache kicks in, and eventually the lights go out.

Aside from the last scene, that is not much different from what happens in migraines. The smiling grocer, the kid who delivers your pizza, or even the waiter at your favorite restaurant brings you foods that seem perfectly innocent. But if you have food sensitivities, they act like subtle poisons, building up in your system with debilitating effects. One person's morning grapefruit is another person's migraine.

PAIN-SAFE FOODS

Pain-safe foods virtually never contribute to headaches or other painful conditions. These include

Brown rice

Cooked or dried fruits: cherries, cranberries, pears, prunes (but not citrus fruits, apples, bananas, peaches, or tomatoes)

Cooked green, yellow, and orange vegetables: artichokes, asparagus, broccoli, chard, collards, lettuce, spinach, string beans, summer or winter squash, sweet potatoes, tapioca, and taro (poi)

Water: plain water or carbonated forms, such as Perrier, are fine. Other beverages—even herbal teas—can be triggers.

Condiments: modest amounts of salt, maple syrup, and vanilla extract are usually well-tolerated.

COMMON TRIGGERS

Common triggers often cause headaches in susceptible people.[6] Some of them might surprise you. Citrus fruits or wheat, for example, seem like perfectly healthful foods. But just as some food sensitivities manifest as a rash on your skin, migraine sufferers have a reaction that is internal— in the blood vessels and nerves. Here are the common food triggers, also known as the dirty dozen, in order of importance:

1. dairy products*	7. nuts and peanuts
2. chocolate	8. tomatoes
3. eggs	9. onions
4. citrus fruits	10. corn
5. meat**	11. apples
6. wheat (bread, pasta, etc.)	12. bananas

  * Includes skim or whole cow's milk, goat's milk, cheese, yogurt, etc.
 ** Includes beef, pork, chicken, turkey, fish, etc.

Certain beverages and additives are also among the worst triggers, including alcoholic beverages (especially red wine), caffeinated drinks (coffee, tea, and colas), monosodium glutamate, aspartame (NutraSweet), and nitrites.

Foods that are on neither the pain-safe list nor the common trigger list should be considered possible, but unlikely, triggers. Almost all common foods, other than those on the pain-safe list, have triggered migraines in an isolated individual in a research study, so they cannot be considered completely above suspicion, but they are far from the most likely culprits.

THE TWO-WEEK TEST

The first step in tackling your migraines is to check whether any of the common triggers are causing them. To do this, you simply avoid these foods. At the same time, include generous amounts of pain-safe foods in your routine, and see whether migraines occur, and, if so, how often.

Here is how to start with antimigraine foods. For two weeks:

1. Have an abundance of foods from the pain-safe list.
2. Avoid the common triggers *completely*.
3. Foods that are not on either list can be eaten freely.

The key is to be careful in avoiding the common triggers. The recipes on pages 234–254 are designed to make this easy. During your two-week test, don't skip meals, and be careful about sleeping in and missing breakfast, because prolonged hunger can trigger migraines.

By the way, although wheat is a common trigger, this does not mean that you cannot have bread or pasta. Health food stores carry breads and pastas made from rice, millet, quinoa, and other grains. Check the ingredient labels.

CONFIRM YOUR FOOD TRIGGERS

If your diet change makes your headaches disappear or become much less frequent, resist the temptation to celebrate with a bottle of red wine and a cheese pizza. The next step is to confirm which foods are your triggers. To do this, simply reintroduce the eliminated foods one at a time, every two days, to see whether any symptoms result. Start at the bottom of the list (bananas) and work your way up to the riskier foods, skipping any that you do not care for. If you wish, you can then check the beverages and additives on the common triggers list.

As you do this, have a generous amount of each new food, so you will know whether or not it causes symptoms. If it causes no problem, you can keep it in your diet. Anything that causes a headache should be eliminated again. Then, after a week or two, try the suspect food once again for confirmation. Keep your diet simple so you can detect the effect of each newly added food.

Meats, dairy products, and eggs are best left off your plate permanently. Aside from being among the worst migraine triggers, they also tend to disturb your natural hormone balance, which contributes to migraines, as we will shortly see. Their cholesterol, fat, and animal proteins are linked to serious health concerns, so there is no need to welcome these problem foods back onto your plate.

LOOKING FOR OTHER FOOD TRIGGERS

If two weeks on the basic antimigraine diet does not reduce your headaches, the next step is to check whether a food that is not on the list of common migraine triggers may be causing your symptoms. This occasionally happens, and in fact, some people are sensitive to several different foods. An elimination diet will help you sort this out.

A SIMPLE ELIMINATION DIET

The elimination diet is designed to track down any unusual pain triggers. It is used for many other conditions as well, particularly arthritis and digestive problems.

The idea is simple. You simply start by building your menu entirely from the pain-safe foods, avoiding all others for the moment. (For recipes, see pages 234–254.)

Once your symptoms have gone or diminished, which may take a week or so, you can add other foods one at a time, every other day, to see which ones cause symptoms. Again, have a generous amount of each new food so you can see whether it causes symptoms. If not, you can keep it in your diet. Hold off adding any foods on the dirty-dozen list and any of the beverage and additive triggers until last.

Here are some tips to help you identify triggers:

- Foods that have caused headaches were usually eaten within three to six hours of the attack.
- The offending foods can be ones you are fond of, perhaps even foods for which you have cravings.[4] They may be the ones you might least suspect.
- Sometimes the headache will not show up until a large amount of the culprit is eaten, perhaps over a few days.

- If you are affected by several foods, eliminating only one may make no difference at all. This sometimes leads people to believe that foods are not the problem.[4]
- You might find that you can have a small amount of a trigger food without getting a headache, while a larger amount brings on the headache.
- Your tolerance might be different at different times. For example, a woman might normally be able to eat half a box of chocolates with no problem, but as she approaches her period, a single piece might trigger the migraine. The reason, presumably, is that the natural changes in hormones that occur over the month affect her sensitivity.[8]
- Your triggers can change over time.
- Your doctor can arrange special blood tests to detect food sensitivities. They can be rather expensive, but are faster than elimination diets. Information is available from Serammune Physicians Lab, 1890 Preston White Drive, Reston, VA 22091, 800-553-5472. Typical skin-patch tests are of little use for migraine triggers, since they detect only certain kinds of allergies.

WHY IS CHOCOLATE SO CRUEL?

How can chocolate or a glass of red wine look so friendly and appealing and then suddenly stab you in the back—or, more accurately, in the side of your head? Two reasons. First, chocolate, red wine, and many other foods contain chemicals that affect blood flow to the brain and encourage inflammation. Second, our bodies sometimes react to the proteins in certain foods with strong symptoms, including pain.

Chocolate contains *phenylethylamine* (PEA), an amphetamine-like chemical that may be part of the reason why it is so addicting. PEA, which is also found in red wine and many cheeses, disturbs normal blood flow in the brain.[9-11]

Wines also contain natural flavonoids that come from the skins and seeds of grapes, as well as sulfites, all of which are under scrutiny for their contribution to migraines.

More importantly, red wine contains a huge amount of *histamine,* which is famous for the sneezing, runny nose, and sinus problems it can cause and that are treated with *anti*histamines. Histamine has a major effect on blood flow, which is probably why it contributes to migraines.[12] Histamine is also found in champagne and other wines, beers, cheese, fish (especially tuna, mackerel, and mahimahi), sausage, and pickled cabbage.[10]

Red wine does seem to be among the most potent triggers. Although some have been skeptical about the link, London researchers tested eleven subjects who believed that red wine triggered their headaches. They tested them with a glass of disguised Spanish red wine and also with a vodka-lemonade mixture. None had a headache from vodka, but nine of the eleven developed a headache from just one glass of red wine.[9]

SHOULD WE CALL HIM SAINT CONRAD?

Chocolate was not invented in Switzerland. The cocoa tree is native to South America and was brought to Mexico by the Mayas. Aztecs used it to make a beverage, a rather bitter ancestor of hot cocoa, which they shared with the Spanish conquistadors. Europeans sweetened it with sugar and added vanilla, nuts, and other flavorings.

Nothing resembling modern chocolate existed until 1828, when a Dutchman named Conrad van Houten invented a machine that could press cocoa butter from cocoa beans. By concentrating cocoa butter and adding it to ground beans, a smooth chocolate was produced that could be sweetened with sugar and molded into enticing shapes.[13]

The history of chocolate has some odd twists, as recounted by Martha Barnett in her book *Ladyfingers and Nun's Tummies*. German chocolate cake's name does not come from Europe at all, but from Samuel German, who worked for an American chocolate factory. The factory was founded by Dr. James Baker, from whom Baker's chocolate gets its name. A New York confectioner, Leo Hirschfield, named his popular chocolate rolls after his daughter Clara, known affectionately as Tootsie. The daughter of another New York candy maker was less fortunate. Her father thought of her when he named his chocolate squares filled with nuts and raisins Chunky.

HISTAMINE IN WINE AND BEER[10]

BEVERAGE	MICROGRAMS/LITER
Red wine	1,010
Champagne	670
Dessert wine	280
Sparkling wine	46
Rosé	40
White	37
Beer (Budweiser)	28
Beer (Tsingtao)	21
Beer, nonalcoholic	26

Histamine does not only come in foods, however. It is also made inside your body. If you are sensitive to dust, pollen, or any foods, your body makes extra histamine, which then adds to the histamine that you got from foods.[14] In 1988, researchers reported a case of a nineteen-year-old woman with a particular sensitivity to beef. One serving tripled the amount of histamine in her blood, and her migraines quickly kicked in.[15]

If you have been exposed to any allergen, histamine is coursing through your veins, working its mischief. If you then drown your sorrows with a glass of burgundy, its load of *extra* histamine adds to that already in your blood.[10] This is why allergy season can make you more sensitive to histamine-rich foods, and conversely, these foods might make you more sensitive to environmental allergens.

Of course, we do not really need to know why any given food causes migraines, any more than we need to know exactly why stings from a swarm of bees can be poisonous. We just need to get out of the way.

Most people find that their migraines are greatly reduced or eliminated by eating generous amounts of pain-safe foods and avoiding any food triggers to which they are sensitive. If your migraines persist, however, four supplements are worth considering: feverfew, ginger, magnesium, and calcium. Their effects differ for different individuals; you will likely find that one helps and another does not. My advice is to simply try them one at a time, using the dosages described below, and see which ones help. Using them in combination is fine. However, I recommend trying them separately at first so you can identify their effects. I encourage you to do this in consultation with your doctor, not because these supplements are dangerous, but because the diagnosis and treatment of headaches require both medical expertise and lifestyle changes.

USING COFFEE TO TREAT MIGRAINES

Coffee is a paradoxical drink. It can trigger migraines for some people. And if you are a regular coffee-drinker, *not* having coffee for a day is likely to give you a caffeine withdrawal headache. But it can also cure headaches.

Surgeons used to puzzle over the fact that so many patients got headaches after surgery. They blamed their anesthesiologists, blamed various medications, and worried that one of their assistants might be leaning an elbow on the patient's forehead. But the answer turned out to be much simpler. The people who got headaches after surgery were those who were not allowed to eat or drink anything the day of the operation. Their headaches simply meant that they had missed their morning coffee. A caffeine tablet before surgery solved the problem.[16]

If your daily routine includes just one cup of coffee or two cups of tea or two colas, all of which hold about 100 mg of caffeine, you can get a headache as early as eight hours after your last dose.[16,17]

Caffeine has a good side, however. It actually has analgesic properties that can be used to fight headaches.[18] It is often added to aspirin, acetaminophen, ibuprofen, and ergotamine to enhance their effects. Ironically, this analgesic effect may actually be the reason why caffeine withdrawal causes headaches: caffeine's painkilling action may suppress your natural defenses to pain, and withdrawal leaves you with less than your normal resistance to pain.

If you tend to get headaches, it is best to avoid coffee, but when a migraine actually hits, you can use it as a treatment, having one or two cups at the first sign of an attack. Avoid it if it is a migraine trigger for you.

FEVERFEW: THE ANTIMIGRAINE HERB

Feverfew is a wild plant with yellow-green leaves and daisylike flowers. It is native to the Balkan peninsula and has spread to much of Europe, where it can be seen in hedgerows, on walls, and wherever no one has mowed recently.

Its name comes from the fact that the ancient Greeks and many later societies used it as a treatment for fever. It has also been used to treat arthritis, gynecological problems, and many other conditions. It was all but forgotten in modern times until it reemerged as a popular migraine treatment in Britain in the late 1970s.

It works. Researchers at the City of London Migraine Clinic found that feverfew eliminated about two-thirds of migraines in a selected group of headache patients, which is similar to the effectiveness of most migraine drugs.[19] However, while some people get a pronounced effect, others get none at all. Averaging everyone together, it eliminates about one-fourth of all headaches.[20] This does not mean that it will eliminate precisely one-fourth of *your* headaches. It will more likely either have a much more noticeable effect or no effect at all.

Feverfew is sold at all health food stores. The amount that has been shown to prevent migraines in research studies ranges from 50–114 mg per day. However, most practitioners use capsules containing about 250 mg of a standardized-potency feverfew, recommending one capsule per day taken on an empty stomach. If you find fresh leaves, the usual dose is two to three leaves per day.[19–21]

Do not expect to see drug companies promoting it, however. As a naturally occurring plant, it cannot be patented. That means that no single pharmaceutical company can get an edge on the competition or elevate its price. There is a much bigger profit margin in patented prescription drugs.

How safe is feverfew? Thousands of people have used it over long periods with no apparent ill effects, and research studies have shown no serious risks.[20,21] However, there has been little effort to systematically look for side effects over prolonged periods. I would encourage you to avoid it if you are (or might be) pregnant; there is no indication that it causes birth defects, but not enough data are in to be sure.[21] Also, people with clotting disorders or who are taking anticoagulant medicines should consult with their doctors about taking feverfew. Otherwise, our best information suggests that you can stay on it indefinitely.

GINGER

In 1990, Danish researchers reported the case of a woman who began to have migraines at age twenty-six. At first, the headaches were not too bad: a colored zigzag aura lasting two to three minutes, followed by a three-to-four-hour mild headache, occurring only once every month or two. As time went on, however, the headaches became more painful and more frequent, arriving two to three times per month and persisting for longer periods. Her doctor put her on dihydroergotamine, which helped some but was a far-from-perfect solution.

Ginger has been used for centuries by Indian Ayurvedic practitioners to treat neurological conditions, including headache, nausea, and even epilepsy, and has more recently been used to treat motion sickness, for which, by the way, it has worked well in placebo-controlled trials using a single, one-gram dose.[22,23]

The woman learned about it and decided to give it a try. When the visual aura hit, she stirred 500–600 mg (about one-quarter teaspoon) of powdered ginger into a glass of water and drank it down. Within thirty minutes, the headache was gone. To keep the headache at bay, she continued to take ginger every few hours for a day or two, totaling 1.5 to 2 grams per day. She started to use ginger as a spice in her daily diet and found that her headaches decreased from two to three times per month to no more than once every two months. When they did occur, a dose of ginger knocked them out.[24]

Why did it work? Presumably because ginger blocks histamine and also inhibits prostaglandins—chemicals that play a role in inflammation, as we will see in chapter 5.

Rarely, a person can be sensitive to ginger and could conceivably have a migraine triggered by it. So far, all the evidence favoring ginger in migraines is based on traditional medicine and observations in individuals. Controlled studies are needed to establish its efficacy.

The amount typically used in research studies is about one-half to one teaspoon (one to two grams) of powdered ginger each day. It has no adverse effects, other than the warming sensation it causes as it goes down.

MAGNESIUM VERSUS MIGRAINES

Magnesium has been shown to have migraine-fighting power in several research studies. No one knows exactly why it works, but migraines are less frequent when your diet is rich in magnesium. One of the reasons why emotional stress contributes to migraines may be that it depletes your body of magnesium.[25]

Researchers have found that 200 mg per day of elemental magnesium, added to the magnesium in the foods you eat, helps prevent migraines. In three thousand people treated with magnesium, 80 percent got at least partial benefit from it.[26] Although researchers typically use supplements, it is easy to get plenty of magnesium from foods alone (see the chart on page 18). In fact, if your diet is so low in magnesium that you are considering a supplement, that is a sign that you need to add more vegetables, legumes, and grains to your routine.

Foods rich in magnesium include whole grains (grains with their natural fiber intact), such as brown rice, barley, and oats; dried noncitrus fruits, such as figs; and green vegetables, especially broccoli, spinach, and chard. All of these are pain-safe foods.

Nuts and wheat are also rich in magnesium, but they are migraine triggers for some people, so they are not recommended until you have assessed how they affect you. The same is true for soybeans, and for other beans to a lesser extent. Meats and dairy products are low in magnesium, as well as being common migraine triggers.

The recommended dietary allowance for magnesium is 280 mg for women and 350 mg for men, including that from foods and any supplements you may be taking. However, this minimal amount only prevents a frank deficiency. Researchers believe that the ideal range for optimal health is 400–700 mg per day for adults.[27]

Magnesium can be particularly helpful in premenstrual headaches, used along with 50–100 mg of vitamin B_6. This combination is most effective when used daily, but can also be used for just five days per month, as the menstrual period approaches.[28,29] Doses of vitamin B_6 of 200 mg or above should be avoided, as they are suspected of causing nerve problems.

USING CALCIUM AND VITAMIN D AGAINST MIGRAINES

Calcium and vitamin D help prevent migraines. Like magnesium, exactly why they work is not clear. You can use supplements if you like, but the best calcium sources are green, leafy vegetables and legumes or, as you might say, "greens and beans." As we saw in chapter 1, a plate of baked beans has more than 100 mg of calcium. A cup of wax beans straight out of the can has 174 mg. Milk and other dairy products do contain calcium, but milk is among the worst migraine triggers, and its calcium is not as well absorbed as that in most vegetables. It should be avoided completely.

More important than eating high-calcium foods, however, is keeping the calcium in your body. Most people in Western countries are losing calcium much more quickly than they need to, and happily, that is something you can correct quite easily. As we saw in chapter 2, certain factors cause calcium to be pulled from the bones, to pass into the bloodstream, and then through the kidneys into the urine.

Calcium losses are dramatically cut when you avoid animal protein and excess salt and sugar. If you drink more than two cups of coffee, the decaffeinated brands help, because caffeine increases calcium's passage through the kidneys. Calcium losses are also increased by smoking and physical inactivity. Controlling these losses helps you keep calcium in your body without a calcium supplement. If you decide to take one for whatever reason, the amount shown in research studies to prevent migraines is 1,000 to 2,000 mg of elemental calcium daily, or try calcium citrate, a highly absorbable form.

Your ability to absorb calcium from foods is controlled by vitamin D, which is naturally formed from sun exposure on your skin. Ten minutes of sun on your face and arms each day is usually more than enough. If you are using a vitamin D supplement, the recommended dietary allowance is 200 IU (5 mcg) per day. The amount used in research studies for migraine prevention is 50,000 IU once per week, which greatly exceeds the RDA, is potentially risky, and should only be used under a doctor's supervision.

FOODS THAT CALM HORMONE SHIFTS

During a woman's monthly cycle, the amount of estrogens (female sex hormones) in her blood rises and falls like a roller coaster. It drops quickly just before her period, and about half of women get their migraines at that time. Just as withdrawal from caffeine causes a headache, a rapid drop in estrogens seems to do the same thing.

Estrogen shifts may make you headache-prone. That is apparently why migraines often begin at puberty, diminish after menopause, occur three times more often in women than men, and all but disappear during pregnancy, when estrogen's effects are countered by progesterone.[30-33]

Foods can smooth out estrogen shifts. Certain foods prevent the amount of estrogen in your blood from climbing too high, so that it does not have so far to fall. This is described in more detail in chapter 8, but here is how it works in a nutshell:

- When you avoid animal fat and keep vegetable oils to a bare minimum, your body makes less estrogen.
- At the same time, high-fiber foods help your body eliminate excess estrogen more easily.

Your estrogen levels will be both lower and more stable when the main sources of fat (animal products and cooking oils) are taken off the menu and, at the same time, generous amounts of fiber-rich vegetables and grains are in your routine. You may feel the result as a reduction in menstrual cramping and are also likely to reduce your risk of breast cancer and to help protect your bones, in addition to helping against migraines.

We can take a lesson from Asia. Traditional Asian diets are not based on the meats, dairy products, or greasy fried foods that are common in Western countries. Their dietary staple is rice, along with generous amounts of vegetables. If animal products are consumed at all, they are used in small amounts, essentially as flavorings. The result is a very low-fat, high-fiber diet that keeps estrogen levels more modest throughout the cycle. And if estrogen does not climb too high, it cannot fall so dramatically. The hormone roller coaster stays on a much flatter plane.

Just about every health problem related to estrogen shifts is less common in Asia: hot flashes, breast cancer, and—yes—migraines. In

America, 6 percent of men and 18 percent of women have a history of migraines. In Hong Kong, where diets are somewhat westernized but still retain much of their Asian heritage, migraines affect only 3 percent of men and 7 percent of women. If you were to venture into rural China, where the Western diet has not yet made any inroads, migraines are much rarer still. They are similarly rare in parts of Latin America where beans, rice, and tortillas are still the order of the day.[34-37]

Hormone shifts are a bigger problem for women than men, at least for migraines. But men benefit from the same diet change. A case in point is Athos, a small peninsula in northern Greece, where fifteen hundred monks live. The monks never eat meat or milk, and they fast frequently. Migraines are only half as common on Athos as in the United States.[38] Should we give the credit to the lack of food triggers, a hormone-balancing effect, or something else? Happily, it does not really matter. An optimal diet helps in all these ways.

You don't have to choose one menu to avoid food triggers and another to change your hormones. The pain-safe foods, such as brown rice and vegetables, are rich in fiber and are extremely low in fat, unless you have added fat in cooking, so they also happen to be among the best at reducing hormone shifts. To do this right, however, it is important not only to avoid animal products but also to keep vegetable oils to a minimum. This is a helpful step.

A natural, nonprescription hormone, called natural progesterone, may also help counteract hormone shifts. It can help women with migraines, at least those who get their migraines around the time of their periods.[39-42]

Natural progesterone is derived from wild yams, and in chapter 1 we looked at its remarkable ability to protect bones. For migraines, John Lee, M.D., a leading progesterone proponent, recommends using a nonprescription, transdermal (skin-applied) progesterone cream, such as Pro-Gest. Starting with a two-ounce jar, you spread a bit on thin skin each day so that you use up one to two ounces over the ten days before your period. Dr. Lee also suggests trying it as a treatment when a migraine hits, using one-quarter to one-half teaspoon of progesterone cream every three to four hours until symptoms subside. Sublingual drops of progesterone in vitamin E oil are also available and may be more rapidly absorbed.

USING FOODS TO FIGHT MIGRAINES

1. Emphasize pain-safe foods: brown rice; cooked vegetables, such as broccoli, collards, spinach, and chard; and cooked or dried noncitrus fruits.

2. Avoid the common trigger foods completely. If your migraines have diminished or ceased, you can reintroduce the trigger foods one at a time to assess their effect.

3. If steps one and two did not diminish your migraines, an elimination diet can help you identify whether an unusual trigger is causing your problem.

4. Minimize hormone shifts by avoiding animal products, keeping vegetable oils minimal, and keeping the natural fiber in grains, beans, vegetables, and fruits.

5. Try these supplements, in consultation with your doctor:

   Feverfew: 250 mg per day or two to three fresh leaves.

   Ginger: one-half to one teaspoon (one to two grams) of fresh powdered ginger per day.

   Magnesium: 400–700 mg per day total (foods plus supplements, if used) or 200 mg per day as elemental supplement alone.

   Calcium: Reduce calcium losses by avoiding animal protein, caffeine, tobacco, and excess sodium and sugar. If you wish, you can take 1,000–2,000 mg per day of elemental calcium, with 200 IU (5 mcg) of vitamin D. Regular physical activity will keep calcium in your bones where it belongs.

IF A MIGRAINE HITS

If a migraine occurs, try the following:

• Although caffeine can be a migraine trigger for some people, for others it works as a treatment. The dose is one to two cups of strong coffee at the first sign of an attack.

• Have a starchy food, such as rice, potatoes, crackers, or bread. Yes, wheat products are migraine triggers for some people, but if you can tolerate them, they might actually help. Some people find that they actually crave starchy foods during migraines and that digging into toast, crackers, pasta, potatoes, or other starchy foods reduces the headache or nausea and can even shorten the attack.[43] Experience will tell you whether these foods help.

• Fresh powdered ginger, 500–600 mg (about one-quarter teaspoon), in a glass of water has been helpful in anecdotal reports. It can be repeated every few hours, up to about two grams per day.

• Calcium might be able to treat migraines as well as prevent them. Researchers reported a case of a woman who was able to stop an early migraine by chewing 1,200 to 1,600 mg of elemental calcium.[44,45] Again, avoid the temptation to get calcium from milk, yogurt, or any other animal source. It causes much more trouble than it is worth.

• Lie down in a quiet, dark room, and sleep if you can. Use hot or cold compresses and massage the blood vessels at the temples.

• Biofeedback is a technique for controlling blood flow through relaxation, and it helps both migraines and tension headaches. The biofeedback instructor will put a temperature monitor on your index finger that will signal you when you have relaxed enough to open up blood flow to your fingertips. Believe it or not, you will be able to influence the blood flow to your brain, and the result can be more control over your headache.[46] Biofeedback training is available at the psychiatry or psychology departments of university medical centers, or look in the yellow pages under psychologists, biofeedback, or physicians specializing in psychiatry.

• Acupuncture has been helpful for many people as well. Practitioners are listed in the yellow pages.

DRUGS FOR TREATING MIGRAINES

If you have carefully followed the above steps and you *still* have some pain, you are no doubt wondering whether you should take pain-relieving medicines. Don't use medications as the mainstay of your approach to headaches if you have not first done a good search for food triggers and followed an optimal diet. Otherwise, you'll be trying to put out a fire while pouring on gasoline at the same time. Medicines do not replace a nutritional approach, but they can supplement it, if necessary. Here is a quick guide to antimigraine drugs and their main side effects:[1,47]

• Aspirin helps for mild to moderate attacks. The main drawbacks are gastrointestinal irritation, bleeding, and allergic reactions. In children, aspirin should be used only under a doctor's supervision, because of the risk of Reye's syndrome.

• Nonsteroidal anti-inflammatory drugs, such as ibuprofen (Motrin, Nuprin) or naproxen (Naprosyn), are similar to aspirin. Gastrointestinal side effects are their main disadvantage.

• Acetaminophen (Tylenol, paracetamol) can also help mild to moderate attacks. Chronic use, however, can cause liver or kidney problems.

• Ergotamine and dihydroergotamine constrict dilated blood vessels and help most people—although not all—if taken early in the migraine. Their big danger is that, when they are used daily, they are habituating and can suppress your body's natural defenses against pain. If you then stop the drug, you will likely have severe, chronic rebound headaches.[48] They do not help tension headaches.

......

PAINKILLERS CAN HELP, BUT . . .

Overuse of simple analgesics or ergotamines can suppress your painkilling endorphins. This reduces your natural defenses against pain, often resulting in a chronic daily headache. If this happens, your doctor will help you taper off the medicine gradually and may recommend using vitamin B_6 to increase your resistance to pain during withdrawal.[53]

How much is too much? Aspirin or other simple analgesics taken every day, combination drugs taken more than three times per week, or ergotamine (for migraines) more than twice a week.[54] If you are taking aspirin to prevent heart attacks, you may wish to speak with your doctor about minimizing your dose.

A drug that treats a tension headache may do little or nothing for a migraine, and vice versa. This is one reason why I encourage you to be evaluated by a physician, not to mention the fact that some medications are available only by prescription.

The pros and cons of medications should always be discussed with your physician, especially if you are (or may be) pregnant.

......

• Sumatriptan (Imitrex) relieves both migraines and cluster head-aches. It apparently works by narrowing the blood vessels to the brain and retains its effectiveness when used over the long term. Overuse and abuse are rare.[2,48–50]

• Lidocaine in a 4-percent topical solution knocks out migraines in about half the people who try it. You lie back on a bed or table with your head tilting backward over the edge and rotated toward the side of the headache. One-half milliliter of the lidocaine solution is dripped into the nostril over thirty seconds. If the headache is on both sides, the same is done with the other nostril. A second dose can be given after two minutes, if necessary. In a fair percentage of cases, the relief is only temporary. Lidocaine apparently works by acting on a nerve bundle that is just under the nasal mucosa.[51]

• Metoclopramide (Reglan) is often used with oral pain relievers to improve their absorption and relieve nausea.

DRUGS FOR PREVENTING MIGRAINES

If your migraines are disabling or occur more than three times a month in spite of your efforts to perfect your diet and your use of feverfew and the other preventive steps described above, you might consider preven-tive medications. They will not eliminate all migraines, but they will cut down on their frequency. Allow a good month or two to see if these med-ications work, and be sure to have a solid diagnosis first; most will not help tension headaches.

• Propranolol (Inderal) and metoprolol (Lopressor) will greatly reduce migraines in about a third of migraine sufferers and have a more modest effect in another third. They are safe for most people and have been used over long periods. You should not take them, however, if you have asthma or diabetes. Also, because propranolol tends to prevent your heart from beating quickly, be sure to discuss your exercise plans with your doctor.

• Calcium channel blockers are sometimes used to prevent migraines, particularly in Europe. Doctors are growing more reluctant to use them, however, due to side effects.

• Serotonin blockers, such as methysergide (Sansert), work about as well as propranolol, but have more side effects when used long-term, particularly fibrosis in the chest and abdomen.

• Amitriptyline (Elavil) is an antidepressant that also helps prevent migraines. It is generally safe, although dry mouth, constipation, and drowsiness are common side effects, and it is important not to exceed the prescribed dose.

• Valproic acid (Depakene, Depakote) is an antiseizure medicine that can help prevent migraines. Occasional side effects include weight gain, hair loss, and tremor.

• Aspirin may help you avoid some migraines. Taken every other day, it was found to reduce migraine frequency by 20 percent in a study of physicians. This modest improvement has to be weighed against its side effects, described above.

If you are (or might be) pregnant, your doctor will be reluctant to prescribe medications, particularly ergotamine, dihydroergotamine, sumatriptan, and valproic acid, and will encourage you to try to wait it out, since migraines tend to go away during pregnancy. Doctors may recommend antinausea medications to help you get through it.[52]

CHAPTER 4

Foods for Other Kinds of Headaches

In the last chapter, we focused on using foods to prevent and treat migraines. In this chapter, we will take a look at chemical-induced headaches, cluster headaches, sinus headaches, and—what is by far the most common type—tension headaches. Food and lifestyle changes can play important roles in all of them.

CHEMICAL HEADACHES

A surprising number of chemicals reach us in foods, in the air, or in the workplace, and some of these can contribute to headaches. Here are the main ones to look out for:

• Monosodium glutamate, or MSG, is the well-known flavor enhancer often used at Chinese restaurants. In about one in three people, it causes headaches and a feeling of tightness around the face about twenty minutes after it touches your lips.[1,2] Chinese food is usually cooked to order, so it is usually a simple matter to ask that MSG not be used. If your appetizers were prepared without MSG, they will sometimes slow the absorption of MSG in other foods to the point where you may feel no symptoms.

• Aspartame (NutraSweet) is implicated in some headaches. It has long been a subject of debate among toxicologists because it contains phenylalanine, a chemical that causes brain damage in susceptible individuals. It is also implicated in some seizures.

Toxicologists still disagree as to whether aspartame deserves the blame it has received. However, it is not a necessary part of anyone's diet and has not proved itself to be especially helpful for losing weight or for anything else, for that matter. So instead of trying to choose between a regular soda sweetened with sugar or a diet soda sweetened with aspartame, why not have sparkling water or mineral water instead? They have no sugar and no chemical sweeteners.

• Nitrites are used to cure bacon, ham, hot dogs, other luncheon meats, smoked fish, and some cheeses, and they can cause a dull headache pain and a flushed face.[2,3] There is no shortage of reasons for steering clear of these products, since they are loaded with fat and cholesterol and may increase the risk of cancer.

• Sulfites are used as preservatives in salad bars and shellfish bars. They are also found in wines, both red and white. If you have allergies, you may also react to the sulfites in wine, particularly when you are exposed to pollens or other allergens at the same time.[4]

• Benzoic acid and tartrazine, a food coloring listed as FD&C yellow #5, can also contribute to headaches.[2]

• Tyramine is a chemical that leads to headaches in some people, especially those taking antidepressants called *MAO inhibitors,* sold under the brand names Parnate (tranylcypromine) and Nardil (phenelzine). Tyramine is found in aged cheeses, sour cream, wine, beer, liver, fermented sausages, pickled herring, broad beans, chocolate, coffee, licorice, pickles, sauerkraut, salted or pickled herring, lox, raisins, canned figs, and yeast.

• Environmental chemicals. If you get a headache at work that goes away when you are home over the weekend, the reason might not be stress; it might be a chemical exposure. A useful clue comes from timing of the headache, which usually begins between one and four hours after exposure. Be especially suspicious of solvents, such as those used for painting or cleaning, formaldehyde, ammonia, pesticides, and diesel exhaust.[5]

CLUSTER HEADACHES

Cluster headaches are perhaps the cruelest form of headache, not only for their intensity, but also for their timing. They are often triggered, not by tension, but by relaxation. After a long, hard workweek, you've cast aside all your cares and have planted your easel by a quiet pond where you are going to paint a relaxing scene. Just as you dip your brush into the pigment, a stabbing pain shoots through your eye with an intensity beyond anything else you have ever felt. It can happen as you arrive home from work or start a long-awaited vacation, or even as you change from dreaming and rapid eye movement (REM) sleep to non-REM sleep.[6]

These headaches get their name from the fact that they occur in clusters, arriving every day—often at the same time of day—for up to three months, after which they simply vanish for months at a time. In a bad case, your cluster can drag on for more than a year. It will affect the same side of your head during the entire cluster, reddening the eye on that side and making it water. You may also have an eyelid droop and narrowing of the pupil, and your nose will get runny or congested.[7]

Cluster headaches seem to be due to inflammation and pressure in the veins inside the brain, and there may be hormonal contributors, as they strike men five times more often than women, unlike migraines, which are more common in women.[8]

Alcohol is the only firmly established dietary trigger for cluster headaches. Any alcoholic beverage can do it; red wine is not singled out as it is in migraines. You might get away with the occasional sip between clusters, but alcohol is a surefire trigger when you are in a cluster period.[9]

Food sensitivities have not been well studied in cluster headache, which is unfortunate, because there are good reasons for being concerned about them. First of all, as we saw in the previous chapter, a chemical called histamine is found in alcoholic beverages and various foods, and it is also released into your bloodstream when you are exposed to any allergen. Histamine has long been known to play a major role in cluster headaches.[10] In fact, doctors used to diagnose cluster headaches by injecting a small amount of histamine under the skin and waiting for the headache to start about a half hour later.

To track down whether any foods contribute to cluster headaches, you can avoid the common migraine triggers and then, if necessary, use an elimination diet, as described in the previous chapter. This technique is used for many other health problems when a food trigger is suspected.

If cluster headaches tend to arrive just when you are relaxing, that does not mean that you will need to stay at work twenty-four hours a day, never take a vacation, and lie awake for fear of a sleep-induced headache. But you can be aware of times when you are vulnerable to headaches and take preventive action, which for some people may mean medications.

Lithium prevents attacks in about 40 percent of patients. Ergotamine can be used, taken at bedtime or every twelve hours, but it carries the risk of dependency, as noted in the previous chapter. When a cluster headache hits, it can be relieved by sumatriptan, ergotamine, or lidocaine drops. Pure inhaled oxygen also works for some people.[8,11]

Perhaps the oddest cluster headache treatment is the hot ingredient in chili peppers, called capsaicin. Capsaicin depletes substance P, the neurotransmitter chemical that nerve cells use to send pain signals. In an unusual experiment, a special capsaicin preparation was put into both nostrils in fifteen patients treated during an acute headache. Symptoms disappeared completely for seven, and three more had a 75 percent reduction in pain. With once-a-day dosing, several had headaches disappear for as long as twenty-eight to forty days.[12] Capsaicin treatments are described in more detail in chapter 5.

TAKING ACTION AGAINST CLUSTER HEADACHES

- Avoid alcohol.
- Avoid food triggers.
- Be aware of times of vulnerability to cluster headaches.
- Use medications as needed for prevention or treatment.

FOODS AND SINUS HEADACHES

Allergens cause sinus headaches. That goes for pollens or dust, of course, because the same swollen mucous membranes that cause congestion or a runny nose also cause pain in the sinuses that are in the forehead and around the eyes.[13]

Foods are often allergens, too, and they enter your body in many times the dose that dust or dander could ever deliver. They can easily contribute to sinus problems. Even if environmental allergies or frequent bacterial infections would seem to account for your sinus problems, consider whether food sensitivities might be aggravating the problem by causing mucus production and setting the stage for infections.

Sadly, many people live with food-related sinus problems for years, never recognizing the cause of their symptoms. Dairy products, for example, are a notorious cause of mucus production, which is why opera singers generally avoid them. From your throat and bronchi to your ears and sinuses, dairy products can make your mucous membranes boggy and congested. The reason may not be a typical allergy, however, and routine skin tests are not likely to show a sensitivity. But clearly, a mild, allergy-like syndrome occurs in many milk drinkers, and it is the first place to look when you have chronic respiratory or sinus conditions. The culprit in milk is the protein, not the fat, so skim milk is just as much a problem as whole milk. A single dose may have no noticeable effect, while exposure over a few days elicits a gradually worsening response.

Other foods can contribute, particularly wheat. Beer and jalapeño peppers can also cause a gradually increasing congestion when consumed daily by a sensitive individual. You can identify food sensitivities in the same way as described for migraines in the previous chapter, focusing on the common triggers. If your symptoms abate when you avoid them, you can reintroduce them gradually, checking for the return of symptoms as you go.

RELAXING A TENSION HEADACHE

Tension headaches are by far the most common type. While they are usually fleeting and mild, they can be more intense, sometimes masquerading as migraines. But you can tell them from migraines and other headaches by the following features:[14]

- a pressing or tightening quality
- mild to moderate intensity
- on both sides of the head, rather than just one
- not aggravated by routine physical movement
- not accompanied by nausea, vomiting, or unusual sensitivity to lights or sounds

Most doctors describe tension headaches as being caused by tense muscles—in the forehead, above the ears, or at the back of the head—

cutting off blood flow in the arteries. This is an oversimplification, but it is a useful way to think about them, because it shows what you need to do to get rid of them. The solution is to relax these muscles, and this becomes quite easy with a bit of practice.

Here is a useful approach to tension headaches:

• First, make sure your diagnosis is right, and rule out other things that might be causing your headache, such as caffeine withdrawal, dental or sinus problems, lack of sleep, lack of food, or any of the other conditions noted in chapter 3.

• Second, try the relaxation techniques described below and in chapter 17. They are quick, and they really work. The more you do them, the more powerful they become. Use them whenever you feel emotional tension turning into muscular tension. Before long, the relaxation response becomes automatic, and your headaches may become only a memory. Biofeedback can be helpful, too, as it is for migraines.

• Third, it is important to get adequate rest. When you are not sleeping well, you will not handle stress as well as you would normally. Be careful about short-term solutions to stress that many people use instead of the rest they really need. Coffee, alcohol, and tranquilizers can, over the not-so-long run, make things worse.

• Fourth, exercise helps melt stress away. A half-hour brisk walk every day or so really helps.

• Fifth, try the basic antimigraine diet, avoiding the major headache triggers as described in the previous chapter, for three weeks. For reasons that have never been clear, it can help headaches that have nothing to do with migraines. The most important foods to avoid are meats, dairy products, and fatty and sugary foods. I suspect that this helps for several reasons. Lower-fat foods improve the circulation to your head and neck by reducing the viscosity (thickness) of the blood. Avoiding animal protein allows your body to have more vitamin B_6 available for other purposes, which may improve your pain resistance. (Vitamin B_6 is consumed in the metabolism of proteins.) Also, steering clear of dairy products obviates a common, if unrecognized, sensitivity.

• Be careful about using pain relievers. They can suppress your body's natural ability to control pain. You will find that, as relaxation techniques give you control over the muscular tension in your head and neck, pain relievers are not usually necessary.

• When simple methods fail, people with recurrent tension headaches often find that antidepressants provide great relief. This does not necessarily mean that you are depressed. Rather, it may mean that the same kinds of chemical imbalances that cause depression can also lead to headaches, and antidepressants are designed to correct those problems.[15] Don't even think about them, however, until you are following a healthy diet and using relaxation techniques to full advantage.

LETTING TENSION GO

There are only four sets of muscles to work on:

- the forehead muscles that raise your eyebrows and wrinkle your brow
- the muscles at the back of your neck
- the muscles at your temples on both sides

You can relax them externally through massage or "internally" by becoming aware of tension and letting it go. Close your eyes and try to feel the muscles in your forehead. Slow your breathing down and imagine that every breath of air carries relaxation into these muscles, and every exhalation carries tension out of your body. Move your eyebrows up and down a bit. Any tension here? Consciously try to let go of any tension you feel.

Then focus your attention on the back of your head, just where the large neck muscles attach to the skull. Move your head slowly forward and back and in a circle. Let go of any tension you feel, and let slow and steady breathing carry it out of your body.

Then direct your attention to the muscles just above your ears on both sides. These muscles help dogs, cats, and deer move their ears forward and back to listen for danger, and some people use them to wiggle their ears to entertain friends. They are also involved in chewing, so they have developed a fair amount of strength, which will turn against you when they tense up. Try to be aware of their tension, and let it go. Let each breath bring relaxation in, and let tension pass out of your body as you exhale.

You will find many more tension-reducing exercises in chapters 16 and 17.

FEELING LIKE YOURSELF AGAIN

If frequent headaches have made you miss out on many things you wanted to do or made you feel as if a ton of bricks were hanging over your head, ready to drop at any moment, you now have the best possible ways of making that threat vanish. The right food choices can take away the pain and put you on your own private island, looking out at calm, clear waters, having forgotten that you ever had headaches.

CHAPTER 5

Cooling Your Joints

W e saw in chapter 3 that some foods tend to bring on headaches, while others help prevent them. Foods affect your joints in much the same way.

Starting in the early 1980s, reports began to appear in medical journals of individuals who had been essentially cured of arthritis by changing their diets. At first, these cases appeared to be unusual, but they were dramatic.

In 1981, the *British Medical Journal* reported the recovery of a woman who had suffered from rheumatoid arthritis for twenty-five years. It turned out to have been a sensitivity to corn. When all corn products were eliminated from her diet, her symptoms disappeared. She looked and felt younger than she had in years.

Six weeks after her remarkable recovery, however, her joint pain came back. Her doctors began to suspect that her startling improvement had been nothing more than a temporary placebo effect—until they discovered that the cook preparing her food had started using cornstarch as a thickening agent. They eliminated the cornstarch, and almost immediately her symptoms disappeared again.[1]

Later, research teams learned how to identify which foods affect which people. Not everyone has identifiable food triggers, and corn is only one of several common culprits. But, as this case illustrates, even simple diet changes can sometimes be powerful.

In this chapter, I will show you how to plan your own antiarthritis menu and, if you need more help, how to use nutritional supplements that fight pain much like anti-inflammatory drugs, but without side effects. For example, researchers at the University of Pennsylvania showed how the natural oil in borage seeds reduces arthritis pain, stiffness, and swelling. Likewise, ginger has been used for thousands of years as an anti-inflammatory medicine in Asia, and modern science is starting to tease out why it works.

You can use the diet change approach, the supplement approach, or both, if you need them. We will also look at some totally unexpected findings. For example, some cases of arthritis are caused by a bacterial infection, meaning that the best treatment might not be aspirin; it might be antibiotics, as was recently discovered for ulcers (see page 97).

TAKE TWO ASPS AND CALL ME IN THE MORNING

My father has had osteoarthritis in several joints and ended up with so many joint replacements that he calls himself the Bionic Man. He found that typical anti-inflammatory drugs did nothing for him. If you have arthritis, you have no doubt found that pain medicines are a less-than-perfect solution. Sometimes they help enormously, but too often they leave you with significant pain, and they do nothing to stop the worsening damage to your joints.

Of course, there are worse things than anti-inflammatory drugs. The Chinese arthritis treatment called snake wine, for example, is made by soaking one hundred dead snakes in five liters of red wine with various herbs for three months and adjusting the alcohol content to 40 percent. The arthritis sufferer drinks it three times per day. It is intoxicating, but it does nothing for your joints.

While Advil, Motrin, Naprosyn, and other typical anti-inflammatories are better than snake wine, they have plenty of side effects, including stomach pain and bleeding, among other problems. Your doctor may have prescribed even stronger drugs with increasingly toxic side effects, while the damage to your joints get worse and worse.

In this chapter, we will focus on new approaches to rheumatoid arthritis, osteoarthritis, gout, and temporomandibular joint syndrome, using foods as our main prescription. If your problem is back pain, see chapter 1.

USING FOODS AGAINST RHEUMATOID ARTHRITIS

Rheumatoid arthritis is among the most aggravating of joint problems. It causes pain and stiffness, and over time it deforms the joints. But it is not caused by old age, and it does not have to be a one-way street. For many people it responds remarkably well to a change in the menu. The pain, swelling, and stiffness in your joints can improve or even go away.

Doctors call rheumatoid arthritis an autoimmune disease, which means that your own body is attacking you. Specifically, your white blood cells are attacking the tissues that line your joints. These cells are supposed to be fighting against bacteria, viruses, and cancer cells, but somehow they have turned against your own sensitive joint membranes.

Certain foods encourage this dangerous reaction. While it is odd to think that foods could affect the inside of your joints, imagine for a moment that you are allergic to strawberries. You could break out in a rash. What if the reaction were not on your skin, but in the tender membranes inside your joints? Food sensitivities in arthritis are a bit different from a typical allergy, but nonetheless, certain foods lead to a painful reaction in susceptible people.

When researchers began to suspect that foods played a role in arthritis, some eliminated the problem by putting patients on a supervised fast for several days. As it turns out, it works well. The vast majority of patients improve, and the relief is often striking.[2] Other researchers have used elimination diets, much like those used in migraine research, to identify which foods are the most common offenders.

I am not speaking of undocumented cases in folklore. Rheumatologists' case reports of food sensitivities published in medical journals led to double-blind, controlled food challenges that have clearly established the role of diet in arthritis. Not all patients have shown food sensitivities, but for many, identifying food sensitivities has made an enormous difference. Some of these patients had suffered with arthritis for years, never realizing that simple diet changes could help.

By 1991, the issue was settled beyond any reasonable dispute. A team of researchers in Oslo, Norway, published a breakthrough research report in the *Lancet,* a prominent British medical journal. They had carefully eliminated foods believed to be common arthritis triggers in a group of twenty-six arthritis patients. The results were dramatic. Joint stiffness melted away, swelling and tenderness decreased, and grip strength improved. The average pain score fell from over five, on a scale from zero to ten, to under three. (This was an average, meaning that some patients got a much greater effect while others got less.) Most importantly, when they checked the patients a year later, the benefits were still there.[2]

Other research teams in many different countries have studied how foods affect arthritis. Problem foods vary somewhat from person to person, although it is clear that certain foods are frequent offenders while others are nearly always safe.

The percentage of people with arthritis who benefit from a diet change varies depending on which research study you read. Supervised fasting yields objective benefits in well over half of participants. Similarly, if testing is done with sufficient care, dietary sensitivities show up in anywhere from 20 to 60 percent of subjects. Pure vegetarian (vegan) diets appear to benefit about half of arthritis patients, including some who did not identify a specific diet trigger.[2-6]

An especially memorable case concerned an eight-year-old girl with juvenile rheumatoid arthritis, reported in the *Journal of the Royal Society of Medicine.*[7] She was admitted to the hospital with pain and swelling in her wrist. The pain spread to her hands, feet, hips, and knees, and over the next six years, she was hospitalized nine times. Her symptoms subsided for three months when she went on a vegetarian diet, but her doctor advised her not to continue the diet for reasons that turned out not to be very sound. She went back to her old way of eating, and her pain soon returned.

Later, she consulted with other doctors, who came to suspect that foods were contributing to her symptoms. They gave particular attention to milk products, which have turned out to be among the most common triggers for arthritis patients. They asked her to avoid all dairy products, and within one week, her joint swelling was gone. In three weeks, her pain was gone.

After a two-week vacation, however, her pain and swelling returned.

A review of the foods she had eaten turned up two Kit Kat bars made of milk chocolate. After resuming a strict nondairy diet, the pain again went away. Two months later, while staying with her grandmother, she had cereal and milk for breakfast each morning, and her joint pain returned. After again omitting milk for her diet, her pain subsided and she stayed well for the next six months.

You might imagine that, by this point, her doctors would have been convinced that milk played a role in her symptoms. But they decided to put it to the test. They asked her to have milk products twice a day. She did so, and within about three weeks, the inevitable happened. Swelling and pain recurred, only to stop within ten days of stopping dairy products. She went back to sports and aerobic dancing and felt well until eighteen months later, when her inexplicably skeptical doctors asked her to try the milk test again. Within ten days, the pains returned and she refused to continue the test.

Many doctors responded to such studies with great skepticism. Richard S. Panush, chairman of the Department of Medicine at Saint Barnabas Medical Center in New Jersey and a leading expert on arthritis, set out to disprove the theory that foods can cause arthritis symptoms.

He began to test patients. Most seemed to have no special reaction to foods. But, as it happened, some did. One woman strongly believed that her joint flare-ups were caused by milk, meat, and beans, so Dr. Panush devised a test in which he gave her capsules containing various freeze-dried foods. She had no idea which foods were in which capsules.

The culprit soon became painfully obvious. Within twenty-four to forty-eight hours of ingesting capsules containing milk, her joints became sore and stiff. Avoiding milk made the symptoms go away. In repeated tests, milk caused her symptoms.

As slow as some doctors have been to acknowledge the role of foods in joint problems, some arthritis organizations have been even slower. The Arthritis Foundation holds that "research, however, has not shown to date that specific foods or nutrients make major forms of arthritis better or worse."

The truth is that no single food or nutrient helps everyone with arthritis, but research studies have clearly shown that certain foods do, in fact, trigger symptoms for a great many people, and other nutrients can ease symptoms, as we will see.

This lethargy on the part of some within the medical community has been tragic for people with arthritis. In the late 1980s, I attended a conference where arthritis patients who had been essentially cured by changing their diets were presented. After returning home, I ran into a medical student who had been struggling for years in a losing battle with arthritis. Even with extensive medical care she had suffered deformities of her hands and other joints. I encouraged her to look into whether dietary factors might help her. She told me that she had already brought it up with her doctor, who told her that foods have nothing to do with joint pain and that a change in her diet was a waste of time. She swept away the suggestion with hands that ached with every motion.

This would be more understandable if typical arthritis treatments were more effective. But given that medicines do not stop the progressive damage to the joints and often do not do much for the pain and stiffness, we should welcome better solutions.

THE ANTIARTHRITIS MENU

The first step in using foods against arthritis is simply to avoid foods that are common joint-pain triggers and to emphasize those that are pain-safe. This is easy to do, particularly with the pain-safe recipes in the back of this book.

Pain-safe foods tend not to encourage inflammation, which is why they are useful for many painful conditions. The list of pain-safe foods for arthritis is nearly identical to that for migraines. The only difference is that apples are not restricted in arthritis, since no studies, to my knowledge, have implicated the proteins in apples or apple products in joint problems.

The list of foods that trigger arthritis was compiled from research studies that have examined limited numbers of patients since the early 1980s. This list also has similarities to its counterpart for migraines. Dairy products and citrus fruits, for example, are common triggers for both. There are some differences, however. Red wine and chocolate are among the worst migraine triggers, but are not such a problem for arthritis. On the other hand, corn and wheat are often implicated in arthritis; less commonly so in migraines.*

Other foods have triggered symptoms in some individuals. While they do not appear to be triggers for most people, that could change as more patients are studied. These include alcoholic beverages, bananas, chocolate, malt, nitrites, onions, soy products, spices (cardamom, coriander, and mint), and cane sugar.

THE FOUR-WEEK ANTIARTHRITIS DIET

For four weeks, include generous amounts of foods from the pain-safe list in your routine.

At the same time, scrupulously avoid the major triggers. It is important to avoid these foods *completely*, as even a small amount can cause symptoms.

Foods that are not on either list can be consumed, so long as you are emphasizing the arthritis-safe foods and scrupulously avoiding the major triggers.

You may well experience benefits earlier than four weeks, but for some people it can take this long for chronically inflamed joints to cool down.

---

*Wheat's versatility accounts for its popularity, which is well deserved, given that it has little fat and no cholesterol at all. Unfortunately, its proteins spark reactions in some people, particularly joint pains and digestive problems.

The grain's linguistic roots deserve mention, as told by Martha Barnette in her book *Ladyfingers and Nun's Tummies*. The word *wheat* comes from Old English and Germanic words meaning "white." Its transformation into pasta brought us *vermicelli* (little worms), *linguini* (little tongues), and *pasta putanesca* (whore's pasta). *Lasagne* comes from the ancient Greek word *lasanon*, meaning "chamber pot." The Romans applied this label to a large cooking pot, and it eventually came to signify its edible contents. *Penne* comes from a Latin word for feather, hence "quill" or "pen." *Tagliatelle* and *fettuccine* mean "ribbons." In 1914, Italian restaurateur Alfredo Di Lelio cooked fettuccine with butter, cream, and Parmesan cheese, immortalizing his name and earning the condemnation of cardiologists everywhere.

PAIN-SAFE FOODS

Pain-safe foods virtually never contribute to arthritis or other painful conditions. These include

Brown rice

Cooked or dried fruits: cherries, cranberries, pears, prunes (but not citrus fruits, bananas, peaches, or tomatoes)

Cooked green, yellow, and orange vegetables: artichokes, asparagus, broccoli, chard, collards, lettuce, spinach, string beans, summer or winter squash, sweet potatoes, tapioca, and taro (poi)

Water: plain water or carbonated forms, such as Perrier, are fine. Other beverages—even herbal teas—can be triggers.

Condiments: modest amounts of salt, maple syrup, and vanilla extract are usually well-tolerated.

After four weeks, if your symptoms have improved or disappeared, the next step is to nail down which one or more of the trigger foods has been causing your problem. Simply reintroduce the foods you have eliminated back into your diet one at a time, every two days.

Have a generous amount of each newly reintroduced food, and see whether your joints flare up again. If so, eliminate the food that seems to have caused the problem, and let your joints cool down again. Then continue to reintroduce the other foods. Wait at least two weeks before trying a problem food a second time. Many people have more than one food trigger.

I do not recommend bringing meats, dairy products, or eggs back into your diet. Not only are they major triggers, but they also encourage hormone imbalances that may contribute to joint pain, as we will see below, and also lead to many other health problems.

If eliminating the major triggers did not help your joints, it may be that you are sensitive to foods other than those on this list. You can still track down your joint pain triggers by using the elimination diet described on page 48. It is done exactly the same way for arthritis as for migraines. It takes some time, but is easy to do and will forever change the way you think about foods. Finding a food trigger is a wonderful feeling, like breaking free from a heavy chain that has kept you in pain.

If you still have some remaining symptoms, the next step is to add special foods that fight inflammation.

....

AVOID MAJOR ARTHRITIS TRIGGERS

1. Dairy products*	6. Citrus fruits
2. Corn	7. Potatoes
3. Meats**	8. Tomatoes
4. Wheat, oats, rye	9. Nuts
5. Eggs	10. Coffee

* All dairy products should be avoided: skim or whole cow's milk, goat's milk, cheese, yogurt, etc.
** All meats should be avoided: beef, pork, chicken, turkey, fish, etc.

....

FOODS THAT FIGHT INFLAMMATION

When you cut your finger or scrape your foot, the injured area turns red and warm, swells, and gets sore. This reaction—called inflammation—is your body's way of increasing blood flow to an injury, bringing in nutrients that heal and white blood cells to swallow germs.

Sometimes inflammation starts unexpectedly. Your joints get hot and painful, not because they have been injured, but because your natural injury response was inappropriately triggered, like a person mistakenly shouting "Fire!" in a crowded movie theater. Inflammation also contributes to headaches, digestive problems, menstrual cramps, psoriasis, eczema, temporal arteritis, and other conditions.

Common painkillers, such as aspirin or ibuprofen, work by blocking inflammation. They are useful, but their relief is often less than complete and side effects are frequent.

Two natural fats that come from plants act like anti-inflammatory medicines, without the side effects of drugs. For some patients, they work dramatically; for others their effect is more modest.

The first, called alpha-linolenic acid, or simply ALA, is found in many common foods: vegetables, beans, and fruits, and in a concentrated form in flaxseed oil, as well as in canola, wheat-germ, and walnut oils. It is in the omega-3 family of fatty acids, the group that also includes fish oils.

The second, called gamma-linolenic acid, or GLA, is much rarer. It is found in only a few unusual seed oils: borage oil, evening primrose oil, black currant oil, and hemp oil.

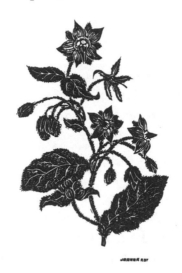

Both of these natural fats can be used to fight inflammation, as researchers have repeatedly shown. At the University of Pennsylvania in 1993, patients with rheumatoid arthritis were given four capsules of borage oil each day, while a control group took placebo capsules made of cottonseed oil. Six months later, the researchers checked the patients' symptoms. Joint swelling and tenderness were reduced by about 40 percent in the borage oil group, morning stiffness was down by 33 percent, and pain was reduced by about 15 percent. Overall, the results were moderate, but considering that the placebo group gradually worsened over the same period, the turnaround in pain, swelling, and stiffness was a welcome change.[8]

Tests at other medical centers showed much the same result with borage oil, evening primrose oil, black currant oil, and flax oil.[9,10] You cannot get the same effect from olive oil, corn oil, sunflower oil, safflower oil, lard, butter, or other common fats or oils.[11] They simply do not have any anti-inflammatory action.

NATURAL OILS

ALA CONTENT[12,13]		GLA CONTENT	
Canola oil	11%	Black currant oil	17–18%
Flaxseed oil	53–62	Borage oil	24
Linseed oil	53	Evening primrose oil	8–10
Soybean oil	7	Hemp oil	19
Walnut oil	10		
Wheat-germ oil	7		

To see how ALA and GLA put the brakes on pain and inflammation, it is important to understand what controls the heat inside your joints.

Inflammation is controlled by various chemicals in your body, the most important of which are called *prostaglandins*. One of them, called prostaglandin E_2, is like gasoline on a fire. If you are injured or if an infection takes hold, prostaglandin E_2 responds with lightning speed. In the blink of an eye, it is manufactured by the cells in your joints, sparks local inflammation, and disappears. Its mission is to help you attack invading bacteria and get the healing under way. Unfortunately, it can attack your own tissues just as quickly. Each molecule of prostaglandin E_2 survives only an instant, but if it keeps being released from your cells, it is like a constant spray of sparks that keep your joints hurting.

Prostaglandin E_2 is made from fat, especially the fat found in meats and cooking oils. When you eat these foods, some of their fat is stored within the outer membrane covering each of the cells of your body. There, it waits, ready to turn into this potentially dangerous chemical.*

Two different prostaglandins have the opposite effect: they work to stop inflammation. Called E_1 and E_3, they are like a stream of cool water on hot joints. They block the swelling, pain, redness, and heat.

These technical-sounding names are not important. What is useful to

---

*The inflammatory prostaglandin E_2 is made from arachidonic acid, which is found in meats (the average omnivore ingests between 200 and 1,000 mg of arachidonic acid each day) and can also be made from another fat called *linoleic acid*, which comes from cooking oils, particularly corn, sunflower, safflower, and cottonseed oils.[14] Plants have no arachidonic acid at all, because they do not have the enzymes that make it.

Typical Western diets include twenty times as much linoleic acid as ALA, or even more, in addition to a hefty dose of artery-clogging saturated fats. These diets program every cell in our bodies toward inflammation. An optimal diet omits meats, dairy products, and added oils and is based entirely on plant foods.

know is that, if you take a supplement of borage oil, evening primrose oil, or black currant oil, the GLA in them turns into prostaglandin E_1 and cools down your joints. Likewise, if there is ALA in the foods you eat, it turns into prostaglandin E_3 and turns on its own anti-inflammatory effect.

The fats that you eat determine which of these prostaglandins will be produced. If your diet is rich in animal fats or cooking oils, you will be packing inflammatory fats into the cell membranes surrounding the cells of your body. On the other hand, if you have more GLA or ALA, these helpful oils take their place, ready to provide natural anti-inflammatory compounds. You will not lose your normal ability to produce prostaglandin E_2 or to mount an inflammatory response to injuries, but you will be better able to avoid excessive and inappropriate inflammation.

GLA is available at any health food store without a prescription. It is most concentrated in borage oil, which gives you the most benefit with the least oil. You can also order GLA-rich oils from the same source that supplies research teams, a company called Health From the Sun in Sunapee, New Hampshire (800-447-2229). Borage oil comes in a mild-tasting liquid (one-quarter teaspoon supplies 300 mg of GLA) or capsules containing an equal amount of GLA.

It can take several weeks for these oils to work, and up to six months to see their full effect. Side effects, such as loose stools, are usually mild and transitory. Even so, I would encourage you to use anti-inflammatory oils under a doctor's supervision, as they really act like medicines, and while they seem to be quite safe, the possibility of side effects after long-term use should not be ruled out. Avoid GLA if you are or may be pregnant, since it may increase the possibility of miscarriage.

A typical arthritis regimen includes *each* of the following every day, usually with the evening meal:

1. Borage, black currant, or evening primrose oil, containing 1.4 grams of GLA.
2. Flaxseed oil, one tablespoon (or four capsules).
3. Vitamin E, 400 IU, or the IU for people with high blood pressure. Vitamin E protects against oxidation of the oils.

Some people use fish oils for their anti-inflammatory omega-3s. However, plant-derived oils have none of the fish odor that can be apparent in the perspiration of people using fish oil. They also tend to be more chemically stable, so they do not oxidize as quickly. They are also lower in saturated fats. Between 15 and 30 percent of fish oil is saturated fat, which is about double that of plant oils. The fact is, fish make their oils from ALA in plankton, just as mammals, including humans, synthesize them from land plants.

NATURAL ALA IN FOODS

While GLA is rare in nature, ALA is common. It is found in green, leafy vegetables, beans and other legumes, and fruits. These plants do not have much oil of any kind, and what they have is heavily balanced toward ALA, as opposed to other kinds of fats.* Only so much fat or oil can fit into the membranes of your cells, and if your diet is rich in these foods, your cell membranes will take up plenty of ALA.

Unfortunately, a diet rich in meats, dairy products, shortenings, and cooking oils (e.g., corn oil or cottonseed oil) means that unfriendly fats get packed into your cell membranes instead of ALA. The unhealthful fats in a piece of chicken or hamburger easily overwhelm the good fats in vegetables and crowd ALA out of your cells. They tie up the enzymes that normally use ALA and, in the process, encourage inflammation.[13–16]

The good news is that, even after years of burgers and fries, you can push these unhelpful fats out of your cells. Just as you can change the oil in your car, you can do essentially the same thing in your cells. It takes longer, but you can do it.

Let's say you've been eating a fairly typical North American or European diet of chicken, beef, eggs, and foods prepared with cooking oils. Your cell membranes contain the fats from these foods. If you were to have a spoonful of flaxseed or linseed oil every day, their omega-3s would gradually replace the other fats in your cells, and your tendency toward inflammation would be reduced.[17] About half the fatty acids in flaxseed and linseed oils are ALA, in contrast to corn oil, cottonseed oil, and butter, which are only about 1 percent ALA.

If you eat generous amounts green, leafy vegetables, beans, and fruits

---

*While most plant foods are low in fat, nuts are an exception. In one hundred grams (about four ounces) of walnuts, there are fifty-seven grams of fat, of which seven grams are ALA.

and avoid the animal fats and concentrated cooking oils that compete with them, your cells will gradually reflect the good balance of fats they hold.

....

PLANT FOODS RICH IN ALA

Vegetables: purslane, lettuce, broccoli, spinach, etc.
Legumes: navy, pinto, or lima beans, peas or split peas, etc.
Citrus fruits are rich in ALA and can be used if you have established that they are
    not pain triggers for you.
Oils: flaxseed, linseed, canola, and walnut oils are richest, followed by wheat germ
    and soy oils. Typical oils, such as corn, safflower, sunflower, or cottonseed, are
    low in ALA.

A TINY AMOUNT GOES A LONG WAY

Your car needs gallons and gallons of gasoline because it is burning it for power. But it needs only a bit of oil to keep friction from overheating the engine. Similarly, your body needs the calories in starchy foods, such as rice, bread, beans, potatoes, and other vegetables, for energy. But only about 3 to 4 percent of your calories need to come from fats or oils. Most of us get ten times that amount, and the fats we get tend to be in poor balance. You can restore a better balance by including generous amounts of vegetables, legumes, and fruits in your daily routine.

YOU REALLY ARE WHAT YOU EAT

Believe it or not, if you were to stick a needle into your abdomen or thigh and pull out a little fat sample and analyze it, it would show the kinds of fat you had been eating over the previous year or two.[18,19] Fish fat, olive oil, beef fat—they all get packed into the membranes of your cells, and they tend to stay there until other fats push them out. People on plant-based diets have much less body fat overall, and the fat they do have tends to favor ALA and the other omega-3s that are made from it, and they have less of the inflammatory fats that are common in meat-eaters.[14]

    If food triggers cause joint pain for you, eliminating them is likely to bring much more rapid and striking benefits than adding "good" fats.

However, changing the amount and type of fat you consume can be an important added step.

A WORK IN PROGRESS

While we know that natural oils such as GLA help cool down hot joints, our explanations as to how they do this are far from complete. In fact, before 1982, omega-3 oils were not believed to be needed in the diet at all. A six-year-old girl changed that. She had been the victim of a gunshot accident in which she lost most of her intestinal tract. Because she could not digest food normally, she had to be fed intravenously. Gradually, she developed symptoms of nerve abnormalities, including numbness and blurred vision, and eventually became unable to walk. The problem was a lack of ALA in her feeding solution. Her doctors added it, and her symptoms soon disappeared.[20]

Vegetables and fruits have an added benefit—they are loaded with natural antioxidants, which may have some ability of their own to counter painful processes, as we will see below.[21–23] If you are tracking down your food triggers, you will want to have most of your vegetables and fruits in their cooked form at first. However, as you learn which foods are not triggers for you, I would encourage you to have more and more fruits and leafy vegetables raw.

GINGER

We think of spices as taste enhancers. But many also have health benefits that may account for why our taste buds so often demand them. Garlic is probably the most famous because it has been proven to lower cholesterol levels, but it is hardly the only flavoring with health benefits.

Several spices show anti-inflammatory effects in test-tube experiments, and perhaps the best studied of these is ginger. Ginger blocks enzymes that would otherwise make inflammation-producing prostaglandins. Indeed, it has been used in traditional Indian Ayurvedic medicine for centuries as an arthritis treatment.

A team of researchers in Denmark who have been studying ginger since the late 1980s accidentally triggered a natural experiment on its effects. One of the researchers mentioned to a newspaper reporter that ginger blocks inflammation in the test tube and that it might prove useful for arthritis or other inflammatory diseases. Many readers decided to try it, and they began to call the research lab to report their results.[24]

A fifty-year-old man with rheumatoid arthritis found that his pain vanished after taking fresh ginger daily for about one month. A woman with osteoarthritis had reduced swelling and better range of movement in her joints. In all, twenty-eight patients with rheumatoid arthritis and eighteen with osteoarthritis reported on their experiences. The vast majority had substantial reductions in pain and swelling.

The most interesting report came from a person who had eaten a generous serving of Crabtree & Evelyn Ginger with Grapefruit Marmalade, which is 15 percent ginger. An anti-inflammatory effect persisted for several days.

Blood tests on human volunteers show that ginger modifies the actions of enzymes in the human body, blocking the production of inflammatory compounds, as it does in the test tube.[25] Still, controlled tests comparing ginger against a placebo have not been done and may well never be, since no manufacturer is likely to pay to test a product that cannot be patented and is already available everywhere.

However, doctors can get around this lack of controlled tests with what are called "n of 1" studies. The *n* is an abbreviation used in research studies to indicate the number of subjects participating. In an n of 1 study, the doctor and patient agree that the doctor will provide the active compound (in this case, ginger) or an identical placebo at different times, and the patient will note the effects. If, say, three months on the active compound produce a noticeable change in the joints that disappears when the placebo is used, the result can be confirmed by repeating the test as many times as necessary. If done carefully, such tests provide statistically meaningful results.

The amount of ginger usually used is one-half to one teaspoon (one to two grams) of powdered ginger each day, although some people have used up to four times this amount. Allow four to twelve weeks for benefits to appear. No adverse effects of ginger have been reported, and the U.S. government includes it on its generally recognized as safe (GRAS) list.[24]

Other spices, including clove oil, garlic, turmeric, and cumin, show similar effects in the test tube.[25-27] In India, turmeric is applied to the skin or taken orally in doses up to five grams per day as an anti-inflammatory agent. None of these spices has been subjected to clinical tests, however.

A NEW TREATMENT FROM AN OLD VINE?

A surprising experimental treatment has emerged from an entirely unexpected source. The thunder-god vine is a woody, rambling shrub that grows in southern China. Its leaves, flowers, and even the skins of the roots are poisonous. In fact, they are so poisonous that they have been used as an agricultural insecticide. Even ingesting honey that contains pollen from the plant can be fatal.

However, someone in the distant past somehow managed to discover that the interior of the roots of this toxic plant make an effective arthritis treatment, and it has been widely used in rural China.[28]

The modern history of the thunder-god vine begins in the Chinese Cultural Revolution of the late 1960s, when Chairman Mao ordered China's increasingly westernized doctors to leave the cities and become "barefoot doctors," learning about traditional Chinese medicine in rural areas. Many of them were intrigued with the vine's efficacy against inflammatory diseases, including arthritis. Many started to study extracts of the vine, and in the late 1980s, controlled research studies found that it effectively reduced joint stiffness, swelling, and tenderness, compared to a placebo. In fact, it worked better than typical nonsteroidal anti-inflammatory drugs.[29] That brought the vine to the other side of the Pacific, where University of Texas researchers are testing it in arthritis patients.[28]

Although it is a natural plant product, it does have potential side effects. It can cause a rash, gastrointestinal symptoms, temporary loss of menstrual periods, and reductions in blood counts. These effects will not rule it out as an arthritis treatment, however, because drugs typically used for arthritis pain also have significant side effects. Stay tuned.

STOPPING THE DAMAGE

We do not just want to stop the pain of arthritis. We also want to stop the damage to our joints. On a molecular level, the damage is caused by free radicals, extremely unstable and destructive molecules that are waste products made by your cells—the biological equivalent of factory exhaust. Free radicals are also made by your white blood cells for use as weapons against bacteria. Unfortunately, these molecular toxins end up attacking your own body tissues and are believed to be what actually causes the damage of inflammation.

Free radicals are an especially serious problem in joints that are already inflamed. In a swollen knee joint, for example, the blood flow is cut off momentarily with every pounding step. As the joint relaxes again, blood rushes in, and this ebb and flow of blood encourages the production of extra free radicals that assault the joint. To protect yourself, you need to neutralize these free radicals.

The cells that line your joints, like every other cell in your body, are surrounded by a thin cell membrane that has built-in antioxidants to knock out free radicals. Among the best-known antioxidants is beta-carotene, which is what gives carrots and sweet potatoes their orange color. It sits in the cell membrane, waiting to neutralize free radicals as they approach.

Vitamin E and the mineral selenium, found in grains, beans, and vegetables, join beta-carotene on the cell surface as important parts of your antioxidant defenses.

Fruits and vegetables contribute vitamin C, which patrols your bloodstream and the watery spaces between cells, looking for free radicals that have not yet reached the cells' surfaces. Vitamin C also repairs vitamin E that has been damaged in the battle against free radicals.

Vitamin supplements can be useful. But they are no substitute for antioxidant-rich foods. After all, a beta-carotene pill contains only beta-carotene. Carrots, sweet potatoes, and spinach, on the other hand, contain hundreds of other carotenoids in the balance that our bodies are designed to accept, something no vitamin pill can match.

ANTIOXIDANTS IN FOODS (MG)

	VITAMIN C	BETA-CAROTENE	VITAMIN E
Apple (1)	8	0.04	0.80
Broccoli	116	1.30	1.30
Brussels sprouts	96	0.67	2.00
Carrot (1)	7	12.00	3.00
Cauliflower	68	0.01	0.10
Chickpeas	2	0.02	5.10
Grapefruit (1)	94	0.38	0.64
Navy beans	2	0	4.10
Pineapple	24	0.02	0.16
Rice, brown	0	0	4.00
Soybeans	3	0.01	35.00
Spinach, fresh	16	2.30	1.10
Strawberries	85	0.02	0.18
Sweet potato (1)	28	15.00	5.90

Serving sizes are one cup, except as otherwise noted.
Sources: J. A. T. Pennington, *Bowes and Church's Food Values of Portions Commonly Used*, 16th ed. (Philadelphia: J. B. Lippincott, 1994), and P. J. McLaughlin and J. L. Weihrauch, "Vitamin E content of foods," *J Am Dietetic Asso* 75 (1979): 647–65.

THE DANGERS OF OIL AND IRON

Two parts of your diet can accelerate the damage of free radicals. The first is oils. We noted above that traces of certain natural vegetable oils help stop inflammation. However, in excess, oils cause more free radicals to form. Fish oils are the worst in this regard, but the same is also true of all oils. This is one reason why I generally encourage you to focus on improving the *balance* of your fats, rather than adding extra oils, except as a temporary measure. This is also why vitamin E is typically added to supplemental oil regimens. It is intended to protect against free radical production from the oils.

Iron aggravates free radical attacks. It acts as a catalyst for the production of free radicals and also increases the damage they do.[30] Of course, you need a tiny bit of iron in your diet for your red blood cells to carry oxygen. But iron is unstable, which is why it rusts so quickly.

Most of us get far more iron than our bodies need, partly because it is in vitamin supplements, but also because the meat-based diets most of us were raised on contain enormous amounts of a highly absorbable form of iron. The excess iron that accumulates in our bodies simply waits, ready to cause damage. It is easy to check how much iron is stored in your body and, if it is excessive, to get rid of it. Here is what you do:

1. Check your iron status with these blood tests. A doctor can order them for you, and in some locations, a clinical laboratory can run them without a doctor's request. Results should always be interpreted by a physician.

- Serum ferritin (normal values are 12–200 mcg/1)
- Serum iron
- Total iron-binding capacity (TIBC)

Serum iron should be checked after an overnight fast. The serum-iron measurement is divided by TIBC. The result should be 16–50 percent for women and 16–62 percent for men.

Results above these norms indicate excess iron. Results below these norms indicate too little iron. If the result suggests iron deficiency, your doctor may request an additional test, called a red cell protoporphyrin test, for confirmation. A result *higher* than 70 mcg/dl of red blood cells suggests insufficient iron. To diagnose iron deficiency, at least two of these three values (serum ferritin, serum iron/TIBC, or red cell proto-porphyrin) should be abnormal.

2. If your blood tests show excess iron, as they do for most adult men and postmenopausal women, you can bring your iron level back to normal with regular exercise and, believe it or not, donating blood. Regular visits to your local blood-donation center can help you unload excess iron, while helping someone in need.

3. To keep your iron in balance, get your nutrition from grains, beans, vegetables, and fruits. They contain plenty of iron, but it is in a form that your body can easily regulate. When you need more, your body absorbs more, and when you already have plenty, your body absorbs less.

4. Avoid meats. They contain a type of iron, called heme iron, that your body cannot regulate. Even if you already have excess iron in your body, it simply barges through your digestive tract, into your blood-stream, like an uninvited guest at a party.

FIGHTING ARTHRITIS WITH ANTIBIOTICS

Strange as it may sound, the best treatment for some forms of arthritis may be antibiotics. Doctors have long known that certain bacteria, such as salmonella, campylobacter, or yersinia, which are common contaminants in raw chicken and beef, can cause arthritis symptoms. Sometimes the joint pains linger on for months or even years.[31,32]

Salmonella infections are common—much more common than is recognized or reported—and most people never get treated for what they imagine to be nothing but the "flu." However, in at least one case in seven, joint symptoms come along with the intestinal illness, typically affecting the knees, fingers, and shoulders.

Sometimes bacteria actually invade your joints, but in other cases the problem seems to be that your body reacts to the bacteria in your digestive tract by making antibodies that then travel in your bloodstream to your joints.

Infectious bacteria are found on about 30 percent of chicken packages at the retail store and on about 15 percent of beef carcasses. Cooking kills them, but does not kill the bacteria that dribble out of the chicken package onto your kitchen counter or that soak into your kitchen sponge.

Other bacteria may get into the act, as well, a further reason why antibiotics are emerging as a potentially important, albeit controversial, treatment for arthritis. Bacterial infections have been suspected of playing a role in arthritis for decades, and the question now is not whether they cause joint symptoms, but how often. Your doctor can advise you on current antibiotic regimens.

OSTEOARTHRITIS

Osteoarthritis, also called degenerative joint disease, can be thought of as an effect of wear and tear on the body. If you could look inside the joints of your hands, wrists, hips, knees, feet, shoulders, or spine, you would find bony spurs and damaged cartilage.

Injuries and repetitive motions at work contribute to osteoarthritis, although, oddly enough, running does not seem to.[33-37]

The most important step in osteoarthritis is to lose excess weight.

Every ten pounds of excess weight increases the risk of osteoarthritis in the knees by 30 percent.[33,38]

The reason is not just that excess weight puts chronic stress on your knee joints. Being overweight even increases the risk of osteoarthritis in your hands.[38,39] No one knows exactly why, but one possible reason is that fat cells make estrogen, and that excess estrogen is somehow involved in joint damage. Support for this idea comes from the observation that women have more osteoarthritis than men, especially if they have had symptoms of estrogen excess, such as uterine fibroids.[40,41]

Happily, the best way to lose weight is also the best way to get your hormones into better balance. If you avoid fatty foods (meats, dairy products, fried foods, and vegetable oils) and emphasize grains, vegetables, fruits, and beans in your routine, excess weight tends to melt away even if you are not counting calories.

At the same time, when your diet is low in fat and high in fiber, the amount of estrogen in your blood quickly drops to a healthier level. For more details on the hormone-adjusting effects of these foods, see chapter 8.

Vitamin E relieves pain and improves mobility in patients with osteoarthritis.[42] A typical dosage regimen is 400 IU each day, or 100 IU for people with high blood pressure.

Some individuals with osteoarthritis have found that avoiding common diet triggers has brought tremendous benefits. Regrettably, however, researchers have not studied the role of dietary factors in osteoarthritis as they have for rheumatoid arthritis, nor is there sufficient information on the role of essential fatty acids in treating osteoarthritis. However, both the basic antiarthritis diet and essential fatty acid supplements described above are healthful and safe, and it may well be worth trying them to see whether they work for you.

TOPICAL CAPSAICIN FOR OSTEOARTHRITIS PAIN

An unusual treatment for pain comes from hot chili peppers, believe it or not. You do not have to eat them. Their "hot" ingredient, capsaicin (pronounced *cap say' a sin*), is mixed into a cream that is applied to the skin over the painful joint. Inside the nerves, this strategy is like fighting fire with fire. A brief stinging sensation stimulates the pain nerves and then shuts them down as capsaicin depletes a chemical called *substance P,* which nerves use to transmit pain signals. This is an old pain remedy, having been used as long ago as 1850 to treat toothaches.[43]

In controlled studies, patients report that capsaicin reduces osteoarthritis pain by more than 70 percent.[44] Because it is used topically, it has no drug interactions and no serious toxicity. The main side effect is a mild to moderate burning sensation on the skin that lasts about two hours after application during the first ten days or so of use. The painkilling power continues to increase week by week, presumably as substance P is being used up, although you will notice most of the benefit within the first two weeks of use. It is most useful for people with one or two painful joints and can be used for both osteoarthritis and rheumatoid arthritis.

You will find capsaicin in drugstores under the brand names Dolorac and Zostrix. The easiest and most effective regimen uses Dolorac (0.25 percent) cream twice a day directly on the affected joint. Zostrix is a more dilute cream that is usually used on a more frequent regimen.

GOUT

Gout is an excruciating pain that begins in the big toe and eventually spreads to other joints. Hospital treatment is usually necessary. If you were to insert a needle into one of your joints and pull out a sample of joint fluid, you would find the cause: it would be full of uric acid crystals.

Most animal species do their best to get rid of uric acid. They have enzymes in their bodies to quickly break it down and eliminate it. However, humans, insects, birds, and reptiles actually save uric acid, apparently because it is a powerful antioxidant, rather like vitamin C. In some people, it builds up in the joints, or in chalky deposits in the skin of the ear, the forearm, the elbow, or the Achilles tendon. There, white blood cells attempt to engulf it, triggering inflammation, pain, and joint damage.

Two common parts of the diet—animal products and alcohol—make gout more likely. The worst contributors are shellfish, sardines, anchovies, organ meats (e.g., liver and kidneys), and beer.[45] However, high-protein diets in general tend to encourage gout.[46] While the reason for their contribution is not entirely clear, avoiding them is certainly a good idea. If your nutrition comes from a variety of grains, beans, vegetables, and fruits, you will get adequate protein while avoiding excesses.

People with a tendency toward gout are more likely to have an attack during times of dietary change, so if you are on medication, continue it through the transition in your diet, and discuss with your doctor the issue of whether and when you can get off your medicines.

TEMPOROMANDIBULAR JOINT PAIN

The temporomandibular joint (TMJ) is where your lower jaw attaches just in front of your ear. It has an enormous job to do, supporting the stresses of biting and grinding the food we eat, with hundreds of forceful movements every day. However, with well-aligned teeth and no unusual trauma, these joints are usually pretty resilient.

However, one out of every three or four people develops TMJ symptoms: reduced range of motion, difficulty closing the jaw properly, pain, and tenderness to the touch.

The usual cause is trauma, e.g., auto accidents, falls, or prolonged hyperextension of the jaw during medical or dental procedures.[47] Many other conditions can mimic TMJ disorder, however, including migraines, intracranial tumors or aneurysms, and even Lyme disease, so a careful diagnosis is important.

When it has been diagnosed, most patients can be comforted by the fact that TMJ disorder will go away without any drastic treatment. It sometimes lingers for a year or two, but it usually runs its course and disappears. Typical treatments include anti-inflammatory medicines, exercises, and one form or another of intra-oral splints, which help in at least three-fourths of cases.

The main role of food in TMJ disorder is to eat softer foods and take smaller bites to take the stress off the joint. Pain clinics sometimes use vitamin B_6, which is also used in carpal tunnel syndrome, diabetic pains, and other conditions. The usual dose is 100–150 mg of B_6 per day.[48]

A broader role for food is suggested by the fact that some cases of TMJ disorder are manifestations of rheumatoid or osteoarthritis, although nailing down specific food triggers or using essential fatty acids as treatments awaits future research.

Some investigators hypothesize that estrogens may play a role. Like osteoarthritis, TMJ disorders occur much more often in women than men, and estrogen receptors have actually been found within the joint itself. Estrogens are believed to encourage the production of inflammatory compounds within cells.[49] So if a TMJ problem begins with trauma, estrogens may aggravate it.

If estrogens do indeed contribute, low-fat, high-fiber foods that reduce estrogen levels (see chapter 8) may help reduce the incidence of TMJ problems. For the moment, however, the main value of such foods as oatmeal and applesauce seems to be their ability to ease the jaw's workload.

Your joints work hard, and it does not take much for things to go wrong. However, by avoiding foods that trigger symptoms and taking steps to reduce your inflammatory response, many people can ease their symptoms and recover much better function.

CHAPTER 6

Curing Stomachaches and Digestive Problems

Digestive problems are a drug company's dream: a virtually endless stream of miserable people arriving at drugstores to buy antacids, acid suppressants, laxatives, fiber supplements, anti-gas preparations, and dozens of other remedies whose relief is short-lived, sending them back for more.

You do not have to be part of it. While many people accept digestive pains and constipation as part of life, foods can have a rapid and decisive effect on these symptoms. In Crohn's disease and ulcerative colitis, genetics play a role, but are by no means the whole story, and a menu change can often make a huge difference. On the other hand, ulcers have long been blamed on foods, forcing people to turn away from spicy meals and their favorite cup of java, but today foods get a not-guilty verdict. Ulcers are actually caused by a bacterial infection in most cases, and a brief course of antibiotics cures them, usually permanently.

THE REAL CAUSE OF ULCERS

An ulcer is a small eroded spot in the lining of your stomach or the first part of the intestine, called the duodenum *(doo a dee' num)*. Some ulcers are caused by aspirin and other anti-inflammatory drugs. The rest were blamed, until recently, on excess stomach acid, presumably as a result of stress, spicy food, or too much black coffee. Doctors advised their patients to try to relax, eat bland food, and take antacids or acid-suppressants, products that are still popular.

However, in 1983, an Australian physician named Barry Marshall discovered that doctors had been wrong.[1] Ulcers are not caused by hot peppers, Indian curry, income tax forms, or cappuccino. They are a bacterial infection, like a strep throat or pneumonia. The culprit, called *Helicobacter pylori,* can be knocked out by two weeks' worth of antibiotics, and 95 percent of ulcers never return. Once you eliminate the infection, your stomach is not the frail, sensitive organ it is now, and you can enjoy that jalapeño salsa again.

Helicobacter also causes gastritis and is implicated in other digestive problems. Where do these bacteria come from? We pick them up as children, presumably from contact with others in the home or from contaminated water, and we carry them for the rest of our lives, unless we are treated.

Roughly half of older adults in the United States and Europe are infected with helicobacter. Infection is more common where children live in crowded or less than hygienic conditions, and improving hygiene has reduced infection rates for younger generations.[2] These bacteria usually remain dormant for years before causing symptoms.

Helicobacter can be detected with blood, saliva, or breath tests. If your stomach pains are accompanied by weight loss, difficulty swallowing, bloody or black stools, or other puzzling or worrisome symptoms, your doctor will want to take a look at your stomach with an endoscope and will take a small tissue sample to test for helicobacter.

All these tests occasionally yield "false negatives," that is, they indicate that bacteria are not present when, in fact, they are. This is especially true if you have recently been treated with antibiotics or if you are over sixty-five, but it can happen at any age.[3] For this reason, doctors sometimes recommend going ahead with antibiotics without bothering with diagnostic tests, since the treatment is generally safe.

The regimen is easy. A typical prescription consists of the following combination taken for ten days to two weeks:

tetracycline, 500 mg four times a day

metronidazole (Flagyl), 400 mg three to four times a day

Pepto-Bismol, 1–2 tablets four times a day

Other regimens are used as well, and you will want to talk with your doctor about the best choices to maximize effectiveness and minimize side effects. Once the bug is eliminated, it is usually gone forever.[4]

The discovery of helicobacter's role revolutionized ulcer treatment. It also led to other, even more surprising, leads. Patients with a form of stomach cancer called gastric lymphoma were found to have a high prevalence of helicobacter infection. In a recent research study, doctors treated the infection with antibiotics, and the cancers actually shrank.[5] Treating cancer with antibiotics is an obviously novel idea. However, this type of tumor appears to grow in response to an irritant, in this case helicobacter.

LICORICE PROTECTS THE STOMACH

When stomach pain is not caused by helicobacter, a useful treatment comes from licorice. Licorice does not kill bacteria or soak up acid. It works by increasing the number of mucus-secreting cells that form the stomach's protective layer. Various licorice extracts have been used to ease stomach pains, including duodenal and stomach ulcers, but have had occasional side effects. A newer and well-tolerated product, called deglycyrrhizinated licorice or DGL, is sold at health food stores as a chewable tablet. DGL can help protect against many kinds of stomach irritation, including that caused by nonsteroidal anti-inflammatories.

USING FOODS TO EASE HEARTBURN

The stomach makes strong acid to digest food and has a special lining that allows it to withstand the acid. However, when acid sneaks up into the esophagus, it causes heartburn. A muscular sphincter is supposed to stop this from happening, but the muscle can be weakened by several factors, some of which are on your plate.

Fatty foods, alcohol, chocolate, and peppermint tend to relax the sphincter and allow reflux. If you have heartburn, you will want to avoid them. You will also want to steer clear of citrus juices, tomato products, coffee, and alcohol, all of which can irritate the esophagus directly, with or without stomach acid.

It often helps to have smaller meals in the evening.[6] A helicobacter infection can also contribute to heartburn, but is easily treated, as noted above.

IRRITABLE BOWEL SYNDROME

Irritable bowel syndrome, also called spastic colon, is an annoying condition in which your intestinal tract seems unable to function properly. Sometimes you get diarrhea. Other times you become constipated. Much of the time your abdomen is bloated, gassy, and painful.

Normally, your digestive tract moves food along in a proper sequence, with food in the stomach signaling the large intestine to allow its contents to move forward. It is an orderly process, like squeezing toothpaste from the end of a tube toward the opening. In irritable bowel syndrome, the intestinal movements are uncoordinated, like squeezing a tube of toothpaste on both ends at once.

As a sufferer from irritable bowel syndrome (IBS), you are not alone. About 15 to 20 percent of people in North America have IBS symptoms. To diagnose it, doctors normally rely on your history, asking about gassiness, a distended feeling, altered bowel habits, and abdominal pain that is relieved by a trip to the bathroom. Doctors will check for Crohn's disease, ulcerative colitis, diverticulitis, malabsorption, diabetes, and hyperthyroidism and will also ask whether antibiotics, antacids, or laxatives are contributing to your problem. They also usually check for infections, such as amebiasis or giardiasis. All of this can be done with simple blood tests, a stool sample, sigmoidoscopy, and a barium enema.[7] While some gastroenterologists conduct endless additional diagnostic tests to rule out other conditions, most will spare you the trouble, as the condition is a familiar one.

There are simple steps that can help enormously. Many people need go no further than to take advantage of foods that calm down the digestive tract and to avoid those that send it into spasms. Some, however, have specific food sensitivities, which are also not difficult to address. If you have persistent problems, you may wish to regulate your digestive function with natural peppermint oil or ginger. Each of these steps is described below.

FOODS THAT CALM THE DIGESTION

Certain foods soothe your digestive tract. You will want to emphasize them in your diet. Of course, sensitivities can occur with just about any food, so skip any that seem to cause problems for you.

Rice is nutritious and usually well tolerated. If you have IBS or just a temporary bout of diarrhea or constipation, rice can be helpful. It is extremely low in fat, with proteins and complex carbohydrates that are easily digestible. It returns the digestive tract to regular function.

Brown rice is best, because it retains its natural fiber coating. On page 238, I'll show you my simple way of cooking it that preserves its texture and flavor. Rice cakes can be kept in your desk drawer as an emergency supply. Choose the plain, unsugared varieties.

Oat products are rich in soluble fiber, that is, plant roughage that dissolves in water, in contrast to *insoluble* fiber, found in wheat and many other grains. Soluble fiber made oat bran famous because it lowers cholesterol levels. It also helps your digestion.

If travel tends to upset your digestion, oatmeal can be your salvation. Hotels often stock a supply, or you can carry a few packets of instant oatmeal in your luggage. Serve it without milk.

If your digestive problems are caused by celiac disease, a condition in which grain proteins are not digestible, you will unfortunately need to avoid oats and all other grains, except for rice and corn.

Vegetables are also rich in soluble fiber, and most are well tolerated, provided they are prepared without added fat and are well cooked. Beans, peas, and lentils are loaded with soluble fiber, but their digestibility varies from person to person, as noted below.

There is no fiber at all in animal products or in refined sugars, and you are better off avoiding these products completely. When your digestive tract has to cope with sugary foods, fish, poultry, meat, milk, yogurt, or cheese, it has less fiber than it needs for optimal digestion, and you know the results. Because animal products are the center of the diet in Western countries, constipation is commonplace. It is easily cured when the plant products our digestive tracts are designed for are returned to the diet.

FOODS THAT TRIGGER IRRITABLE BOWEL SYMPTOMS

Fatty foods are key contributors to bowel symptoms.[6,8] A hamburger, greasy fries, potato chips, or a drumstick can stir up serious digestive problems that can persist for hours. The reason is that any kind of fat can stimulate intestinal movements by simply *touching* the stomach and duodenum, even before it is absorbed.[8] This does not mean a faster digestion. If these intestinal movements are uncoordinated, they cause a bloated, crampy feeling, rather than diarrhea.

The digestive tract is richly supplied with nerves that sense what has been ingested in order to trigger digestive secretions and intestinal contractions. When olive oil, for example, touches the stomach and duodenum, these nerves trigger intestinal movements. In experiments, researchers have numbed these nerves by infusing an anesthetic into the stomach and found that olive oil then has no effect. Fats and oils do not just work on one small part of your digestive tract at a time; they actually trigger reflexes that send waves affecting all of your digestion.

The effect of greasy food changes depending on how much of it you eat. Researchers fed bread to a group of volunteers and then used hydrogen breath tests to measure how thoroughly it was digested. Adding two teaspoons (11 grams) of butter to the bread reduced its digestibility. However, with five teaspoons (26 grams) of butter on the bread, the effect was different. The load of fat was large enough to slow down the passage of food through the small intestine, probably by triggering a reflex that disrupted the intestinal movements.[9]

CUTTING THE FAT

Fatty foods can disrupt the normal movements of the digestive tract.

- Avoid meats, poultry, and fish. They all have hidden fat and never contain any fiber.
- Steer clear of potato chips, french fries, onion rings, and other fried foods.
- Nonstick cookware allows you to avoid cooking oils.
- Instead of sautéing vegetables, braise them in a small amount of water in a saucepan.
- Use nonfat toppings on baked potatoes, e.g., salsa, Dijon mustard, steamed vegetables, a spoonful of baked beans, etc.
- Use nonfat dressings or a squeeze of lemon juice on your salad instead of oily dressings.
- Replace margarine or butter on toast with jam, or simply enjoy the hearty taste of fresh whole-grain bread.

Between one-half and two-thirds of people with irritable bowel symptoms react to specific foods. Of these, the worst offenders are dairy products, wheat, corn, coffee, tea, and citrus fruits, although individual experiences vary tremendously.[10,11] These and other foods are discussed in more detail below.

Dairy products present two problems. Milk sugar, called lactose, is a common cause of digestive symptoms, and milk proteins can elicit reactions as well.

Young children can nearly always digest lactose, because they have plenty of the *lactase* enzyme that splits it into smaller sugars, called glucose and galactose, which are then absorbed. However, the lactase enzyme begins to disappear after infants are weaned, and most adults have little of it left, which is why a glass of milk can cause indigestion and gassiness.

This is not an abnormality or illness. The disappearance of the lactase enzyme is completely normal, and the discovery of this fact is actually one of the more embarrassing chapters in recent nutrition history.

Until the mid-1960s, American and European dietitians believed that cow's milk caused digestive symptoms in only a small minority of people. However, in 1965, researchers at Baltimore's Johns Hopkins University tested sixty hospital patients and found that, while only about 15 percent of white adults had digestive symptoms from cow's milk, the figure for African-Americans was 70 percent.[12] Other researchers then went to the Maryland House of Correction and offered twenty white prisoners and twenty African-American prisoners extra canteen money in exchange for participating in lactose challenge tests. Only 10 percent of the whites developed symptoms, but 90 percent of African-Americans did.[13]

Researchers set out to study populations in Africa and Asia and found that the vast majority of individuals lose their lactase enzymes as they grow out of childhood. If they had more than about one cup of milk, they soon regretted it, and some could not tolerate even that much.[14] The same turned out to be true of Native Americans.

Symptoms after ingesting milk are common among those whose ancestry is African, Asian, Native American, Arab, Jewish, Hispanic, Italian, or Greek.[15] As the *American Journal of Clinical Nutrition* reported, "It rapidly became apparent that this pattern was the genetic norm, and that lactase activity was sustained only in a majority of adults whose origins were in Northern European or some Mediterranean populations."[16] In other words, Caucasians tolerate milk sugar only because of a genetic mutation that occurred in their distant ancestors. Researchers and dietitians studying lactose who were of European ancestry themselves had assumed that drinking milk without symptoms was normal.

Overall, about 75 percent of the world's population, including 25 percent of those in the United States, lose lactase enzymes after weaning.[14] While those who could not digest milk were once called "lactase deficient" or "lactose intolerant," they are now simply called normal, and those adults who retain the infant enzymes that digest milk are more properly called "lactase persistent."

Why would Mother Nature take away enzymes that digest milk sugar? The answer, apparently, is that nature "designed" milk with the right nutrient mix for an infant. But just as a rocket drops its boosters shortly after launch, mammals no longer need milk after infancy, and all mammals stop drinking it as soon as they are able to meet their nutrition needs otherwise. If you have associated loss of lactose-digesting enzymes with a disease or problem, rest assured it is as natural as losing your baby teeth and baby fat.

Milk's fat, growth factors, and sugars are essential for infants, but are not appropriate for adults and may even pose dangers. Long-term exposure to milk sugars is linked to increased risk of cataracts, infertility, and ovarian cancer. The culprit appears to be galactose, the simple sugar that is released from lactose by an infant's enzymes and also exists freely in dairy products (e.g., Lactaid) that have been treated to "help" people who do not digest lactose. Galactose can enter the lens of the eye, which may be why there is a strong epidemiologic correlation between milk consumption and cataracts. Its effect on the ovaries is worrisome, given that ovarian cancer is often aggressive, and is a matter of ongoing research. Milk consumption is also linked with higher breast cancer risk, presumably due to growth factors in milk.[17]

The sugar in milk is not its only problem. Some people are sensitive to milk proteins, which can cause diarrhea and vomiting, in addition to more typical allergic symptoms, such as a runny nose, skin conditions, or asthma.

Doctors can test your ability to digest milk sugars with a breath test, because milk sugars that are not digested are fermented by bacteria that produce hydrogen. However, if the test shows that you are able to digest lactose, there is still no advantage to doing so, as you are then subjected to the galactose that comes from it.

If you want something to splash on your cereal, try soy or rice milks instead, and choose the lower-fat brands. Some are calcium-fortified. For more information about good sources of calcium without milk, see page 18.

Wheat. While most people tolerate wheat with no symptoms, accounting for its ubiquitous use in breads and pasta, it causes adverse reactions for some, either because they lack the enzymes needed to digest wheat proteins, as in celiac disease, or because they have an allergy or sensitivity to them. Wheat-free breads and pastas are available at health food stores.

Even for people who do not have digestive problems, wheat is not completely digested. This depends in part on how much of it you eat; the bigger the serving, the less is digested.[9]

Other grains, such as corn, barley, or rye, sometimes cause problems, too, and are easy to avoid. Rice, the staple of many Asian cultures, is generally well tolerated.

Coffee and tea. About one in five people with irritable bowel symptoms tends to react to coffee or tea. Decaffeinated brands may be less of a problem.

Raw fruits (e.g., citrus fruits, apples, grapes, raisins, cantaloupe, or bananas) often cause digestive problems, as can some fruit juices, particularly citrus, apple, and prune juices.

Try fruits that can be peeled and cooked. If the seeds in strawberries, raspberries, or blackberries bother you, try blueberries. Avocados are an unusual fruit in that they are high in fat and therefore present the same problems of other high-fat foods.

Raw vegetables sometimes cause problems. This is particularly true for cruciferous vegetables (e.g., broccoli, cauliflower, brussels sprouts, cabbage), tomatoes, celery, spinach, peppers, and carrots. Cook your vegetables thoroughly, preferably by steaming or any other fat-free method. Some vegetables, such as spinach, work well pureed. If you have a juicer, try carrots, perhaps in combination with cucumbers or other vegetables. If onions or garlic give you problems, try onion or garlic powder.

It may be that certain vegetables will give you problems no matter how well you cook them. Broccoli or cabbage, for example, is much better tolerated when thoroughly cooked, but will still present difficulties for some people.

Beans and bean products (e.g., tofu) sometimes cause gas. This does not mean you have to avoid them, but you can use small amounts, always thoroughly cooked. There are no al dente beans. You may also find that different kinds of beans have different effects. Navy or pinto beans might cause gas, for example, while chickpeas or black beans do not. Effects vary from person to person and can change over time.

IN PRAISE OF BEANS

Beans are good food. They have no cholesterol and almost no fat. They are loaded with protein, calcium, and iron. They have soluble fiber, which many people associate only with oat bran, and they have omega-3 fatty acids, which we tend to think of in fish oils. About the only thing that beans do not have is a good lobbying group to promote their advantages.

Unlike the modern world, which considers beans a humble food, at least one ancient civilization held them in high esteem, as food historian Harold McGee wrote in *On Food and Cooking*:

"Each of the major legumes known to Rome lent its name to a prominent Roman family: Fabius comes from the faba [or fava] bean, Lentulus from the lentil, Piso from the pea, and Cicero—most distinguished of them all—from the chickpea. No other group has been so honored."[18]

Nuts and nut butters are high in fat (with the exception of chestnuts) and present the same problems as other high-fat foods.

Condiments and flavorings. Be careful about black or red pepper, cinnamon, chili powder, cloves, nutmeg, dried parsley, mustard seeds, grated orange rind, and soy sauce. The sorbitol sometimes used in sugarless gum and jam causes diarrhea if taken in more than modest amounts.

If you are unsure whether any given food is a problem for you, give yourself the benefit of a short test. For a week or so, have generous amounts of rice, cooked vegetables and fruits, and modest amounts of well-cooked beans, peas, and lentils, avoiding any vegetables that you know you cannot tolerate. Eliminate dairy products, meats, fried foods, and added oils. Once your digestive tract settles down, you will be able to reintroduce the eliminated foods and recognize which ones cause problems.

If your problems continue, you may wish to try a more comprehensive elimination diet, which is designed to track down more unusual causes of symptoms and is described on page 48.

BACTERIA THAT HELP AND HURT

Bacteria in your intestinal tract help you with digestion. However, if you take antibiotics for any reason, some of these friendly bacteria are killed. After your antibiotic treatment is over, you can replenish these bacteria with supplements of normal flora that you will find at any health food store or drugstore. Some people use yogurt for this purpose, because yogurt is made by adding bacteria to milk. However, I would encourage you to buy the friendly bacteria directly and skip the yogurt.

While some species of bacteria are helpful, others are anything but. Salmonella, campylobacter, giardia, *E. coli,* and many other malicious microbes that are common stowaways in raw poultry and meat can cause serious digestive problems. If you have chronic digestive problems, your doctor will check for these common infections. While most intestinal bacterial infections pass on their own, sometimes treatment is necessary.

PEPPERMINT OIL

Most people experience dramatic improvement after eliminating fatty foods, emphasizing natural high-fiber foods, and avoiding problem foods. If you still have some symptoms, however, you may wish to try peppermint oil.

Peppermint is a natural hybrid of the spearmint and watermint plants. Its leaves contain an oil that has been used since the 1700s to soothe digestive ailments. The active ingredient is menthol, which relaxes the muscles of the digestive tract.

Peppermint oil is not just a folk remedy. Controlled research studies clearly show that it works. For example, in a study of sixteen patients with irritable bowel syndrome at Hope Hospital in Manchester, England, all but three improved with peppermint oil, while placebo pills used for comparison yielded no consistent improvement.[19] Some gastroenterologists have even used peppermint oil to relieve spasms in the digestive tract while they are doing endoscopic exams. They simply squirt a bit of peppermint oil through the endoscope tube into the digestive tract, and it relaxes the muscles within thirty seconds.[20] If you were to swallow the oil directly, it could relax the sphincter muscle between the esophagus and the stomach, causing heartburn. With this in mind, manufacturers pack peppermint oil into pills that dissolve further downstream.[21] You will find them at all health food stores. Peppermint oil capsules should be taken on an empty stomach so that foods do not delay their passage. Avoid peppermint oil if you have gallbladder or bile-duct problems.

GINGER

Ginger has been used in traditional Indian Ayurvedic medicine for intestinal discomfort and flatulence, as well as for inflammatory conditions, such as arthritis.

Its value has been specifically demonstrated in motion sickness. Because this is a common problem for navy personnel, pilots, and astronauts, researchers have been interested in finding solutions. In one study, researchers decided to test ginger's effect on sailors heading out to sea for the first time. On the first day of rough water, the sailors were given a capsule that contained either one gram of ginger or a placebo. Those receiving the ginger were much less likely to have vomiting or to be incapacitated.[22]

In another test, researchers put volunteers into a tilted rotating chair that was designed to produce motion sickness. Ginger proved more effective in blocking symptoms than dimenhydrinate (Dramamine), a drug commonly used for motion sickness. The subjects on dimenhydrinate encountered worse nausea, and none was able to last all six minutes in the chair, while half of those on ginger were able to go for the full time.[23] The amount used to calm the stomach is one-half to one teaspoon (one to two grams) of powdered ginger, and it can be taken daily if needed.[24]

IT'S NOT JUST WHAT WE EAT, IT'S HOW

Unhurried eating helps every aspect of digestion. This does not mean you need an extralong lunch break, but taking the time to chew your food thoroughly and avoiding stress while you are eating will get your digestion off to a good start.

Sometimes people complain that something must be wrong with their digestion because they see whole pieces of corn or other undigested material pass right through them. If this has happened to you, the problem was not in your digestive tract; it was at the dinner table.

A snake can swallow a small animal whole and eventually digest it. You cannot. Your digestive tract can only work on foods that are thoroughly chewed, so that natural digestive enzymes can mix with the food and do their job.

Relaxed eating is important, too. Stress causes your body to release hormones that get you ready to fight or to run away. When you are under threat, digesting your salad is not a high priority, so stress-related hormones do nothing to help your intestinal tract. Quite the contrary. They disrupt the normal synchronized contractions of the intestinal muscles, causing cramps rather than an orderly passage of foods.[25]

Some people do better with four to six small meals throughout the day, rather than three large meals. This sort of "grazing" approach is healthy and presents smaller challenges to your digestive tract. Also be aware of the temperature of your foods. For some people, hot soups or beverages stimulate colonic activity, leading to pain or diarrhea. If this is a problem for you, you may wish to serve them at room temperature.

CURING COLIC

Babies get upset stomachs, too. About one in five babies develops colic. Luckily, simple diet changes usually solve the problem. Cow's milk and cow's milk formulas are the most common culprits. A switch to breast-feeding, if possible, or soy-based baby formula, usually solves the problem.

Surprisingly enough, breast milk can cause colic, too, depending on what the *mother* has been eating. For example, if a woman consumes dairy products, some of the cow's milk proteins will pass from her digestive tract into her bloodstream, then into her breast milk. Not so long ago, doctors believed that proteins were completely broken down in the digestive tract, and that it would be impossible for animal proteins to end up in a woman's breast milk. However, in the April 1991 issue of *Pediatrics*, researchers reported finding that intact cow's milk proteins do, in fact, pass through the blood into the milk of milk-drinking women, a phenomenon now known to occur quite commonly.[26]

Several years ago I took a train to New York to give a lecture on children's diets to a group of pediatricians. The train car was nearly deserted, which was lucky, because a couple near the front of the car were struggling to console their wailing baby. By coincidence, I happened to be reviewing some articles on the hazards of cow's milk products for infants, one of which is colic. At the risk of being intrusive, I asked the young couple if they had noticed whether any foods affected their child. "Well, I'm breast-feeding, so all he gets is breast milk," the mother said. "But this happens every time I have either milk, coffee, or chocolate."

Other parents have noticed the same thing. The *Journal of the American Dietetic Association* published the results of a survey of 272 breast-feeding mothers that found that when they eat certain foods, their babies tend to be colicky. The most common offenders: cow's milk, onions, cruciferous vegetables (e.g., broccoli, cauliflower, or cabbage), and chocolate.[27] The solution is to avoid these foods, especially during the first four months of breast-feeding.

Stomachaches in older children are similar to irritable bowel syndrome in adults and are treated in much the same way by pediatricians. Avoiding problem foods, having more soothing foods, and using peppermint oil can all be effective.

DIVERTICULAR DISEASE

Diverticuli are small pouches that form in the wall of the large intestine. When they become inflamed and painful, the condition is called diverticulitis. Doctors used to treat it with low-fiber diets on the theory that compact, low-fiber stools would be easier on the intestinal tract. It turned out that the opposite was true. Small, hard stools are like rocks going through your digestive tract. High-fiber foods hold water and keep stools soft, allowing diverticuli to heal.

High-fiber foods come in four groups: grains, legumes, vegetables, and fruits. Of these, the best for keeping things moving through your digestive tract are whole grains, such as brown rice, oats, and whole wheat bread, and any foods from the legume group, such as beans or lentils.

If you have irritable bowel symptoms along with diverticular disease, you may want to favor soluble fiber, as is found in oatmeal and beans, rather than the insoluble fiber of wheat and most other grains, and may need to keep bean servings moderate.

As noted above, animal products have no fiber at all, and refined carbohydrates, such as white bread or pasta, have had most of their natural fiber removed.

Fiber supplements are also available, but are rarely necessary for people on a diet that eliminates animal products.

CROHN'S DISEASE AND ULCERATIVE COLITIS

In irritable bowel syndrome, your digestive tract acts up in unpleasant ways, but if you could look at it, it would actually look perfectly normal and healthy. That is not true of inflammatory bowel disease, a group of conditions that are exactly what they sound like. The digestive tract is inflamed and damaged.

The common inflammations of the digestive tract are *Crohn's disease* and *ulcerative colitis*. Crohn's disease usually involves the large intestine and the last part of the small intestine, but can occur anywhere in your gastrointestinal tract. It often affects young people, causing pain after meals, along with a low-grade fever and mild diarrhea. Episodes often become more frequent and severe.

Ulcerative colitis occurs only in the colon (that is, the large intestine). Symptoms include rectal bleeding, diarrhea, pain, weight loss, and fever.

The causes of inflammatory bowel disease are poorly understood. It almost surely has mixed causes, including genetics. Identical twins—who have exactly the same genes—always have the same color hair and eyes. However, if one has Crohn's disease, the chances of the other twin's having it, too, are only fifty-fifty. For ulcerative colitis, the chances are lower, around one in five.[28] This means that part of the risk is genetic, but a big part of the risk has nothing to do with genetics and may be subject to control.

Some researchers believe the problem starts when infections or food sensitivities irritate the digestive tract, and then an exaggerated inflammatory response does the damage.[29] A study in southern England identified one type of bacteria, called *Mycobacterium paratuberculosis,* which is sometimes found in livestock, in two-thirds of Crohn's disease patients, providing more evidence that, indeed, infection may be at least part of the cause.[30]

A role for diet emerged gradually, much as it did for other diseases. Like heart disease and diabetes, inflammatory bowel disease is rare in rural Asia, but more common in parts of Asia that have westernized their diets. Similarly, it is rare in Africa, but more common in African-Americans. These studies suggest that an environmental factor, such as diet, plays an important role.

Inflammatory bowel disease is most common in North America and Northern Europe, where high-fat, meaty diets are routine.[31] In addition, the rise in Crohn's disease over the last thirty years has paralleled the increase in other diet-related conditions, such as obesity and some forms of cancer, over the same period.

Diets of people with Crohn's disease tend to be low in fiber and high in sugar. In particular, they are low in fruits and vegetables, compared to others.[32] In a research study in England, doctors asked one group of patients to eat more whole-grain bread, brown rice, fruits, and vegetables, and to reduce the amount of sugar, white flour, and white rice they consumed, while leaving patients in another group to their habitual diets. Over the next five years, thirty-two patients in each group were followed. The diet group had less than one-third the number of hospitalizations, and their hospital stays were shorter; altogether they spent only one-fifth as many days in the hospital, compared to the other patients. Only one person in the diet group needed surgery, compared to five in the regular group, and the one who needed surgery was operated on for a condition that was already present when the diet was introduced.[33]

Fiber increases stool volume. If you have a history of strictures, you should increase the fiber content of your diet gradually, rather than suddenly. Also, always be sure to chew your food thoroughly.

TRACKING DOWN PROBLEM FOODS

When people with inflammatory bowel disease need hospitalization, solid food is usually replaced with an "elemental" diet, that is, a liquid formula in which the nutrients have been broken down into their smallest building blocks. Proteins are broken down into individual amino acids, in order to eliminate the possibility of protein sensitivities. Carbohydrates are given as glucose, and fats are provided only as simple fatty acids.

In a research study in Cambridge, England, researchers treated Crohn's disease patients with an elemental diet, but instead of returning them to their usual diets when the symptoms improved, they added foods back one at a time to see which, if any, might cause symptoms.

Dairy products and wheat turned out to be the most common triggers, causing symptoms in one-third to one-half of patients. Broccoli, corn, yeast, meats, tomatoes, citrus fruits, and eggs were also common culprits. Other studies have indicted essentially the same list of foods. In isolated cases, individuals have reacted to rice, apples, onions, barley, rye, alcohol, and chocolate. Overall, about 70 percent of patients are able to identify one or more foods that trigger symptoms.[34,35] (See table.)

COMMON TRIGGERS FOR CROHN'S DISEASE[34,35]

1. Wheat	6. Yeast	11. Coffee or tea
2. Dairy	7. Tomatoes	12. Bananas
3. Cruciferous vegetables*	8. Citrus fruits	13. Potatoes
4. Corn	9. Eggs	
5. Meat, poultry, or fish	10. Peanuts	

*The cruciferous vegetable group inclues broccoli, cauliflower, and brussels sprouts.

The foods that contribute to Crohn's disease are surprisingly similar to those that trigger migraines and arthritis. Dairy products and wheat are again strongly implicated. For some patients the problem with milk is the milk sugar, lactose, just as we saw for irritable bowel syndrome. But for more patients, the problem with dairy products appears to be a reaction not to the lactose sugar but to the milk proteins.

Decades ago, when this fact was beginning to be appreciated, researchers reported unusual cures from simple diet changes. Researchers in Copenhagen described the case of a farmer who had been having ten to twenty watery stools per day. He had applied for disability benefits because of extreme fatigue. He was hospitalized and put on a lactose-free diet. Within two days, his stools became normal. Over the next two weeks he gained fifteen pounds and insisted on leaving the hospital, because he had to go home to sow his fields.[36]

In research studies, when milk is removed from the diet—even in patients who show no signs of lactose intolerance—symptoms often diminish or go away. In one study, this was true of about one-fourth of patients with ulcerative colitis, and one-third of patients with Crohn's disease.[36] Further evidence against milk comes from the fact that infants who are reared on breast milk, rather than cow's milk formula, have less risk of Crohn's disease.[37] In addition, sophisticated immune tests have shown sensitivities to milk proteins in patients with both conditions.[37,38] Sugar, margarine, and a lack of fiber have also been implicated.[37]

Food sensitivities are not as predictable in inflammatory bowel disease as they are in migraines or arthritis, and they can change over time. Nonetheless, for those who identify their food triggers and avoid them, the relapse rate is only about 10 percent per year. In comparison, the vast majority of untreated patients relapse within the first year or two after an episode.[34,39]

In rare cases, the elemental treatment diets themselves have caused symptoms that disappeared when the doctors switched to a different brand. Some are derived from corn starches and peanut or safflower oil, so a reaction might not be surprising if traces of corn or peanut proteins inadvertently entered the mix.[35]

OMEGA-3'S FOR ULCERATIVE COLITIS

Omega-3 fatty acids may help, too. In chapter 5 we saw how these special oils can fight inflammation. They have been shown to help in about three-quarters of people with ulcerative colitis. They do not make the disease go away, but they do reduce symptoms and the need for medications.

A deficiency of fatty acids is probably not the cause of the disease, but fatty acids can serve to blunt the inflammatory response that does the damage. Omega-3s have not been shown to help in Crohn's disease.[37,40–42]

While some have used fish oils for this purpose, I recommend the more stable (and more palatable) botanical oils, as described in chapter 5. Flaxseed oil is a concentrated source of omega-3 fatty acids; borage, evening primrose, black currant, and hemp oil are rich in gamma-linolenic acid. For dosages and product information, see page 83.

None of this means that inflammatory bowel disease will simply go away. Sometimes it does. But often the goal is to keep it from returning so frequently, allowing you to get on with life rather than worrying about the return of symptoms.

CHAPTER 7

Fibromyalgia

Roughly 3 to 4 percent of women have muscle pain and tenderness over much of their bodies, a condition called fibromyalgia. The cause of the problem is probably not in the painful muscles themselves, but in a nervous system that reacts to normal sensations in unusual ways. Instead of your nerves telling you that someone has touched your arm, for example, they send pain sensations to your brain. Along with the pain comes fatigue, poor sleep, morning stiffness, digestive problems, and depression.[1] Fibromyalgia occurs less often in men—only about one-half of one percent of men have it.[2,3]

Other problems are also common in people with fibromyalgia: tension and migraine headaches, menstrual pain, rheumatoid arthritis, lupus erythematosus, fatigue, irritable bowel, upper respiratory infections, heat and cold intolerance, chronic bladder or vulvar pain, and low-grade fevers. Many have neurological symptoms aside from pain: numbness or tingling in about 80 percent, increased sensitivity to sounds in 70 percent, hearing loss in 27 percent, and subtle disorders of eye movements in 40 percent.[4]

New diagnostic standards call for doctors to ask about chronic pain and check for tenderness at eighteen different points on your body. But if you have fibromyalgia, you have no doubt endured the frustrations of doctors fumbling to diagnose it and unable to treat it. Antidepressants are routinely prescribed; they can help, but are not a complete answer.

The symptoms of fibromyalgia are in many ways similar to those of chronic fatigue syndrome. Aches and pains, fatigue, and depression are common in both, and it is useful to think of the two syndromes as over-lapping and requiring similar treatment.

To diagnose chronic fatigue syndrome, doctors look for persistent or relapsing, debilitating fatigue lasting at least six months that is not caused by any other condition. Additional symptoms include memory or concentration problems, sore throat, tender lymph nodes, muscle pain, joint pains, headaches, poor sleep, and prolonged fatigue after exercise.

The cause of chronic fatigue syndrome remains as obscure as that of fibromyalgia. Many researchers believe that an infection is responsible, although no culprit has been identified. The Epstein-Barr virus turned out not to be the cause, and no other virus has yet been convincingly implicated. Immune abnormalities are also considered to play a role, but what triggers them remains unknown.

The most common treatments include antidepressant medicines to reduce pain, treat depression, and improve sleep. Anti-inflammatory drugs can help for headaches, and muscle and joint pains.[5,6] But typically the disease lingers on for months and years.

RELEASING YOUR ENDORPHINS

Exercise activates the body's endorphins, natural chemicals that are part of your internal pain-control system. They are made in the pituitary gland and work within the brain and nerves themselves and also travel in your bloodstream to reduce pain. Exercise also improves sleep, which, in turn, reduces pain sensitivity. Studies of healthy people have shown that those who exercise frequently (six hours or more per week) have dra-matically reduced sensitivity to pain.[7]

These facts have not been lost on people with fibromyalgia, who feel much better when they get regular vigorous aerobic exercise, such as bicycling, running, or step aerobics. The keys are frequency and vigor-ousness, but it is important to increase your regimen gradually and stay within your limits.[8-11]

Many people with chronic fatigue syndrome avoid exercise, finding that they easily become worn-out and even laid up by exertion. However, if they start with brief, simple exercises and gradually work their way up to longer exercise periods, they often feel better and more energetic. It might help to know that, although people with chronic fatigue syndrome *feel* weak, tests show that their muscle strength and exercise capacity are normal, except insofar as the illness makes them sedentary.[12]

A study published in the *British Medical Journal* in 1997 found that, if patients with chronic fatigue syndrome started out slowly, with just five to fifteen minutes of walking, five days a week, they tolerated it well.[13] By adding one to two minutes per day, they could gradually work their way up to a thirty-minute walk. If they preferred, they could substitute any similar exercise, such as swimming or cycling.

After the twelve-week study, more than half the exercising patients reported feeling substantially better. And the benefits continued—a year later, 63 percent of the participants were doing significantly better. In a second group that did stretching and relaxation exercises instead of aerobic exercise, only about a quarter of the participants improved. Aerobic exercise—that is, exercise that gets your heart beating and your lungs moving—seems to be the key.

One important caution: Some people with chronic fatigue syndrome are subject to rapid and unexpected drops in blood pressure while standing or exercising, a disorder called neurally mediated hypotension. They suddenly feel faint, start sweating, and need to sit or lie down to avoid passing out. To guard against this possibility, your physician should evaluate your capacity for exercise and guide you to a safe regimen.

THE ROLE OF FOOD

Nutrition has an important role in at least some cases of fibromyalgia and chronic fatigue. Of all the nutrients, magnesium has gotten the most attention.

Researchers at the University of Texas in San Antonio gave magnesium and malic acid to patients with fibromyalgia. By taking 150 to 300 mg of magnesium, along with 600 to 1,200 mg of malic acid, twice a day, patients noticed a significant reduction in pain and tenderness.[14] The regimen starts at the lower doses and gradually increases as needed.

A 1991 British study found that magnesium was useful in chronic fatigue syndrome, improving energy levels and reducing pain in 80 percent of subjects. The study used an injectable form of magnesium weekly for six weeks, but it can also be taken orally.[15]

Some people with fibromyalgia have found that avoiding certain foods makes an enormous difference. A case in point is Claire Musickant, of Milwaukee, Wisconsin. Her symptoms began one day while she was teaching a class at a local college. Pain started out in her right foot, traveled up her hip to her lower back, and gradually intensified. By the time the class had ended, the pain was excruciating. She could barely make it to her car. In the days that followed, things got worse. Claire became tender to the touch all over her body, and she developed headaches, bowel symptoms, fatigue, anxiety, and depression.

As is often the case with fibromyalgia, it took a long time before Claire Musickant's symptoms were correctly diagnosed, and even longer before they were effectively treated. Eventually it turned out that she was particularly sensitive to sulfites—preservatives used in salad bars, shellfish, wines, and many other foods. She was also sensitive to dairy products, cranberries, melons, and corn.

She read package labels carefully so as to scrupulously avoid triggers. She also began a course of vitamin and mineral supplements to strengthen her immune system, along with a regular exercise regimen. Her pain and fatigue gradually diminished and eventually disappeared completely, and her energy came back better than ever.

The test that identified her sensitivities was developed by Russell M. Jaffe, a former National Institutes of Health researcher who found that, for many patients, sensitivities to foods and environmental chemicals play a major role in fibromyalgia. In a research study of twenty-five fibromyalgia patients, he checked for sensitivities to foods or chemicals, used supplements to correct deficiencies, and recommended regular exercise for three months. Most patients had reduced pain, and some had a complete elimination of pain. Tenderness, stiffness, and fatigue also diminished, depressed spirits lifted, and bowel symptoms improved.[16]

Sensitivities varied from one person to another, and most patients were sensitive to more than one exposure; in fact, most were sensitive to anywhere from fifteen to thirty different items. The most common included monosodium glutamate (MSG), caffeine, food colorings, chocolate, shrimp, and dairy products.

The allergy test, called ELISA/ACT, which stands for the Enzyme-Linked Immunosorbent Assay/Advanced Cell Test, is not the skin-patch test that allergists have traditionally used. It is done by drawing a blood sample and testing to see which chemicals elicit a reaction in the white blood cells. The test can be expensive, but Dr. Jaffe has found it to be a useful guide to exposures that aggravate symptoms.

Like traditional allergy testing, ELISA/ACT has occasional false positives and false negatives. In other words, it may indicate a sensitivity to a food or chemical that is actually an innocent party, and it may also miss a true sensitivity. If a certain exposure seems to cause symptoms for you, it is worth avoiding it even if testing suggests that it should not be a problem. Your doctor can arrange an ELISA/ACT test by contacting Serammune Physicians Lab, 1890 Preston White Drive, Reston, VA 22091, 800-553-5472.

Claire Musickant began the program in 1991, and her symptoms have stayed in remission. At age sixty-four, she walks two miles per day and only has a recurrence of symptoms if she violates her diet for a few days. Fatigue and pain return, which go away when she resumes her diet.

A LOW-FAT, VEGETARIAN DIET

When we began our study of a low-fat, vegetarian diet for menstrual pain, one of our research participants who had had symptoms of fibromyalgia and chronic fatigue syndrome for years found that, as she began the vegetarian diet, she started to feel much better.

The diet we used was a *pure* vegetarian diet, meaning that it excluded all dairy products, along with all other animal products. Our goal was to reduce estrogen levels, but in the process, we ended up eliminating some of the most common food sensitivities. We also kept vegetable oils to a bare minimum, which can improve immunity.

The diet is surprisingly practical, once participants learn how to integrate it into their routine, and it would be useful to test its effects in more people with fibromyalgia and chronic fatigue.

CAN FOODS INCREASE YOUR PAIN RESISTANCE?

What is actually happening in the nerves or the brain that causes pain? Many fibromyalgia symptoms could be explained by a lack of *serotonin*, a brain chemical that suppresses pain.[4] Serotonin is also essential for regulating moods (which could explain why depression hits about 40 percent of people with fibromyalgia) and plays a role in sleep, which is also often disturbed in fibromyalgia. Sleep deprivation can reduce pain resistance even in people without fibromyalgia.[4,17]

Serotonin is made from *tryptophan,* which is one of the amino acid building blocks of protein. When researchers test the blood of people with fibromyalgia, they often find low levels of tryptophan.[4]

Tryptophan supplements have been shown to reduce experimentally induced pain in volunteers.[18] Tryptophan was taken off the U.S. market after several people developed an unusual blood disorder, apparently caused by a contaminant. However, foods can boost serotonin naturally. Foods that are high in carbohydrates—breads, pasta, potatoes, or fruits—can increase the amount of serotonin in the brain.* High-carbohydrate foods also increase a second brain chemical, called norepinephrine, which is also important in pain control and in moods.[4]

SALT

Another potentially useful food treatment emerged for use in chronic fatigue. Researchers at Johns Hopkins University found that adolescents with chronic fatigue tended to have low blood pressure. So, in addition to their other medications, they put them on high-sodium diets to raise their blood pressure and found that, in many cases, it led to a dramatic improvement.[19]

WHAT TO DO

If you have symptoms of fibromyalgia or chronic fatigue, let me encourage you to:

1. See your doctor for an accurate diagnosis and to rule out other

---

*For the technically minded, tryptophan is an amino acid, that is, one of the building blocks of protein. It is found in many different foods, but it has trouble getting from the bloodstream into the brain because it has to compete with many other amino acids also trying to enter the brain. High-carbohydrate meals cause the body to release insulin, which, among other things, drives competing amino acids from the blood into the cells of the body. With these competitors gone, tryptophan can easily get into the brain, where it is quickly converted into serotonin.

causes of pain and fatigue (a long list, including many different kinds of infections). Your doctor should also check your ability to exercise safely.

2. Low-impact aerobic exercise is helpful. This can include riding a bicycle, swimming, walking, or whatever you are most comfortable with. Start slowly, especially if you have symptoms of chronic fatigue. Start out with three or four minutes of exercise five times a week and gradually lengthen your exercise periods. Don't overshoot your capacity.

3. Magnesium, 150 to 300 mg taken twice per day, has been shown to help fibromyalgia patients. Use it under your doctor's supervision.

4. Brief cognitive-behavioral therapy is offered at some medical centers to help people reduce stress and manage pain and fatigue. It can be beneficial. You may also benefit from reducing stress with massage, relaxation, or acupuncture.[20]

5. Track down whether foods are contributing to your symptoms. The foods that seem to be implicated in some cases of fibromyalgia are similar to those that have been identified for migraines (see page 46). I would suggest that you avoid these foods for eight weeks or so and see how you feel. The pain-safe recipes in the back of this book will help you. You may also wish to use the ELISA/ACT test to help identify sensitivities.

6. Antidepressant medications can be used along with any other aspects of your treatment. They are helpful for many people, often at low doses. Although they help with the depression that is common in fibromyalgia, they are mainly used to reduce pain sensitivity. Amitriptyline is a common first choice. If it causes dry mouth, constipation, or other side effects, as it often does, other drugs can be substituted.

PART III

HORMONE-RELATED

CONDITIONS

CHAPTER 8

Using Foods Against Menstrual Pain

A few years ago, a young woman called me to ask for painkillers. Her menstrual cramps were so excruciating she was unable to work. She was actually unable to do much of anything except lie in bed and wait for her pain to go away. Her mother had had the same problem and needed Demerol, a narcotic painkiller, for a few days every month in order to function.

I told the young woman that I would be glad to prescribe painkillers for a few days, but I also suggested that she try a diet change, just as an experiment, for the next four weeks. She agreed, and a month later she called again. She felt wonderful. The disabling pain that was such a regular feature of her life had simply not come back.

At the time, I was not entirely sure that my suggestion would work, because we did not know then what we know now about how foods affect hormones. But, as it turned out, an educated guess worked wonderfully.

I described this episode in a previous book, *Food for Life*, and some months later I received a letter from Ellen Moore of Houston, Texas. She had tried the nutrition approach I recommended, and she had lost four dress sizes and her energy level increased. "The greatest benefit of all, however, is that since January I have not had to take even one extra-strength Tylenol for menstrual cramps," she wrote. "This is a miracle of the first order. As a teenager, I can recall having cramps so severe that not even Percodan or Demerol provided complete relief. Now I finally am able to live a normal life."

WHAT CAUSES THE PAIN?

Nearly half of all women live with menstrual pain, and in up to 10 percent it is severe enough to interfere with work and other activities for one to two days every month. Sometimes it diminishes after childbirth, but for many it continues.

In the 1960s, it became clear that chemicals called *prostaglandins* are a central part of the problem. In chapter 5, we saw that these chemicals are made from traces of fat stored in cell membranes and that they promote inflammation. They are also involved in muscle contractions, blood vessel constriction, blood clotting, and pain.

Shortly before your period begins, the endometrial cells that form the lining of the uterus make large amounts of prostaglandins. When these cells break down during menstruation, prostaglandins are released. They constrict blood vessels in the uterus and make its muscle layer contract, causing painful cramps. Prostaglandins also enter the bloodstream, causing headache, nausea, vomiting, and diarrhea.[1]

Researchers have measured the amount of prostaglandins produced by the endometrial cells in women with menstrual pain and found that it is higher than for other women.[2] The concentration of prostaglandins circulating in the blood is higher, as well.[1]

This helps explain why nonsteroidal anti-inflammatory drugs work for menstrual pain. Ibuprofen (Motrin), naproxen (Anaprox), and other NSAIDs reduce the production of prostaglandins.

For most women and their doctors, that is the end of the story. For a few days each month, painkillers battle with prostaglandins. The problem, however, is that for many women the relief is far from complete. They find themselves taking more painkillers than recommended without getting the relief they need.

USING FOODS AGAINST PAIN

There may be a more fundamental approach. Rather than focus on the prostaglandins themselves, it may help to focus on the cellular "factories" that make them. After all, we know that birth control pills reduce menstrual pain, apparently by reducing the growth of the endometrial cell layer. The smaller this layer of cells is, the less tissue there is to make prostaglandins.

In every monthly menstrual cycle the amount of estrogens in a woman's body rises and falls.* Estrogens are female sex hormones. You can think of them as a sort of hormonal fertilizer, making the cells of your body grow. Estrogens are responsible for breast development at puberty, and each month, they cause the lining of the uterus to thicken in anticipation of pregnancy.

If you measured the amount of estrogens in a woman's bloodstream as her period ends and a new cycle begins, you would find that it is gradually rising. For about two weeks, it rises toward a peak, then falls quickly around the time of ovulation. It rises again in the second half of the month and then falls just before her next period. The uterus sheds its lining in a menstrual flow, accompanied by crampy pain.

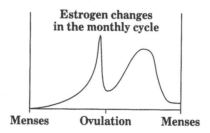

Estrogen changes in the monthly cycle

Menses   Ovulation   Menses

When the young woman called to ask for help with menstrual cramps, I simply helped her choose foods that would keep her estrogen level from rising so high. The goal was simply to smooth out the hormone roller coaster, so that the changes in her uterus would not be so dramatic.

HOW FOODS CHANGE HORMONES

The amount of estrogen in your blood is constantly being readjusted. Some foods push hormone levels up. Others bring them down.

Here's how it works. Fat drives estrogen levels up. Any kind of fat will do it: chicken fat, fish fat, beef fat, olive oil, canola oil—you name it.

---

*The term *estrogen* actually refers to a group of hormones, including estrone, estradiol, and estriol. To keep things simple, I will refer to them collectively as estrogens.

It does not matter if it is animal fat or vegetable oil; the more of it there is in your diet, the more estrogen your body makes.

If you cut the amount of fat in your diet, the amount of estrogen will be noticeably reduced within the first month. Cancer researchers have taken a great interest in this phenomenon, because lowering the level of estrogen in your blood helps reduce the risk of breast cancer. Less estrogen means less stimulation for cancer cell growth. If a woman eating a Western diet cuts her fat intake in half, her estrogen level will be about 20 percent lower.[3] If you reduce fat even more, your estrogen level will drop further.

When I suspected that a change in estrogen level got the credit for the newfound comfort that many women experience when they changed to a very low-fat diet, I discussed these findings with Anthony Scialli, M.D., a gynecologist at Georgetown University Medical Center. We decided to see whether the benefits I had seen in individuals would hold up in larger numbers of women. We tried diet modification with a group of nineteen women who suffered from moderate to severe menstrual pain. Every Tuesday evening, when they came to the office of the Physicians Committee for Responsible Medicine, we discussed how foods affect the body and how to change the diet to reduce hormone production. Jennifer Raymond, who produced the recipes for this volume, gave cooking classes. We asked everyone to avoid all animal products and added oils for two months, and to focus on simple, unprocessed foods, such as rice and other whole grains, beans, vegetables, and fruits, making their diet rich in natural fiber.

As we tracked the results, a few women noticed no change. But most noticed a difference, and for some the change was profound. Their pain was gone or dramatically reduced, something they had not experienced for years. If they needed any pain medicine at all, they needed much less than before.

After two months, we asked part of the group to return to their previous diet so we could compare the effects. To our surprise, many were extremely reluctant to do so. They had less pain, they had more energy, and they had lost weight. Although it had taken a couple of weeks to get used to the new way of eating, they had become attached to it. They began to view meat and other fatty foods as an enemy that had caused their problems.

The diet change was designed to do two things. First, it eliminated all animal fats and nearly all vegetable oils. Less fat in the diet meant that less estrogen was produced, which was a good thing. Second, plant foods also increased the amount of plant roughage (fiber), helping the body get rid of excess estrogens. Estrogens are normally filtered from the bloodstream by the liver, which sends them through a small tube, called the bile duct, into the intestinal tract. There, fiber soaks them up like a sponge and carries them out with the wastes. The more fiber there is in your diet, the better your natural "estrogen disposal system" works. Grains, vegetables, beans, and other plant foods keep waste estrogens headed toward the exit.

Animal products never have any fiber at all. If fish, chicken, yogurt, or other animal products make up any substantial part of your diet, there will be little fiber in the digestive tract. The result is disastrous. Waste estrogens, which should bind to fiber and leave the body, end up passing back into the bloodstream. This hormone "recycling" increases the amount of estrogen in the blood.

So, by avoiding animal products and added oils, you reduce estrogen *production*. And by replacing chicken, skim milk, and other fiberless foods with grains, beans, and vegetables, you will increase estrogen *elimination*.

PUTTING FOODS TO WORK

You can do this yourself. The key is to follow the diet *exactly*, so that you can see the effect it has for you.

Eat plenty of:
* whole grains, such as brown rice, whole grain bread, and oatmeal
* vegetables: broccoli, spinach, carrots, sweet potatoes, Swiss chard, brussels sprouts, or any others
* legumes: beans, peas, and lentils
* fruits

Avoid completely:
* animal products of any type: fish, poultry, meats, eggs, and dairy products
* added vegetable oils: salad dressings, margarine, and all cooking oils

- any other fatty foods: doughnuts, french fries, potato chips, peanut butter, etc.

This sounds like a significant change, and it is. However, we have found that, while everyone feels a bit at sea for the first several days, virtually everyone makes the change in about two weeks. Those who have the best time with it are those who experiment with new foods and new food products and who enlist the support of their friends or partners at home.

As the benefits begin—reduced menstrual cramps, easy weight loss, and increased energy—the diet change is so rewarding that you will only wish you had tried it sooner.

It is important to avoid animal products and oily foods *completely.* Even seemingly modest amounts of them during the month can cause more symptoms at the end of the month.

Be sure to have your foods in as natural a state as possible, choosing brown rice instead of white rice and whole grain bread instead of white bread in order to preserve their fiber.

Give this experiment a careful try for just one menstrual cycle (one month), and you will see what it can do for you. You will likely start to look at the power of foods in a very different way.

CALCIUM BALANCE

Other aspects of diet, aside from the amount of fat and fiber, can affect how you feel. Calcium, vitamin B_6, essential fatty acids, and other factors all play a role. First, calcium.

Evidence suggests that getting into better calcium balance can help reduce both menstrual pain and PMS. Not all women notice an effect, but some do. Calcium may particularly help women with milder symptoms; the benefits for those with more severe symptoms are not yet known.

In a study of thirty-three women, calcium carbonate supplements (1,000 mg per day) reduced both pain and PMS symptoms.[4] In another study of ten women with normal menstrual cycles and only mild menstrual symptoms, a combination of calcium and manganese reduced menstrual pain and premenstrual water retention and also improved mood and concentration.[5]

Although these studies show that improving calcium balance can help, it may be that taking more calcium in the diet or in supplements is not the most important issue. Most of the calcium that we consume ends up being excreted. Some 60 to 70 percent is not even absorbed by the digestive tract and simply passes right through, and a portion of that which is absorbed ends up being lost in the urine.

The key is to reduce calcium losses. As we saw in chapter 1, the amount of calcium your body loses minute by minute is strongly affected by several specific factors.

First of all, animal proteins increase calcium losses by increasing the amount of calcium your kidneys remove from the blood and excrete in the urine. When people avoid animal proteins, their calcium losses are cut to less than half what they had been.[6] Calcium losses can be further reduced by:

- avoiding excess sodium and sugar
- limiting coffee to two cups per day
- avoiding tobacco
- regular exercise
- vitamin D, either from the sun or a multiple vitamin

Having said that, you do need calcium in your diet, and the healthiest sources are green, leafy vegetables and legumes (the group that includes beans, peas, and lentils), rather than milk, which has no fiber at all and has many other ill effects. See chapter 1 for more details.

VITAMIN B₆

Vitamin B$_6$ (pyridoxine) has been shown to reduce pain in some research studies. It has been used to increase resistance to pain in people who are withdrawing from overused pain medications, in carpal tunnel syndrome, in nerve pains of diabetes, and other conditions.[7] It apparently works by increasing the production of neurotransmitters that inhibit pain sensations.

B vitamins also appear to play a role in controlling estrogens by facilitating their removal in the liver. If your diet is low in B vitamins, the amount of estrogen in your blood may rise.[8] Vitamin B$_6$ has also been shown to help with depression, irritability, and other symptoms in some research studies.[9,10]

The usual B_6 dose is 50–150 mg per day. Avoid higher doses, as they can actually cause nerve problems.

To treat premenstrual headaches, some people have used a combination of vitamin B_6 (50–150 mg) and magnesium (200 mg) daily. This combination is most effective when used daily, but can also be used for just five days per month. Pyridoxine has been effective when used with gamma-linolenic acid, or GLA (see below), for premenstrual symptoms.[11,12] Even though research studies show these supplements to be safe in these doses, I recommend they be used under the guidance of your physician, who can monitor your progress and tailor your treatment to your needs.

Vitamin B_6 occurs naturally in whole grains, beans, bananas, and nuts. This is another reason to use whole grains. When they are refined, they lose much of their B_6 along with their fiber. Sources are listed on page 170.

The amount of B_6 that you need may depend on how much protein is in your diet, since this vitamin is used to metabolize protein. The typical European or North American diet is high in protein from meats, dairy products, and eggs, so it can tend to deplete the amount of B_6 you have available. Plant products have adequate protein and help you avoid the excesses.

ESSENTIAL FATTY ACIDS

As mentioned at the beginning of this chapter, prostaglandins are involved in muscle contractions and menstrual pain. Many commonly used painkilling medicines treat menstrual pain by inhibiting the effects of prostaglandins.

Prostaglandins are made from fats stored in your cell membranes. In turn, these fats reflect the contents of your plate. There is not much fat in green, leafy vegetables and legumes (beans, peas, and lentils), and the fat that they have is strongly balanced toward anti-inflammatory *omega-3 fatty acids*, rather than other fats. Omega-3s encourage the production of helpful prostaglandins that inhibit inflammation, rather than those that fan the flames. If your diet is rich in these foods and eliminates meats, dairy products, and added oils, you will get the omega-3s you need.[13] Indeed, women whose diets are balanced in favor of omega-3s rather than other fats tend to have milder menstrual symptoms. You want to make this change anyway, as it helps you to reduce estrogen production; the rebalancing of your diet toward omega-3s is an added bonus.

Some people adjust their fat balance by adding extra omega-3-rich oils, such as flaxseed oil, to their diet to counteract the "bad" fats in meats and dairy products. Another approach is to use an omega-6 fat called GLA, or gamma-linolenic acid, which suppresses the production of prostaglandins that would otherwise encourage inflammation. Doses and sources are listed on pages 82–83.

The disadvantage of this strategy is that it adds five to six grams of fat to your daily diet, while a low-fat, vegetarian diet does the same thing with no added fat. If, however, the remainder of your diet is low in fat, the effect of these added oils on your total fat intake will not be great, and their effect on your prostaglandins will be that much more pronounced, since they will have fewer other fats to compete with.

Some investigators caution that GLA should not be used if you are or may be pregnant, since it may increase the possibility of miscarriage.

PHYTOESTROGENS

Certain foods that are common in Asian and vegetarian diets also have special benefits. Soy products, for example, such as miso soup, tofu, and tempeh, contain weak plant estrogens called *phytoestrogens*, which reduce your natural estrogens' ability to stimulate your cells. (The prefix *phyto* simply means "plant.")

Normally, estrogen attaches to the surface of your cells by hooking onto tiny receptor proteins that allow it to change the chemistry inside the cell. An estrogen molecule is like a jumbo jet that lands at an airport and hooks onto a Jetway. It discharges its passengers through the Jetway into the terminal, which is suddenly a busy, noisy place. Phytoestrogens, being weak estrogens, are like a tiny private plane that has few passengers and no cargo, but can still occupy the Jetway. They prevent your normal estrogen from attaching and acting on the cell.

Plant estrogens do not eliminate all of estrogen's effects, but they do reduce them. The result appears to be reduced breast cancer risk, and possibly reduced menstrual symptoms.

Because phytoestrogens are weak estrogens, however, they may have a different effect in women after menopause, whose bodies make much less estrogen. In these women, phytoestrogens may actually have a slight estrogen effect, which may help reduce hot flashes and other menopausal symptoms.

Although soy products are particularly rich in phytoestrogens, they are also found in many other legumes, vegetables, and fruits. The more of these foods you include in your routine, the better.

NATURAL PROGESTERONE

During the normal monthly cycle, estrogen dominates during the first half of the month, causing the uterine lining to thicken in anticipation of pregnancy. During the second half of the month, a different hormone, progesterone, dominates. Among other jobs, progesterone opposes the actions of estrogen, preventing too much stimulation of the uterus.

Progesterone is only made if you ovulate, i.e., an ovary releases an egg. If that does not happen for whatever reason, there is no progesterone to oppose estrogen.

To restore hormone balance, doctors sometimes prescribe synthetic progesterone derivatives (e.g., Provera). Unfortunately, they have a long list of side effects. An equally effective and much safer form is available without a prescription. The most common and convenient brand, Pro-Gest, is a transdermal cream that releases natural progesterone through the skin. It is available from Transitions for Health (800-648-8211). This progesterone is derived from yams or soybeans and is an exact duplicate of human progesterone.

To use natural progesterone for menstrual pain, use 15–20 mg per day from day twelve of your menstrual cycle through day twenty-six (counting the first day of bleeding as day one), then stop until the next month. Rather than measuring this amount each day, you may find it easier to simply aim to use up one-third of a two-ounce jar over this period.

Simply apply the cream to areas of thin skin, such as the neck, upper chest, abdomen, and the insides of the arms and legs, covering as wide an area as possible and varying the areas to which it is applied. Allow two to three months to see benefits. Stopping the progesterone in advance of the day you anticipate your period will start allows the normal shedding to occur.

If symptoms of premenstrual tension are prominent, you may need a higher dose. Use 30–40 mg per day, from day fifteen to twenty-six, which will consume about half a two-ounce jar each month. After a few months, begin to reduce the dose as symptoms abate. The rationale for the higher dose is that emotional tension is accompanied by the release of the "stress hormone" cortisol, which competes with progesterone for receptors on the cells.

FOODS FOR FIBROIDS

Underneath the lining of the uterus designed to nourish a growing baby is a muscle layer that allows the uterus to contract. Sometimes pockets of these muscle cells overgrow into a knot, called a fibroid or, technically, a leiomyoma.

Fibroids are not cancerous. Most cause no symptoms at all, and small fibroids are present in up to three-quarters of women in the United States. Sometimes, however, they can become large and painful.

What starts this process is not known. We do know that estrogen makes fibroids grow, which is why the usual "treatment" recommended by gynecologists is simply to wait. When menopause arrives, fibroids shrink on their own as the amount of estrogen in your blood naturally drops.

As you know by now, you do not have to wait for menopause to get estrogens under better control. The low-fat, high-fiber diet described above reduces estrogens dramatically and is a good first step in addressing fibroids.

In addition, you may wish to consider using natural progesterone, which counteracts the effects of estrogen and can be used to keep fibroids from growing, and perhaps even to shrink them. A typical regimen calls for 15–20 mg per day from day twelve to day twenty-six of your menstrual cycle, which means using up about one-third of a two-ounce jar per month.

ENDOMETRIOSIS

Sometimes there are specific, identifiable causes of menstrual pain. One of the most common is endometriosis, in which some of the lining cells from the inside of the uterus end up in the wrong place. They attach to the ovaries, intestinal tract, bladder, or elsewhere. And just as the cells inside the uterus swell and are shed each month, these misplaced cells do exactly the same thing. They swell and bleed, causing pain and infertility.

More than 5 million women in North America have been diagnosed with endometriosis, which is about 10 percent of women in their reproductive years.[14] It runs in families to a degree, but genetic factors are not strong. If you have endometriosis, there is about a 4–5 percent chance that your mother or a sister will also have had it.[15] After menopause, endometriosis is rare, except in women who take supplemental estrogens as part of hormone "replacement" therapy.

Endometriosis starts with cells that are wandering in the wrong direction. Normally, the uterine lining cells pass down and out of the body during menstruation, but sometimes these cells slip through the fallopian tubes that lead to the abdominal cavity. From there, they can end up virtually anywhere.

This happens to some extent in all women, but ordinarily the immune system spots these out-of-place cells and calls in white blood cells to eliminate them. If they somehow evade your immune defenses and attach in your abdominal cavity, the result is endometriosis. Occasional microscopic clumps occur in women with no symptoms at all. When they are more than minimal, the inflammation and pain can be severe and nearly disabling.[16–18]

The only way to diagnose endometriosis is by making a small incision below the navel and actually looking into the abdominal cavity with a slim tube called a laparoscope. Doctors who have not done this test sometimes dismiss the pain or misdiagnose it. The Endometriosis Association, based in Milwaukee, reports that 70 percent of women diagnosed with the condition were first told by their doctors that there was no physical reason for their pain. Among black women, 40 percent were told that their pain was caused by a sexually transmitted disease.

DO FOODS CAUSE ENDOMETRIOSIS?

Certain foods appear to make endometriosis more likely. According to researchers at the Harvard School of Public Health, women who have two or more cups of caffeinated coffee (or four cans of cola) per day were found to be twice as likely to develop endometriosis as other women. Why caffeine has this effect is unknown.[19]

Foods tainted with certain chemicals appear to encourage the implantation of cells in the abdomen. Polychlorinated biphenyls (PCBs) were commonly used in electrical equipment, hydraulic fluid, and carbonless carbon paper, and organochlorine pesticides have commonly been used in agriculture. In 1992, German researchers found that women with high blood levels of PCBs had a higher prevalence of endometriosis.[20]

These chemicals presumably do their dirty work by weakening your immune defenses. Indeed, the *natural killer* cells and other white blood cells that are supposed to maintain a constant lookout for any abnormal cells have been shown to be less effective in women with endometriosis.[17] In addition, some organochlorines mimic the effects of estrogens.[14,21]

These toxins tend to accumulate in animal fat, and the major route of human exposure is through food, particularly fish. They also show up in meats and dairy products.[14] Chickens, cattle, pigs, and other animals are fed grains treated with pesticides and sometimes contaminated with other organochlorines, and these compounds tend to concentrate in their muscle tissues and milk. While there may also be organochlorine pesticide residues on nonorganic fruits or vegetables, they are less concentrated and can at least partially be removed by washing or peeling. Organic produce is grown without chemical pesticides.

To measure the concentration of organochlorines in a woman's body, researchers sometimes check samples of breast milk. Breast tissue is a natural target for chemicals that dissolve into fat, and in fact, during breast-feeding, a woman can excrete up to half of all the dioxin she has accumulated in her body tissues.[21] Unfortunately, the recipient of these chemicals is the nursing baby.

A vegetarian diet has obvious advantages. By avoiding fish, other meats, and cow's milk, you avoid the foods that harbor most organochlorines. Indeed, researchers have found that vegetarian women have much lower levels of pollutants in their breast milk, compared to other women.[22] The earlier in life a plant-based diet is begun, the better.

Happily, bans on some of these compounds have caused exposures to decrease since the 1970s, although the amount in your body drops only slowly.

FOODS AS A TREATMENT FOR ENDOMETRIOSIS

Some women with endometriosis improve on their own, although most find that their symptoms continue or gradually worsen. Medical treatments rely on anti-inflammatory painkillers and hormone treatments designed to shrink endometrial tissues: danazol, gestrinone, GnRH agonist analogues, progesterone derivatives, and progesterone-estrogen combinations.

Surgical treatments include removing cell clumps, severing pain nerves, and even hysterectomy, sometimes with removal of the ovaries. Surgery to remove endometrial cells has about the same effectiveness as drug treatments, but both are usually temporary measures, as they do not reliably eliminate all of the troublesome cells.[23,24]

Dietary treatment is based on the fact that, whatever causes endometriosis to start, estrogen keeps it going. Without estrogen, the clumps of cells do not grow each month and soon wither away. This means that the same dietary approach that reduces estrogens can also be used for endometriosis. In my discussions with gynecologists who have tried this approach, it is clear that, for some patients at least, it can make a big difference.

Ronald Burmeister, M.D., a gynecologist in Rockford, Illinois, describes the case of a twenty-four-year-old woman who had had terrible menstrual pain every month since her periods began. She had had laparoscopic surgery twice, but her pain continued. She had tried birth control pills, but they caused depression and other side effects. Hormone-blocking medications were helpful, but the medicine was expensive and, in any case, could be prescribed for only six months without an increased risk of osteoporosis. After it was stopped, her pain returned. A progesterone derivative helped some but did not abolish the pain. One of her doctors recommended hysterectomy, but she wanted to avoid such a drastic solution.

Dr. Burmeister suggested a hormone-balancing diet. Using low-fat, purely vegetarian foods, his patient could reduce her hormone shifts, and unlike medicines or a hysterectomy, it would not interfere with her efforts to get pregnant. He gave her a set of recipes and recommended several books for further information.

Within three months she was noticeably better, and at six months her pain was gone. She stopped the progesterone derivative and set about seeing if she could become pregnant.

Based on this success, Dr. Burmeister made the same recommendation in three other cases and found that it was helpful in reducing pain. One patient reported that if she deviated at all from the diet, by having some dairy products or a bit of chicken, her pain came right back, much like skipping one or two pills can make a prescription fail.

No one has yet conducted a clinical study on the use of a low-fat, vegetarian diet for endometriosis. That should change because, unlike hormone treatments, it does not interfere with efforts to conceive. It is also cheap and safe and provides many other health benefits, too.

Aerobic exercise also helps. Women who run, jog, or work out for two hours per week have only half the risk of endometriosis, compared to other women. The reason, presumably, is the well-established ability of exercise to reduce hormone activity. In fact, women who exercise strenuously and consistently sometimes miss periods altogether.[16] Exercise also strengthens the immune system, making you better able to eliminate errant cells.

Natural progesterone can also be used to oppose estrogen in endometriosis. It is typically used from day eight to day twenty-six of the monthly cycle (counting the first day of bleeding as day one), using up a two-ounce jar each month. This delivers about 40–50 mg per day. Normally, this dose is continued for about four months, then the dose is reduced as the pain diminishes.

IMMUNE-BOOSTING FOODS

If endometriosis is caused by an immune system failure to recognize and eliminate out-of-place cells, immune-boosting foods might help prevent it.

You already want to reduce the amount of fat you eat in order to keep your estrogen level lower. Getting away from fat also helps your immunity.[25] Researchers have found that fatty foods impair the function of white blood cells. This is true for any kind of fat—animal fat or vegetable oil. It is also true of cholesterol. When researchers add cholesterol to white blood cells in the test tube, they find that their immune strength is diminished.[26-28] As we saw in chapter 2, a low-fat, zero-cholesterol diet simply means getting your nutrition from plant sources, rather than animal sources, and keeping added oils to a minimum.

Researchers have studied the effect of different diets on the *natural killer* cells that seek out and destroy abnormal cells, and it is clear that getting away from fat and cholesterol makes a big difference. When blood samples are taken from volunteers and the ability of their natural killer cells to destroy abnormal cells is tested, vegetarians do twice as well as their omnivorous counterparts.[29]

You can get an extra immune boost from beta-carotene, found in orange vegetables, such as carrots and sweet potatoes, from vitamin E, found in grains and beans, and from vitamin C, which is in many fruits and vegetables.

ADENOMYOSIS

Adenomyosis is a condition in which the cells that normally line the uterus are found in pockets within the muscle layer of the uterus. This occurs to some extent in up to 40 percent of women and will probably cause no symptoms at all unless it goes fairly deep into the muscle layer.

As in the case of endometriosis, the stimulus for the growth of these cells is probably estrogen,[30] which again means that reducing estrogen production through diet changes makes good sense. Unfortunately, these diet steps have never been put to the test for adenomyosis. One complicating feature may be that the endometrial cells make *their own* estrogen, and the extent to which diet changes can influence this local production is unknown.[30]

We have good evidence that diet changes can help women with common menstrual pain, and time will tell if these same changes help women with specific causes of pain, including endometriosis and adenomyosis.

There are many other approaches to menstrual pain. Some researchers are beginning to test whether ginger's anti-inflammatory effect helps reduce menstrual pain, when used in doses of one-half to one teaspoon (one to two grams) each day. Unfortunately, unlike motion sickness and arthritis where we have good evidence of its efficacy, tests of ginger for menstrual pain have been limited to individuals.[31] More and more herbal supplements are also available. It helps to keep an open mind, and to see what they might do for you.

The cornerstone of a program to control menstrual pain is a low-fat, vegetarian diet. By avoiding animal products, keeping vegetable oils to a bare minimum, and having plenty of fiber-rich foods in your routine, you will naturally reduce estrogen's effects on the uterus, avoid most chemical pollutants, and boost your immunity.

CHAPTER 9

Breast Pain

The ebbs and flows of hormones during a woman's monthly cycle can affect almost every part of her body. For some women, hormone changes during the menstrual cycle bring breast pain, swelling, or tenderness. The diagnosis your doctor gives you, *cyclic mastalgia,* does not tell you the cause. It is simply a more elaborate way of repeating what you told him or her. The Greek word *mastos* means the breast, *algia* refers to pain, and *cyclic* refers to its being monthly. Still, the term is an improvement on the old diagnosis, "fibrocystic breast disease," which was used for any of a wide variety of normal and abnormal conditions found on breast exams and mammograms.

Breast pain does not mean that you have cancer or any other serious condition. Cancer risk is higher only in unusual cases when doctors find overgrowing or abnormal cells on biopsy.* What is common in women with breast pain is a hormone balance that has tipped too far in favor of hormones that get the breasts ready for lactation, that is, *estrogens* and *prolactin.*

FOODS AND BREAST PAIN

Estrogen stimulates breast cells. It is responsible for breast development at puberty, and a wave of estrogen reaches the breast tissue during every menstrual cycle. As we saw in the previous chapter, the amount of

---

*For information on foods and cancer, and an approach to postmastectomy pain, see chapter 10.

estrogen in your bloodstream increases during the first two weeks after your period, then falls quickly around the time of ovulation. It gradually rises again in the second half of the month and then falls just before your next period.

During the second half of the month, estrogen's effects are counteracted by another hormone called *progesterone.* Researchers have measured the amount of progesterone in the blood of women with cyclic breast pain and found that it is often lower than for other women.[1,2] With less progesterone to oppose its effects, estrogen works overtime, overstimulating the breast cells, and you can feel its effects.

Foods can get you back into better balance. When you reduce fat and increase the fiber in your diet, the amount of estrogen in your bloodstream drops quickly. When a group of young women with cyclic breast pain cut their fat consumption from the American average of 35 percent of calories down to 20 percent for a three-month research study, the amount of estrogens in their blood was reduced by one-third.[3,4]

You will find details on how to do this on pages 129–130. In a nutshell, the first step is to cut out fatty foods—meats, eggs, dairy products, and added oils. With less fat in your diet, your body will make less estrogen. The second step is to eat generous amounts of vegetables, beans, and whole grains. The fiber in these foods speeds up your body's elimination of excess estrogens. The low-fat, high-fiber combination helps bring estrogen excesses under control.

I would encourage you to give this a serious try. This means following the guidelines on pages 129–130 carefully, so that, in a month or two, you can see what it will do for you. The recipes in the back of this book will make this effort a pleasure.

TESTING YOUR REACTION TO CAFFEINE

In 1979, a surgeon at Ohio State University suggested that avoiding caffeine and related chemicals found in coffee, tea, and chocolate could reduce breast pain.[5] In high doses (i.e., more than two cups of coffee or four twelve-ounce colas per day), caffeine causes a variety of hormone changes, including an increase in a type of estrogen called estrone, along with an increase in a protein that binds and inactivates estrogens.[6]

Research studies looking at whether women actually feel better when they avoid coffee have yielded mixed results. Some people find that it helps to avoid coffee and others do not. The most sensible advice, in my opinion, is simply to see whether avoiding caffeine helps you.

If you do eliminate coffee from your routine, you may want to do so gradually, because caffeine withdrawl can cause headaches.

NATURAL PROGESTERONE

Progesterone is nature's way of putting the brakes on estrogen. Through a fluke of nature, an exact copy of human progesterone is found in the wild yam. As we saw in chapters 1 and 8, it is available in a concentrated transdermal cream (e.g., Pro-Gest) that slowly releases the progesterone through your skin and into your blood, ready to counteract estrogen's excesses. Using a two-ounce jar, you spread a bit on thin skin each day so that you use up one to two ounces over the ten days before your period, stopping a day or so before you expect your period to begin.

THE NATURAL ANTI-INFLAMMATORY ACTION OF GLA

If you still have pain, you may wish to try borage or evening primrose oil. About half of women get significant benefit from it. These oils are rich in gamma-linolenic acid (GLA), which has a proven anti-inflammatory effect, as we saw in chapter 5. The dose used in research studies is 3,000 mg of evening primrose oil per day. It may take up to twelve weeks to work.[7] GLA has also been used in combination with vitamin B_6 (100–150 mg per day) for premenstrual symptoms, including breast pain.[8]

Borage oil is less well known than evening primrose oil, but it has an advantage in that it has a much higher GLA concentration, so you get more effect with less oil. The appropriate dose of borage oil is 1,000 to 1,500 mg (which provides roughly 240–360 mg of GLA) per day. A reliable source for ordering these products is Health From the Sun, Sunapee, New Hampshire, 800-447-2229, and they are also found at health food stores. Avoid these oils if you are or may be pregnant, since they may increase the possibility of miscarriage.

If you have pain that does not vary with your menstrual cycle, the above steps may still be helpful, but you will need to get an accurate diagnosis from your doctor. Pain can also come from a kind of arthritis, called *costochondritis*, that occurs where the ribs meet the breastbone. See chapter 5.

To put these steps together, here is a sensible approach to breast pain:

1. First, have an exam by a breast specialist. Although the vast majority of women do not have the cellular changes that indicate increased risk of cancer, it is important to check.

2. Use the hormone-balancing foods described on pages 129–130. This is a vital first line of defense, and a healthy step for many other conditions, too.

3. If pain continues, try additional steps, starting with seeing how you feel without caffeine.

4. Try natural progesterone. Use one to two ounces total (not per day) over the ten days before your period.

5. If you still have pain, try GLA, 240 to 360 mg per day. This is the amount of GLA in 1,000 to 1,500 mg of borage oil or 3,000 mg of evening primrose oil. Black currant or hemp oils can also be used.

CHAPTER 10

Cancer Pain

It is hard to imagine that foods could affect cancer or the pain that can come with it. We tend to think of cancer as something that only surgery, radiation, or chemotherapy can control, and even they often fall short.

Let me share with you the results of research studies that have forced us to think otherwise. We do not have all the answers to this difficult disease—far from it. But it is clear that foods provide intervention we had not expected, power that we are only beginning to put to use.

In this chapter, I will focus on how foods can prevent cancer, prevent recurrence, and extend survival, because our most potent weapons against pain are those that keep cancer itself at bay. Later, I will also share some comments about the use of pain medications.

You may have heard of Anthony J. Sattilaro, M.D., the author of a well-known book called *Recalled by Life*. I first met Tony in 1986. The events I will describe here began several years before.

Tony was a successful physician who had started out as an anesthesiologist and had become president of Methodist Hospital in Philadelphia. One day, during a routine chest X ray at the hospital, the radiologist found a large density in the left side of Tony's chest. This was puzzling, because he had had no symptoms, apart from a chronic backache. Given all the projects he had taken on in his work, he had not given much thought to his health. But this looked potentially serious, and a careful workup had to be done.

The radiologist scheduled a bone scan, which was done the same day.

Before the exam was even finished, it was clear that the results were far from normal. The suspicious area on the X ray turned out to be a large knot of cancer cells in one of Tony's ribs. More clusters of cancer cells were lodged in his skull, sternum, and spine and were slowly growing.

This was not exactly what Tony had had in mind for that day, and he was scared. In a few hours, he had gone from being a busy doctor preoccupied with his work to being a patient with advanced cancer.

His doctors wanted to track down where the cancer had started in order to plan the best treatment. They scheduled him for biopsies to look for cancer cells. The prostate biopsy told the tale.

Prostate cancer is common in older men. When it begins later in life, it often grows slowly—so slowly, in fact, that doctors sometimes recommend no treatment at all. But Tony was just forty-six. At that young age, prostate cancer is extremely aggressive. In his case, it had already spread so widely that there was essentially nothing to be done. Surgical removal was impossible. His oncologist told Tony honestly that he would have to get his affairs in order.

Not long afterward, the pain of cancer cells growing inside his bones took hold. As it worsened, he began to need narcotic painkillers to get through the day. They caused problems of their own, particularly nausea, which, at times, was severe. Between the cancer pain and the side effects of his medications, he struggled to continue his work at the hospital for as long as he could.

Tony Sattilaro had no illusions about the disease, however. He had seen his share of cancer, as any doctor has. Moreover, his own father was dying of lung cancer at the time. Not long after Tony received his own diagnosis, he had to bury his father and had to try to support his mother as best he could.

After the burial, he drove to the New Jersey Turnpike to return to Philadelphia. Two hitchhikers—men in their midtwenties—were looking for a ride. And while they looked a bit scruffy, he picked them up, welcoming the chance to have someone to talk to. He told them of his father's death, and that he himself was now under the same sentence. As it happened, these two young men had just gotten out of macrobiotic cooking school. Very taken with the power of foods, they told him that cancer did not have to be fatal. He could change his diet and make it go away.

This he found thoroughly irritating. Here were two kids, half his age, with no medical background at all and no apparent recognition that he was a trained physician who knew all too well what he was up against. They treated his condition almost casually. But he did not stop them. He let them go on about yin and yang and how foods could affect the energy balance of the body, all of which struck him as complete nonsense. When he dropped them off, they asked for his address in order to send him more information. A few days later, a package arrived, sixty-seven cents postage due. Inside was a book about diet and cancer. It was not much more convincing than the young men had been, except that it included a statement written by a physician—a woman with breast cancer, for whom a macrobiotic diet had made an enormous difference. It had apparently driven her cancer into remission. That rang a bell, because breast cancer is a hormone-related cancer, as is prostate cancer, and here was a physician endorsing a nutritional approach. Still skeptical, but interested in learning more, he found himself on the doorstep of Philadelphia's macrobiotic teaching center.

The word *macrobiotic* means "long life," and the macrobiotic diet is based on grains, vegetables, and beans, which are balanced in certain ways using principles derived from Chinese medicine. Modern macrobiotic diets draw heavily on the traditional Asian foods, with generous amounts of rice and vegetables, and strictly avoid dairy products, meats, and sugary and refined foods.

Tony could find no double-blind studies to show what the diet could do, but he was driven by a mixture of curiosity and desperation. He shared meals at the center, and the staff gave him food to take home. The tastes were a departure from what he was used to, but soon something happened that made it all take on a very different flavor: his pain started to diminish.

He could feel changes day by day. He needed less and less pain medication, and in three weeks his pain was gone. He had no idea whether the diet got the credit for this change, but he was not about to stop it. Each day, he carried his chopsticks into the doctors' dining room and, much to the amusement of his colleagues, followed an Asian peasant's diet—with no Western indulgences whatsoever. His energy returned, and without any need for painkillers, he was able to concentrate on his work again.

A year later, he still felt well, and he decided to ask his treating physician if they could take a look to see what was going on. He wanted to repeat the bone scan that had shown the spread of his cancer. They scheduled the test, and when the results came in, his doctors were shocked. No trace of the cancer was left—not in his spine, not in his skull, or anywhere else. Presumably it was not gone, but it was too small to be seen on the scan. His health continued to improve, and he decided to leave Methodist Hospital to devote himself to exploring the relationship between foods and health, and to writings and lectures. He wrote a book about his experiences that became a best-seller.

When I met Tony, he was living in Florida, studying, writing, and exercising every day. He showed me the scan that had been used to diagnose his cancer and the follow-up scan that documented its disappearance. He had received endless letters from people with cancer seeking advice, to whom he responded saying that he honestly was not sure whether diet had made the difference for him. Certainly, he had had a remarkable recovery, but he could simply not say whether what had worked for him could do the same for others.

Then he told me something that made me nervous. He had decided to stop the diet. Having been free of cancer for close to ten years, he wanted to test himself to see whether the cancer really was gone. He gradually added fish and then chicken back to his routine.

I could not see why he would want to do this. A cancer that has been effectively suppressed is not the same as a cancer that is totally gone. And whether he believed that the diet brought his improvement or not, why rock the boat? His macrobiotic counselors had told him that getting cancer to go away once is enough of a challenge. Letting it return and trying to tame it again is something they did not want to try.

Not long after this, Tony's cancer returned, and the pain that had disappeared for years enveloped him again. He had to resume his narcotic painkillers, and this time there was no going back. During my last conversation with him, his speech was slurred, and he was groggy and unable to concentrate.

After he died, the questions he had posed still remained. Did the diet change make his cancer disappear? Had abandoning the diet caused it to return? There is no way to answer these questions definitively, but a surprisingly large body of evidence shows that foods do indeed influence the hormones that drive cancer and also play a role in determining whether cancer will start and progress.

This does not mean that people with cancer should ignore other treatments. Surgery, radiation, chemotherapy, and hormonal treatments all have important roles. But it does mean that, in addition to the other treatments a cancer patient is receiving, it is important to take advantage of the power that foods do have.

USING FOODS AGAINST CANCER

Cancer begins when one cell starts multiplying out of control. It may be in the prostate gland, the lung, the breast, the digestive tract, or anywhere else. It divides over and over, becoming a mass that invades neighboring tissues. Eventually, some of the cancer cells break off and spread to other parts of the body, a process called metastasis.

One in three adults in Western countries develops cancer. This is a huge increase over statistics from years past and very different from the experience in countries where Western eating habits have not yet taken hold.

The National Cancer Institute has set out to analyze how much of our cancer risk is due to genetics and how much is due to factors that we can potentially control, e.g., smoking, diet, X rays, radon, etc. According to the best assessments, 80 to 90 percent of cancers are attributable to environmental factors, if we define our environment to include our diets and our smoking habits. Thirty percent of cancers are caused by tobacco, including cancers of the lung, mouth, throat, kidney, and bladder. Even more cases—from 30 to 60 percent—are caused by foods. Cancer of the prostate, breast, ovary, uterus, colon, stomach, and even lung, among other sites, are linked to specific kinds of foods that encourage the growth of cancer cells. Food is not the only cause of cancers at these sites, but it contributes along with toxic exposures, radiation, genetic vulnerabilities, and other factors.

Clues about how foods affect cancer come from many different kinds of studies. Researchers have compared cancer rates of various countries where diets differ greatly, for example, Japan and the United

States. To separate diet from genetics, they then studied people who had moved from Asia to the United States and adopted Western eating habits. They also studied the diets of cancer patients and compared them to those of other people living in the same community. It has become abundantly clear that certain foods promote cancer, while others tend to be protective.

We can use this information to reduce the odds of ever developing cancer. And if you have been diagnosed with cancer, we also have information on how foods influence its course, which is vitally important when your goal is to prevent a recurrence, become free of pain, or minimize the effect of the cancer on your life. We know much more about how foods help prevent cancer than about how they influence it after it has been diagnosed, but there is certainly a great deal of important information about both.

The kinds of cancer that are most strongly linked to diet are those that arise in organs that are controlled by sex hormones, i.e., the prostate, breast, uterus, and ovary, and those that begin in organs involved with the digestion of food, i.e., the esophagus, stomach, colon, liver, and pancreas. However, eating habits have been shown to influence other kinds of cancer as well.

If you have been diagnosed with cancer, let me encourage you to work with your doctor to individualize your treatment and to take a long look at how nutrition might help. Not all doctors are comfortable counseling patients on diet, since most have had only scanty nutrition training. However, doctors can refer you to a knowledgeable dietitian and can also be asked to become familiar with the concepts in this book so they may integrate them as appropriate with whatever other recommendations they may make.

PROSTATE CANCER

Prostate cancer is much less common in Asia than in Europe or the United States. A man in Hong Kong is only half as likely to develop prostate cancer as a man in Sweden. Venturing into less westernized parts of China reveals even lower rates.

In population studies, prostate cancer is consistently linked with consumption of animal products, such as milk, meat, eggs, cheese, cream, and butter—foods that have become staples in Western countries.[1-11] Along with oils used in cooking, they contribute a load of fat that stimulates the production of testosterone in a man's body, which in turn fuels the growth of prostate cells, causing benign prostate enlargement, and also encourages the growth of cancer cells.

Prostate cancer is less common in vegetarians and people who consume more rice, soybean products, and green or yellow vegetables.[2,12-16] These foods have two features that help reduce cancer risk. First, they are low in fat, so they tend to reduce testosterone levels. Second, the fiber (roughage) that is natural in plant foods helps carry testosterone out of the body. The mechanism is the same one we saw in chapter 8 for the removal of estrogen. As the liver filters the blood, it removes testosterone and sends it down a small tube, called the bile duct, into the small intestine. There, fiber soaks it up and carries it away with other wastes. Vegetables, beans, and grains keep this testosterone removal system working. On the other hand, since fish, chicken, eggs, and all other animal products have no fiber at all, the more you include these products in your diet, the less fiber there is to bind your waste testosterone. Some of the testosterone ends up being reabsorbed from the digestive tract into the bloodstream, where it again becomes active.

Plant-based diets also help tame testosterone's activity. The richer your diet is in plant foods, the more actively your body makes a protein molecule called sex-hormone binding globulin (SHBG), which holds on to testosterone, keeping it inactive until it is needed. Interestingly enough, the Massachusetts Male Aging Study found that the more SHBG there is in a man's bloodstream, the less likely he is to be overly aggressive and domineering. So presumably, men who eat their vegetables are better able to limit testosterone's not-so-good side. This effect will not make you less macho, but it might make you easier to get along with.[17]

Part of the power that plant foods have against cancer comes from the red pigment lycopene. A Harvard study of 47,000 health professionals found that men who eat plenty of strawberries and tomatoes have less risk of prostate cancer.[18] Those who had ten or more servings a week of tomato juice, spaghetti, raw tomatoes, or other tomato-based foods—even pizza—had up to 45 percent less risk. Tomatoes are rich in lycopene, and cooked tomatoes seem to be more protective than raw tomatoes, perhaps because they release more lycopene. Of course, many people are sensitive to tomatoes and will be glad to know that lycopene is also found in watermelons, pink grapefruit, and guavas.

Foods affect more than just who gets cancer and who does not. They also influence the course of the disease once it has started.

When prostate cancer has been diagnosed, doctors do everything they can to reduce testosterone's effects, using female hormones and, often, castration. As we have seen, foods themselves can help tame testosterone. And statistics show that, although a man in Hong Kong has only half the risk of developing prostate cancer compared to a man in Sweden, he has only one-eighth the risk of dying of it. The reason, presumably, is the effect of a plant-based diet on testosterone.

No one can guarantee that a new diet will work for everyone as it seemed to for Dr. Sattilaro, but it is important to take advantage of what we do know. The basic dietary prescription for reducing the risk of prostate cancer or for slowing its course and, hopefully, reducing cancer pain relies on two principles:

• Avoid all animal products and keep vegetable oils to a bare minimum to reduce testosterone production.

• Emphasize foods that are rich in fiber (grains, vegetables, beans, peas, and lentils) to accelerate the removal of testosterone. Vegetables are also rich in vitamins that are associated with anticancer defenses, as we will see in more detail below.

• To insure complete nutrition, it is important to have a source of vitamin B_{12}, which could include any common multivitamin, fortified soymilk or cereals, or a vitamin B_{12} supplement of 5 mcg or more per day.

• If you would like more information on the macrobiotic diet program Dr. Sattilaro used, write to or call The Kushi Institute (see page 335).

BREAST CANCER

When I was a medical student, among the first patients I cared for were women with breast cancer. Many were surprisingly young. At the time, I was struck by how common breast cancer was. It was, and still is, a leading killer of women in their thirties and forties. The lifetime risk was one in fourteen women, and it has increased to one in eight today.

Studies of patients with breast cancer show a pattern similar to that for prostate cancer. In the 1950s, breast cancer was rare in Japan, where low-fat diets were routine. The staple of the Japanese diet was rice, along with generous amounts of vegetables. Dairy products were virtually never consumed, and if meat was used, it was in small amounts, basically as a flavoring.

Over the past few decades, however, all that has changed. Western influences—heavy on meat and milk—have entered Asian diets, and fast-food restaurants have spread like a virus.

Between the 1950s and the 1980s, the consumption of rice and vegetables in Japan declined dramatically, while meat, poultry, and egg consumption increased eightfold. The use of dairy products is now fifteen times what it was in 1950, and fat intake has tripled.[19] During this time, breast cancer rates have soared. Affluent Japanese women who eat meat daily have more than eight times the risk of breast cancer compared to poorer women who rarely or never eat meat.[20]

Many other studies have examined the diets of populations in which cancer is frequent and compared them to others where it is rare. Researchers have also compared diets of cancer patients to women without cancer. It has become clear that the more fat, particularly animal fat, in the diet, the higher the risk of breast cancer.

As we saw in chapter 8, the more fat there is in the diet, the more estrogen the body makes, and the less fiber there is, the less estrogen your body eliminates.[21-23] Indeed, researchers have found that women with breast cancer tend to have a higher concentration of estrogen in their blood compared to other women.

Animal fats appear to be a bigger problem than vegetable oils. Researchers at New York University compared the diets of 250 women with breast cancer to those of 499 women without cancer from the same province in northwestern Italy. Both groups consumed plenty of olive oil and carbohydrates. What was different about the cancer patients was the amount of animal products they ate. Those who consumed the most meat, cheese, butter, and milk had about three times the cancer risk of other women.[24]

A vegetarian diet has special advantages. It obviously eliminates animal fat and includes plenty of fiber, so vegetarian women have less estrogen in their blood. They also have more SHBG, the protein that binds and inactivates estrogen, just as it does testosterone. Plant-based diets are also rich in *phytoestrogens,* weak estrogens that can displace your normal estrogens from their receptor sites on breast cells, reducing estrogen's effects. Soy products are a particularly concentrated source of these natural compounds, but many vegetables have them as well, which may also contribute to the lower cancer rates in Asian countries.[25]

One surprise is that milk products are linked to breast cancer risk. Studies of different populations show that breast cancer occurs more frequently where milk is commonly consumed, and that breast cancer patients are more likely to have been milk drinkers. Even when the fat content of the diet is about the same, those who consume more milk tend to have higher breast cancer rates.

In a research article published in 1997, my colleagues and I at the Physicians Committee for Responsible Medicine teased apart what it is in cow's milk that might encourage breast cancer.[26] We concluded that the problem is not simply the fat in milk, although that is certainly of concern, since about half the calories of whole milk come from animal fat. However, milk also contains estrogens, because dairy cattle are kept continuously pregnant to maximize milk production. Milk also has growth factors to help a calf grow rapidly. The best known of these, called insulin-like growth factor, or IGF-1, is an even more potent stimulus for cancer cell growth than estrogen.

Alcohol also contributes. Even one drink a day can increase breast cancer risk by more than 50 percent, compared to nondrinkers.[27] Environmental chemicals, which are often dissolved into the fat of meats, fish, and dairy products and occur in somewhat smaller traces on nonorganic produce, are also implicated.

Other factors that are linked to increased breast cancer risk include estrogen "replacement" therapy, which is often (and inappropriately, in my judgment) recommended to women after menopause, oral contraceptives, obesity, radiation, environmental toxins, and in a some cases, genetics.[28–33] Your exposure to environmental toxins is strongly affected by what you eat, as is described in chapter 8.

BREAST CANCER SURVIVAL

More than thirty years ago, Ernst Wynder of the American Health Foundation in New York noticed that not only were Japanese women much less likely than American women to get breast cancer, but when they did get it, they tended to survive longer.[34] Evidence suggests that the effect is at least partly due to the lower fat content of the diet. Numerous studies have shown that the less fat there is in the diet, the better the chances of surviving breast cancer.

Researchers in Buffalo, New York, examined the diets of women diagnosed with breast cancer that had already spread to other parts of the body. They found that their risk of dying at any point in time increased 40 percent for every thousand grams of fat consumed per month.[35] To see what this means in practical terms, if you added up all the fat in a typical American diet over a month, it would total about 2,000 grams for a person taking in 1,800 calories per day. For comparison, a plant-based diet prepared without added fat has only about 600 grams of fat per month. If the research findings hold, this corresponds to nearly a 60 percent difference in whether women lived or died at any point.

This does not mean that a person's risk of dying is 60 percent. It simply means that it is 60 percent higher than it would otherwise have been, assuming the individual is comparable to those studied.

Similarly, a Canadian research study found that postmenopausal women with cancer were more likely to have lymph node involvement if they had a higher intake of saturated fats. (This is the kind of fat that is particularly common in dairy products, poultry, red meat, and even fish—between 15 and 30 percent of fish fat is saturated fat. It is at much lower levels in vegetables, grains, beans, and other plant products.)[36]

More confirmation came from a 1995 study of 698 postmenopausal breast cancer patients published in the journal *Cancer*. Those who ate the least fat had only half the risk of dying, compared to the other women. Nonsmokers also had better survival rates than smokers.[37]

Vegetable-rich diets are low in fat and rich in fiber, complex carbohydrates, and beta-carotene, all of which are associated with a better prognosis. They also help keep you slim, which, in turn, helps prevent cancer and also improves survival if cancer is diagnosed.[36,38-41]

POSTMASTECTOMY PAIN

About 10 percent of women who have undergone mastectomies have continuing pain at the surgery site. It begins immediately after surgery and is sometimes persistent, apparently due to the disruption of the nerves involved.

A helpful treatment has come from an unusual source. As we saw in chapter 5, the "hot" ingredient in red chili peppers, called capsaicin, has a useful feature. When it is mixed into a cream and applied to the skin, it depletes the neurotransmitter chemical *substance P,* which conducts pain sensations. It sometimes stings a bit at first, but this usually abates as the treatment is continued.

Several studies have shown that capsaicin works for postmastectomy pain. One of these involved fourteen women who had been in pain for an average of four years. After using 0.025 percent capsaicin cream for four weeks, eight of them reduced their pain to the extent that it was no more than mild, and four more had at least a 50 percent improvement. In several cases, the best pain relief did not come until three to four weeks of use. Two other studies yielded similar results.[42]

Capsaicin cream is sold at drugstores under the names Zostrix and Dolorac. To use it, simply apply it to the skin four to five times per day for three to four weeks. If it stings too much, you may wish to apply it to a small area at first and gradually cover a larger area, or you can pretreat the area with a lidocaine spray such as Solarcaine. After a week or so of regular use, the stinging usually goes away.

CANCER OF THE UTERUS AND OVARY

The uterus and ovary are strongly influenced by sex hormones, just as the prostate and breast are. Population studies have shown that, indeed, ovarian cancer is more common where people eat higher-fat diets.[1,43] Researchers at Johns Hopkins University found that the higher a woman's cholesterol level—which reflects a fattier diet—the greater her risk of ovarian cancer.[44] High-fat diets and obesity are linked to uterine cancer, as well, although other factors, including estrogen supplements, also play an important role.[1,43,45,46]

Some evidence indicates that milk may increase the risk of cancer of the ovary. Dr. Daniel Cramer of Harvard University compared the diets of hundreds of women with ovarian cancer to a group of women who were similar in age and other demographic variables, but who did not have cancer. The women with cancer consumed noticeably more dairy products.[47]

Dairy products are often high in fat, of course, but that was not the factor that Dr. Cramer was most concerned about. His concern was the milk sugar, lactose. Lactose is made of two smaller sugars, called glucose and galactose, and galactose is potentially toxic to the ovaries. Dr. Cramer had also found that milk consumption is linked with higher rates of infertility.

Normally, enzymes help the body eliminate galactose. Some women have particularly low levels of these enzymes, and when they consume dairy products regularly, their risk of ovarian cancer is triple that of other women. Because galactose comes from the milk sugar, not the milk fat, it is in skim milk, just as in whole milk, and is present in yogurt, ice cream, cheese, and all other dairy products.

We do not yet have good evidence as to whether foods influence survival in cancers of the uterus or ovary, but it is likely that they do because these cancer sites are influenced by the same sex hormones that influence survival in breast cancer. A much needed research study would test a very low-fat, high-fiber vegetarian diet designed to reduce estrogen effects.

SET ASIDE BLAME

When we find evidence that foods increase the risk of cancer, sometimes people with cancer feel that this means that they themselves are somehow to blame for their disease, or that researchers or health advocates are pointing fingers. If you find yourself feeling this way, let me encourage you to set this issue aside. No one could have known in advance what research studies might show, and even now few doctors give their patients the information they need to put the power of foods to work. Blame has no place in cancer research or cancer treatment. As knowledge emerges, it should be used to empower us—to allow us to make choices that help keep us healthy.

....

COLON CANCER

The colon—that is, the large intestine—is in intimate contact with everything you eat. So, it is not surprising that foods have a strong effect on colon cancer risk.

The worst of the lot are meats. In the first place, animal products often harbor cancer-causing chemicals. You are probably familiar with the concern of backyard barbecuers that beef fat dribbling onto hot coals produces smoke that coats the meat with a thin layer of carcinogens. That is true, but you do not have to be using an outdoor grill to be concerned. An even more common source of carcinogens in meat is cooking itself. As animal proteins are heated, they produce cancer-causing chemicals called heterocyclic amines. The heating itself does it, quite apart from the effects of barbecuing or smoke.

While this has long been known to be true for beef, researchers had not tested chicken until recently. A report by the National Cancer Institute shows that the same phenomenon occurs in chicken. In fact, it appears to be considerably worse in chicken than in beef. A well-done hamburger contains 33 nanograms per gram of the carcinogen PhIP and a well-done grilled steak has about the same. But grilled chicken is much worse. It contains 480 nanograms per gram, fifteen times higher than beef.[48]

These dangerous chemicals are most strongly linked to colon cancer and may also contribute to breast cancer. A twenty-four-year Finnish study of nearly ten thousand people showed that fried meat consumption was linked to a higher risk of hormone-related cancers in women (breast, ovary, and uterus), even after adjustment for fat intake.[49]

An even more important factor in colon cancer is what happens to the digestive juices that stream down the intestinal tract. Bile acids are secreted by the gallbladder to help absorb fats. However, bacteria in the digestive tract change these bile acids into cancer-promoting chemicals called secondary bile acids. Meats encourage the growth of bacteria that cause these dangerous secondary bile acids to form, while vegetable-based diets foster the growth of harmless bacteria.

These problems are not theoretical. They show up over and over again in cancer statistics. The Harvard Nurses' Health Study showed that women who eat meat every day have more than twice the risk of colon cancer, compared to those who rarely or never consume meat.[50] A similar study in men, also conducted by Harvard researchers, showed that regular meat consumption more than triples their risk of colon cancer.[51] The same has been found in international comparisons and in studies examining the diets of cancer patients.[12,50,52]

On the other hand, grains, beans, vegetables, and fruits are protective. People who consume plenty of vegetables have a lower risk of colon cancer.[12] Plants have no animal proteins or animal fat, and their roughage speeds the passage of food through the colon, helping you remove carcinogens. Fiber also absorbs and dilutes bile acids and changes the bacteria that populate your colon, so that harmful secondary bile acids are less likely to form.

This is important for anyone who aims to prevent colon cancer. But it is particularly important if you have already been diagnosed with colon polyps, growths that have a tendency to become cancerous. Jerome J. DeCosse, a surgeon at Cornell Medical Center, gave bran to patients with recurrent polyps. Within six months, the polyps became smaller and fewer in number.[53] This does not mean that the answer has to lie in bran supplements, however. Grains, beans, and vegetables are also loaded with natural fiber and are free of the animal fats and cholesterol that encourage colon cancer.

OTHER DIGESTIVE TRACT CANCERS

People who eat plenty of fruits and vegetables have lower rates of many types of cancer, including those arising in the esophagus, stomach, pancreas, and colon.[54]

The esophagus has to cope with some special challenges, particularly alcohol and tobacco, which work synergistically to increase cancer risk. Frequent use of very hot beverages or pickled foods is also linked to a higher risk of esophageal cancer.

Stomach cancer is linked to smoked and salt-pickled foods.[12] This form of cancer is common in Japan, in contrast to traditionally low rates of other forms of the disease, reflecting the common use of smoked and salt-pickled foods.

Cancer of the pancreas has also been studied in international comparisons and is linked to consumption of meat, alcohol, and coffee. As Japan's diet has westernized, the incidence of pancreatic cancer has gradually increased.[12,19]

While the specific contributors vary from one form of cancer to another, two overriding themes are seen again and again in cancer research studies. Diets rich in animal products and other fatty foods tend to increase cancer risk, while vegetables and fruits help reduce it. People who consume the most fruits and vegetables have the lowest cancer rates, and this is true of a surprising number of forms of the disease: lung, breast, colon, bladder, stomach, mouth, larynx, esophagus, pancreas, and cervix.[54] A fifty-five-year-old male smoker whose diet is low in fruits and vegetables has a one-in-four risk of dying of lung cancer in the next twenty-five years. But if the smoker has a high intake of fruits and vegetables, or even vitamin C supplements, his risk drops to 7 percent.[55]

Vegetarians have a 40 percent lower cancer risk compared to meat-eaters. If a vegetarian diet also omits dairy products and fried foods and includes plenty of fresh vegetables, it may well reduce cancer risk even further.

STRENGTHENING IMMUNITY

Recent research indicates that part of the strength of certain foods against cancer comes from their effect on your immune defenses. When cancer cells arise, your white blood cells must recognize that they are abnormal and destroy them. These soldiers work much better when they are well nourished and do not have to cope with a load of fat in the bloodstream.[56-58]

Researchers in New York asked a group of volunteers to reduce the fat content of their diets, cutting down fats from all sources. Three months later, the researchers took blood samples from the volunteers and examined their cells' ability to recognize and destroy abnormal cells. Indeed, their immune function was greatly increased.[56]

Vegetables, fruits, grains, and legumes are not just low in fat. They also contain nutrients, particularly beta-carotene, vitamins C and E, and the mineral selenium, all of which have been shown to bolster immune function.[59-61] This does not mean that you have to eat enormous amounts of vegetables to see a difference. The amount of beta-carotene shown to boost immune function was 30 mg, the amount in two large carrots.[62]

Not surprisingly, vegetarians again have a tremendous advantage. Researchers at the German Cancer Research Center in Heidelberg took blood samples from vegetarians and from nonvegetarian volunteers working at the cancer center. They tested their white blood cells' ability to knock out cancer cells. The vegetarians had more than double the ability to destroy cancer cells compared to nonvegetarians, presumably because their diets were lower in fat and higher in vitamins and minerals.[63]

A healthful diet can be used along with whatever other treatments for cancer you may be using. I would strongly encourage you to plan your treatment carefully with your doctor, making good nutrition an integral part of it.

A WORD ABOUT PAIN MEDICATIONS

In many cases of advanced cancer, pain medicines are essential. Too often, however, they are used in doses that are too small and infrequent. I cannot tell you how many times I have been asked to evaluate cancer patients for depression and listlessness, only to discover that their problem was untreated pain. Narcotic painkillers are routinely used to treat pain, and they work well. Unfortunately, some doctors limit the dose or frequency of their use in a naive attempt to avoid addiction. Sometimes that makes sense, but more often it leads to undertreated pain.

Pain medicines are like antibiotics; you have to use the dose and frequency that knocks out the problem, not some halfway measure, unless the patient specifically prefers to use less medicine. When I was taking care of hospitalized patients early in my medical training, we routinely prescribed painkillers for use every four hours, only to find that they wore off in three hours. Instead, they should be prescribed to give continuous relief.

It is also common for hospital patients to have to request painkillers and then to have to wait, sometimes an agonizingly long time, for the nursing staff to administer them. Sometimes the doctor or nurse will encourage the patient to "tough it out" to minimize the use of medicines. A better strategy is to prescribe pain medicines on a set schedule, to be administered without the patient having to ask, and with no negotiating or moralizing. The patient can decline the medicines if he or she so chooses, but otherwise, they are used on schedule. This assures that pain is adequately treated.

If you or a loved one are receiving medications for chronic pain, I would suggest that you arrange a consultation to evaluate the regimen you are on. Most often, this is done by psychiatrists who specialize in psychotropic medications, and they can be enormously helpful.

PART IV

METABOLIC AND IMMUNE

PROBLEMS

CHAPTER 11

Carpal Tunnel Syndrome

You've been working at the cash register or on your computer keyboard day after day, and you have begun to notice a slight numbness and tingling in your fingers. The tingling gradually turns into pain, and you begin to drop things.[1] Your doctor has no trouble diagnosing the problem. It is called carpal tunnel syndrome, which means that a nerve is getting pinched as it passes along the carpal bones at the base of your hand.

The nerve in question is the median nerve, the main communication line between your brain and your thumb and index and middle fingers. To reach the hand, it has to slip through a slim passage between a band of ligaments just under the skin and the bones beneath them. That would be no problem, except that the nerve is joined by blood vessels and many different tendons that are moving back and forth with every movement of your fingers.

As you can imagine, if you were to type vigorously on a computer keyboard or let loose on the piano, your wrists would have more comings and goings than Grand Central Station. If you touch the fingers of one hand to the tendons of your opposite wrist, you can easily feel how active the wrist is with any movement of your fingers. People whose jobs demand repeated, forceful hand movements are at particular risk for inflammation and swelling. When that happens, the tendons and nerves no longer fit so well, and the nerve gets pinched.[2]

Carpal tunnel syndrome can sometimes just come out of the blue, without any special overwork. It is common in people with diabetes, rheumatoid arthritis, gout, or hypothyroidism, in people who are on dialysis because of kidney problems, as well as in pregnant or middle-aged women.

As illnesses go, carpal tunnel syndrome seems to be quite new. Hippocrates wrote about all manner of diseases that we still recognize today, but his ancient writings never mentioned anything like carpal tunnel syndrome. Neither did those of the medical writers in the Middle Ages. If it existed at all, it escaped notice until 1880, when it was first added to medical textbooks.[3] We really do not know why this condition has emerged as it has, but some researchers have speculated that modern working conditions and modern diets have conspired to stress the nerve and cause the symptoms.

Surgeons have their scalpels sharp and ready to relieve the pressure on the nerve, but you might want to consider other approaches first.

THE PAIN-FIGHTING VITAMIN

The answer to carpal tunnel syndrome could lie in a simple vitamin—vitamin B_6, also called pyridoxine. Its analgesic properties are commonly used to increase resistance to pain for people who are withdrawing from overused headache remedies and for people with nerve pains of diabetes and temporomandibular (TMJ) joint pain.[4]

The use of vitamin B_6 in carpal tunnel syndrome began with the observation that some, although not all, people with the syndrome are low in the vitamin on blood tests.[5,6] That suggested that perhaps correcting the vitamin deficiency might eliminate the pain. And in fact, several studies have shown it reduces swelling and the tingling or discomfort in the hand and sometimes makes the condition go away.[7–14]

In one study of ten subjects and a follow-up study with eleven subjects studied at the University of Texas at Austin, researchers John Ellis, Karl Folkers, and their colleagues found that vitamin B_6 could eliminate carpal tunnel symptoms, although not necessarily rapidly. While some subjects benefited within a few weeks, in others it took up to twelve weeks to work.[15,16]

In a way, the vitamin's benefits come as no surprise. It has long been known that the body uses B_6 to make neurotransmitters, the chemicals that conduct our nerve messages, including those that affect the way we feel pain. Vitamin B_6 is important in the synthesis of serotonin and GABA, two neurotransmitters that inhibit pain impulses in nerves.[17,18]

USING VITAMIN B₆ FOR CARPAL TUNNEL SYNDROME

- Vitamin B_6 is essential for making pain-inhibiting neurotransmitters.
- The usual dose is 50–150 mg per day. Avoid higher doses.
- Allow twelve weeks to see benefits.
- It should be used under your doctor's supervision.
- Use B_6 along with a wrist splint to stop continuing trauma to the wrist.

Vitamin B_6 mainly seems to affect the pain itself, not the underlying condition. When researchers check the nerve *function* of patients with carpal tunnel syndrome or diabetes, vitamin B_6 does not usually have an impact. Its effect is against pain.

The percentage of people who benefit from vitamin B_6 varies depending on which study you read. In general, half to two-thirds of treated patients improve significantly, and less dramatic improvement is seen in the remaining subjects.[11,13,19,20] However, some researchers have not found any benefit from it over placebo treatments, and no one has yet been able to explain why it seems to help some people and not others.[6]

The usual treatment dose is 50–150 mg per day, allowing twelve weeks or so for it to work. The vitamin appears to be safe at these doses. However, at doses above 200 mg per day, it may actually cause nerve symptoms.

Researchers use supplements to boost B_6 because they have more of the vitamin than you will find in any food. However, it may be that consuming natural foods rich in vitamin B_6 can, over the long run, have benefits that are similar to a temporary course of supplements. Whole grains, beans, bananas, and nuts are rich in B_6 and will easily bring you the recommended dietary allowance of 2 mg per day for women and 2.2 mg for men. Supplements are useful if you have acute symptoms, but foods can perhaps act as a preventive.

People in Western countries do not always get the vitamin B_6 they need, for two reasons. First, their diets do not contain much in the way of the whole grains and legumes that provide it. Second, protein tends to use up vitamin B$_6$, and Western diets are far too high in protein, due to the common use of meat, poultry, and fish. Part of the vitamin's job is to convert proteins from one form to another, and high-protein diets demand more of the vitamin than is needed on a lower-protein diet.[20]

HEALTHFUL SOURCES OF VITAMIN B$_6$ (MG)

Avocado (1)	0.85	Navy beans (1 cup, boiled)	0.30
Banana (1)	0.66	Pinto beans (1 cup, boiled)	0.27
Broccoli (1 cup, boiled)	0.22	Potato (1, baked)	0.70
Brussels sprouts (1 cup, boiled)	0.46	Soybean flour (1 cup)	0.57
Chickpeas (1 cup, boiled)	0.23	Spinach (1 cup, boiled)	0.44
Kidney beans (1 cup, boiled)	0.21	Sweet potato (1 cup, boiled)	0.80
Lima beans (1 cup, boiled)	0.30	Vegetarian baked beans (1 cup)	0.34

SOURCE: J. A. T. Pennington, *Bowes and Church's Food Values of Portions Commonly Used*, 16th ed. (Philadelphia: J. B. Lippincott, 1994).

HORMONES AND CARPAL TUNNEL SYNDROME

Other factors play a role in carpal tunnel syndrome. Tobacco increases the risk, in case you needed another reason for avoiding it. Findings on alcohol are mixed. A high intake increases the risk, while modest alcohol use may actually reduce the risk, for reasons that are unknown.[21]

There is also clearly a role for female sex hormones, although exactly what is going on and what we should do about it is not entirely clear yet. The syndrome is much more common in women than men. It often kicks in during pregnancy, especially during the third trimester, just as certain hormones (estriol and progesterone, among others) are reaching a peak, and it usually resolves soon after the baby is born.[5,22] Rarely, it begins with breast-feeding and disappears when breast-feeding is discontinued.[23] In addition, birth control pills, which are mixtures of hormones, increase the risk of carpal tunnel syndrome.[24]

A role for hormones is also supported by the syndrome's rather recent emergence, which parallels that of other hormone-related conditions, all of which have been aggravated by the aggressive spread of high-fat, meat-laden diets and the declining popularity of vegetables, grains, beans, and fruits we have seen during the past 150 years in the Western Hemisphere, and since World War II in Asia.

What are these hormones doing that could cause carpal tunnel syndrome? First, estrogens can cause fluid retention and swelling, which can crowd the median nerve.[24] In addition, birth control pills can apparently reduce the amount of vitamin B_6 in the blood.[25,26]

BRINGING HORMONES INTO BALANCE

Foods can reduce hormone shifts, as we saw in chapter 8. In a nutshell, the more fat there is in the foods you eat, the more estrogen your body makes. Excess body fat does the same thing; fat cells contain enzymes for making estrogen.

In addition, high-fiber foods, such as whole grains, vegetables, beans, and fruits, help the body to eliminate estrogens. Researchers are already studying the use of such diets for reducing breast cancer risk and other hormone-related conditions. Unfortunately, no researcher, to my knowledge, has yet used them for carpal tunnel syndrome.

NATURAL PROGESTERONE

Chapters 1, 3, and 8 describe the use of natural progesterone against osteoporosis, migraines, and menstrual pain. Some experts believe that it is also helpful for carpal tunnel syndrome, although the jury will remain out until controlled studies are done. The use of progesterone in carpal tunnel is paradoxical, because during pregnancy the body makes a large amount of progesterone, yet pregnancy is when carpal tunnel syndrome is particularly common. However, its advocates point out that progesterone counteracts the effects of estrogens and helps correct connective-tissue problems.

Dr. John Lee, the leading proponent of natural progesterone's applications in medicine, recommends using the transdermal natural progesterone cream in a dose of 15–20 mg per day from day twelve to day twenty-six of your menstrual cycle, counting day one as the first day of bleeding. This dose uses up about one-third of a two-ounce jar each month. A postmenopausal woman would use the cream for twenty-five to twenty-six days each calendar month, using up a two-ounce jar during that time, and then stop until the beginning of the next month. It may take a few months to work.

WHAT TO DO ABOUT CARPAL TUNNEL SYNDROME

• First, get a solid diagnosis. Your doctor needs to look for medical conditions that are associated with nerve symptoms. Any treatment should be discussed thoroughly with your physician, and this is especially true during pregnancy and nursing.

• Avoid repetitive movements and awkward positioning of the hands during work, and take rest breaks as needed.

• Try vitamin B_6, 50–150 mg per day, under your doctor's supervision. It typically takes twelve weeks to see benefits.

• Splinting the wrist can help.[27] As symptoms improve, you can begin to use the splint only at night.

• When conservative measures fail, doctors sometimes recommend diuretics, local injections of steroids, or surgery. Surgery is not always curative and should be used only as a last resort, particularly in pregnancy, since the syndrome usually resolves after delivery.

CHAPTER 12

Diabetes

A particular kind of pain occurs in diabetes. When people have had the disease for several years, they sometimes develop sharp, burning sensations in the lower legs and feet. This is a symptom of malfunctioning nerves, which can also manifest as pins and needles or numbness.

This condition, called *diabetic neuropathy,* is presumed to be caused either by poor circulation in the tiny blood vessels that nourish the nerves or by a toxic effect that occurs when blood sugar is poorly controlled. Your nerves need oxygen and nutrients, just like every other part of your body, and if they do not get them because of poor circulation, they cannot function properly. Similarly, circulation problems that commonly occur in diabetes can damage the eyes, kidneys, and heart.

The pain of neuropathy can be physically debilitating and can make you feel that you are on a one-way street to more and more symptoms from which there is no relief. You have probably already tried medications, and they do help some people. Certain antidepressants, for example, have been shown to reduce diabetic pain, apparently by blocking the chemical transmitters in nerves that cause you to feel pain.[1] They do not make the nerves function better, however, and many people get only moderate pain relief, or even none at all. This is where foods come in.

The fact is, by choosing the right foods and adding a simple exercise program, the pain often goes away completely. In fact, diabetes itself can go away in many cases, or at least improve dramatically.

Many researchers have been looking at how foods can help in diabetes. Milton Crane, M.D., focused on the pain symptoms in an important study in Weimar, California. He included twenty-one patients who had developed nerve pains in their legs and feet after having had adult-onset diabetes for many years. They used a special diet and exercise program that went beyond the rather weak diets that are in common use.

It worked wonderfully. In just two weeks, seventeen patients had their leg pains completely disappear, and the other four had partial relief. Five patients stopped all their diabetes medicines, and the remaining patients cut their doses by about half.[2] In this chapter, I'll show you how this kind of diet and exercise program works and how you can use the same powerful steps.

WHAT IS DIABETES?

Diabetes is a condition in which sugar builds up in the bloodstream. Sugar normally comes from starches in the diet and is also released from storage molecules in the liver that act like spare batteries, giving you energy when you need it.

The hormone *insulin* is the doorman for the cells of your body. It escorts sugar from the bloodstream into each cell. In diabetes, however, insulin is not doing its job properly. Rather than helping sugar to go into the cells, it simply lets it build up in the blood. With extra sugar in the blood, some of it passes through the kidneys into the urine, where it can be detected in simple urine tests.

When diabetes occurs in children, it is because the cells in the pancreas that are supposed to make insulin have stopped doing so. These children will need insulin injections regardless of the diet they follow, although the right kinds of foods can help them minimize their doses and reduce the complications of the disease. Diet may also be able to prevent it from occurring in the first place, as we will see.

In the adult-onset (or non-insulin-dependent) form of diabetes, there is still insulin in the blood, but it is simply not working well. This form of diabetes often improves or goes away with the right kind of diet and exercise.

Traditional "diabetic diets" are not very powerful. Older diets were based on the theory that, since starches release sugars, most starches should be eliminated from the diet. Unfortunately, that eliminates some of the most healthful grains, beans, and vegetables and leaves the patient with foods that are high in fat or protein. Fat in the diet makes insulin function even worse, and excess protein accelerates kidney damage and other problems.

Newer diabetic diets use a set of "exchange lists" that rigidly prescribe certain amounts of milk, fruit, vegetables, starch, meat, and fat to be eaten to keep the diet fairly constant day after day. This makes it easier to gauge the amount of medicine you will need to regulate your blood sugar. This is an improvement over the older diets, but it still does not get most patients off their medicines. It is not very effective at preventing serious complications, and most people on such diets find themselves in a downward spiral with more symptoms, more prescriptions, and more medical treatments.

Hints that there might be a better way came in research studies in the early 1980s that threw out the exchange lists and focused on foods that help insulin to do its job better. Many research subjects were able to get off their medications completely, and others needed much less medication. But only now are we discovering how powerful this approach really is.

A REVOLUTIONARY APPROACH

When researchers design modern diets to improve diabetes or make it go away, they use three keys that improve insulin's ability to function and prevent a sugar buildup.

1. *Low-fat foods help insulin work better.* Insulin is sensitive to fat. If there is much fat in the blood or if you have excess body fat, insulin has trouble getting sugar into your cells. It is as if insulin's hand keeps slipping on a greasy doorknob, and the doorway to the cell never opens. Sugar builds up in the blood, and insulin cannot do much about it.

The less fat you eat, the better. This is a powerful step, and one that the exchange lists do not take full advantage of, because they include butter, meat, oils, and other foods with much more fat than the body needs.

2. *Complex carbohydrates release their sugars gradually.* The starchy part of beans, vegetables, and grains is *complex carbohydrate,* which means natural sugars that are chemically linked together in a chain. During digestion, these sugars gradually come apart and pass into the blood a bit at a time, rather than all at once. Your body can then use these natural sugars for energy.

On the other hand, when you have table sugar, a candy bar, or a soda, its sugar enters your bloodstream abruptly. The same is true for some fruits, whose sweetness comes from simple fruit sugars that can quickly pass from your digestive tract into your blood.

3. *Fiber keeps the absorption of sugar slow and steady.* Fiber simply means plant roughage. It is in the outer coating of grains, which is retained in whole wheat bread and brown rice, but has been eliminated in white bread and white rice. There is also plenty of fiber in beans and vegetables. Animal products never have any fiber.

By using these three principles together, we can see which foods will help insulin to work better. Whole grains, such as brown rice and whole grain bread, are extremely low in fat. Only 5 percent of the calories in brown rice come from fat. Grains also have plenty of complex carbohydrates. And so long as they are not refined into white rice and white bread, they have plenty of fiber, too. Beans and vegetables are similar. Most are between 4 and 10 percent fat, and all are high in complex carbohydrates and natural fiber.

Fruits are low in fat and high in fiber, but their fruit sugars are absorbed more quickly than those that would come from starchy plants.

Animal products are no help at all. As we saw in chapter 2, all meats—even chicken breast without the skin—contain a significant amount of fat, much more than in plant foods. And no animal products—meats, dairy products, or eggs—have any complex carbohydrate or fiber.

Vegetable oils should be avoided, too. They are better for your heart than animal fats, but their effect on insulin is not so different.

When researchers have tested diets with generous amounts of vegetables, grains, and bean dishes, while generally avoiding animal products and added oils, they have found that they do not need exchange lists to keep blood sugar under control. And there is no need to limit portion size.

Studies using this kind of diet, along with regular walking, cycling, or other exercise, showed that 90 percent of adult-onset diabetics using oral medications could stop them in less than a month. Of those who had been taking insulin, 75 percent no longer needed it. The benefits hold up over the long term, and for many patients, the disease simply goes away.[3,4]

Other researchers found that the combination of a plant-based diet and exercise not only gets blood sugars under control, it dramatically reduces the risk of eye, kidney, and nerve complications.[5-7]

VEGETARIAN FOODS ARE BEST

At the Weimar Institute, Dr. Crane followed the same principles. He used a vegan (pure vegetarian) diet of vegetables, grains, and beans, eliminating all animal fat and keeping vegetable oils to a bare minimum. The result was that diabetes came under much better control and leg pains disappeared. Results were rapid, even for people who had been suffering for years.

We assume that plant products work to stop nerve pains by bringing diabetes under better control, because high blood sugar levels can make you more sensitive to pain. Researchers at the Veterans Administration Medical Center in Minneapolis tested pain tolerance in eight healthy young men. They placed an electrical clip on the web of skin between the first and second fingers on each volunteer. As one of the researchers gradually turned up the voltage to the clip, they asked each subject to say when he could feel any pain and when it became unbearable. They found that when they gave the subjects an intravenous infusion of sugar (glucose), their pain sensitivity increased markedly. They were aware of the pain sooner and experienced it more intensely.

They then tested people with diabetes, who, of course, generally have higher than normal blood sugars. They found the same thing. Their pain sensitivity was much higher than that of people without diabetes.[8]

However, vegetarian diets have another effect that may play a role, too. Complex carbohydrates stimulate the brain to make two chemical neurotransmitters that are involved in mood and pain control: noradrenaline and serotonin. These are the same chemicals that antidepressants are designed to increase, and as we have seen, antidepressants can be helpful in treating diabetic nerve pain. The noradrenaline boost is sufficient to measurably increase your calorie-burning speed for more than two hours after the meal. Whether or not this helpful adjustment of body chemistry gets some of the credit for the disappearance of leg pains is still unconfirmed.

To take things a step further, a research study conducted by my colleague Andrew Nicholson, M.D., at the Physicians Committee for Responsible Medicine, along with the Georgetown University Medical Center, looked at what foods can do *without exercise*. I should emphasize that exercise is important for good health and especially so for people with diabetes, but for research purposes, we wanted to see what foods could do by themselves.

We found that their power is extraordinary. Like Dr. Crane, we used a vegan diet without added vegetable oils, but we did not recommend any exercise program at all. The patients' blood sugars dropped fully 54 points on a vegan diet, compared to less than half this amount on the traditional diabetic diet. Subjects were not counting calories, but even so, the average weight loss over the three-month study was sixteen pounds, compared to only eight pounds on the usual diabetic diet. Kidney abnormalities also improved dramatically.[9]

In summary, standard diabetic diets based on exchange lists are not very powerful. If you use a low-fat, unrefined vegetarian diet, the results can be dramatic. And if you add exercise to the regimen, your benefits will be greater still because working muscles pull sugar out of the blood, even with little insulin present.

Let me share with you what this can mean to an individual. Bruce Burdick, of Lenexa, Kansas, had learned about the approach I recommend and wrote me the following letter:

> My daughter Heather, who owns a health food store, wanted me to try your program for just three weeks. At the time, I was a diabetic with high blood pressure and blood serum that looked like sausage gravy. I was 72 pounds overweight.
>
> Something told me it was the right thing to do. I convinced my wife, Mary, to join me in a 21-day program as a vegetarian. We did not consciously restrict our calorie intake in any way. We ate lots of beans, rice, pasta, fruits, and vegetables. We also got a bread machine, so we had fresh bread every day. In addition, we started a mild exercise program; we walked at the mall every day for 30 to 45 minutes.
>
> The results were fantastic. The first three weeks flew by. We discovered all kinds of new recipes. Over the past six months, I

have lost 47 pounds, and my shirt size has come from 3X to 2X to XL to L. My blood pressure came down from 160/100 to 130/80. Also, I am controlling my blood sugar to the point that I no longer have to take insulin.

I could go on and on about how good I feel and how great I look (that is what my friends are saying). Thank you so much for sharing your knowledge and information.

Bruce's experience is not unusual. Although it feels miraculous to be able to cut down on medications or get off them completely, to have pain disappear, and to feel healthy again, it is something that we have come to expect when the diet changes are the right ones.

OTHER TREATMENTS

In chapter 11, we saw how vitamin B_6 can help stop the nerve pains of carpal tunnel syndrome. It also helps in diabetes. It can reduce pain, although it may not improve the function of the nerves.[10] Like medications, B_6 should be viewed as an adjunct to a low-fat, vegetarian diet and exercise for those who need extra help, not as a replacement for them. The usual dose is 50–150 mg per day, and it typically takes several weeks to see benefits. Higher doses should be avoided, as they may actually cause nerve problems.

Capsaicin, the "hot" ingredient in hot peppers, is mixed into a cream that is useful for some patients with postmastectomy pain, arthritis, and shingles. It has also been tested in patients with diabetic neuropathy. Investigators in a multicenter research study tested 0.075 percent capsaicin cream, recommending that it be applied to the painful areas four times per day. It helped 70 percent of patients. In this study, however, a placebo treatment helped 53 percent of patients, so capsaicin's advantage, while present, is less impressive than for some other conditions.[11]

My opinion of vitamin B_6 and capsaicin for diabetic pains is that they may be useful adjuncts to a low-fat, vegan diet and exercise program. If you have not yet tried the diet and exercise program, however, that should be your first priority, as it can change the fundamental course of your illness.

THE APPROACH TO DIABETES

1. Follow a low-fat vegan (pure vegetarian) diet, avoiding all animal products and added oils. In the recipe section, you will find many choices that put these principles to work in the most delightful possible way. If this kind of diet is new for you, resolve to try it very strictly for three weeks. This gives you plenty of time to experiment with different foods, without the daunting feeling of a long-term commitment.

2. Focus on foods that are rich in complex carbohydrates and fiber: beans, vegetables, and whole grains, rather than those whose fiber has been removed (e.g., white bread, pasta, and white rice).

3. Exercise regularly, within the limits prescribed by your physician. A half-hour walk every day or an hour three times per week is a good regimen for most people, and you can do more as your exercise capacity increases. Exercising muscles pull sugar out of the blood.

4. To insure complete nutrition, a source of vitamin B_{12} is important. This could include any common multivitamin, fortified soymilk or cereals, or a vitamin B_{12} supplement of 5 mcg or more per day.

5. If nerve pains continue, try vitamin B_6, 50–150 mg per day, in consultation with your physician, who can monitor your progress.

DOES COW'S MILK CAUSE DIABETES?

Cow's milk has come under scrutiny as a possible cause of childhood-onset diabetes. Many studies have suggested that cow's milk proteins elicit the production of antibodies that can damage the insulin-producing cells in the pancreas. In 1992, the *New England Journal of Medicine* added new evidence suggesting that cow's milk exposure was indeed a contributor to the disease. Of 142 children with diabetes, every single one had high blood levels of antibodies to a particular cow's milk protein.[12]

While it may seem odd to think of milk proteins causing any sort of health problem, it is useful to remember that nature never figured on humans drinking the milk of a cow. Cow's milk has the perfect nutrient mix for a newborn calf, but it is not at all nutritionally correct for a human infant. In this case, the problem stems not from the fat or the lactose sugar, but from the milk proteins, which can cause the human body to produce antibodies. These antibodies are believed to damage the pancreas. Cow's milk proteins are also the main cause of colic, which affects one baby in every five, and they are among the most frequent triggers for migraines, arthritis, and digestive problems.

At the time that the *New England Journal of Medicine* article appeared, cow's milk had already been shown to contribute to iron deficiency and other health problems in children. Unfortunately, parents are often told that milk is a good source of calcium, but are rarely told of its disadvantages or of healthier calcium sources.

With the new evidence of an additional health concern, the Physicians Committee for Responsible Medicine held a press conference with child-health expert Benjamin Spock, M.D., Frank Oski, M.D., the director of Pediatrics of Johns Hopkins University, and other health experts who joined me in recommending that parents be advised about the potential risks of dairy products.

Needless to say, the dairy industry fought back, trying to dismiss the findings. However, shortly thereafter, the American Academy of Pediatrics convened a panel to examine the issue. It concluded that exposure to cow's milk protein may indeed be an important factor in the development of diabetes. Based on the more than ninety studies that had addressed the issue, the Academy reported that avoiding cow's milk exposure may delay or prevent the disease in susceptible individuals.[13] More evidence continues to weigh in on the issue, including a recent article in the *Lancet* that again suggested that milk may contribute to diabetes in children.[14]

Finding out that milk may cause juvenile-onset diabetes will not be of much comfort if you already have it. But I share this information because, even though it has received a tremendous amount of research attention, it is still all but unknown among parents, who continue to be deluged with milk advertisements.

Regardless of whether you have the childhood- or adult-onset form of diabetes, the right food choices can be tremendously powerful. If you have pain, it may well go away. Your need for medication can be reduced, and if you have the adult-onset form, the disease itself could well disappear.

CHAPTER 13

Herpes and Shingles

Viruses are so small, it is amazing that they do so much mischief. The various members of the herpes family of viruses cause cold sores, genital sores, and shingles.

Foods can affect your immune strength against viruses, and one amino acid in particular, called lysine, has been tested for its ability to prevent and treat herpes viruses. In this chapter, we will look at lysine and other allies in the fight against these intruders.

COLD SORES AND GENITAL HERPES

Cold sores are caused by the herpes simplex virus type 1 (HSV-1). The virus spreads easily from person to person, and worldwide, about 90 percent of people have it. Usually, it lies dormant, but it can emerge in cold sores, usually where skin meets a mucous membrane, for example, at the corner of your mouth.

Its first cousin, the herpes simplex virus type 2, causes genital herpes, which is acquired through sexual contact. The sore is reddened at the base, topped with a cluster of blisters that burst, leaving a painful ulcer that takes two to three weeks to heal. Like HSV-1, HSV-2 can simply lie dormant for long periods. In fact, 40 percent of people never have another sore. Stress or immune suppression can make the sores recur.

LYSINE VERSUS HERPES

Beginning in the early 1970s, scientific reports began to show that, for some people, lysine helped prevent recurrences of herpes sores and sped up healing.

Lysine is an amino acid, that is, a small molecule that is one of the building blocks of proteins. Our bodies do not make it. It is an *essential* amino acid, meaning that we have to get it from food to build the proteins that make up our bodies. One of the many happy differences between us and herpes viruses is that herpes tend to choke on lysine. That is to say, it inhibits their ability to multiply.[1]

On the other hand, the virus needs a second amino acid, called *arginine*. If it does not have it, it cannot make the proteins it needs to replicate. It does not die, but at least it cannot multiply.

These two amino acids compete with each other, and you can use this fact to your advantage. Lysine interferes with the absorption of arginine in your digestive tract and encourages your kidneys to eliminate it in the urine. It also tends to deplete the arginine from your cells, so herpes viruses have less arginine available.[2]

··

LYSINE TO PREVENT AND TREAT HERPES

If you are using lysine, the following guidelines may be helpful.

1. Use L-lysine. There is also a D-lysine, which is biologically inactive.

2. Use the lowest dose that works for you, between 500 and 3,000 mg per day. The first studies that showed effectiveness used 500 mg to prevent attacks, and double that amount to treat sores once they emerge.[6] Later research studies have used a preventive dose of 1,000 mg three times per day, taken with food.[3] Doses at this level appear to be safe, but the safety of higher doses is unknown.[7]

3. Avoid arginine-rich foods, such as nuts, seeds, chocolate, and gelatin.

4. Work with your doctor. Lysine can be used along with the antiviral medicines your doctor may be prescribing.

··

In a 1987 study, Richard Griffith of Indiana University prescribed lysine to people who had cold sores or genital herpes. At the same time, he asked them to avoid high-arginine foods, particularly nuts, seeds, chocolate, and gelatin. He compared the lysine treatment to a placebo and found that lysine reduced both the number of attacks and the time needed for sores to heal. Some people found that they could even stop an emerging sore by taking 3,000–4,000 mg of lysine for several days.[3]

As other researchers have studied lysine, it appears that it helps some people but not others.[4,5] So far, there are no reports of any dangers of lysine within the doses used.

CANKER SORES

Lysine seems to help for canker sores, too, as suggested by a 1983 user survey.[8] Operating on the theory that a herpeslike virus may be the cause of canker sores, researchers provided lysine to twenty-eight patients and found that, in nearly every case, lysine helped prevent the sores from beginning and also hastened their disappearance.[9] The dosage was 500 mg per day, which could be doubled if the initial dose was not effective at preventing them. If a canker sore started, the dose was raised to 1,000 mg every six hours until the sore disappeared.

SHINGLES

Herpes zoster, also called shingles, is a painful rash on your abdomen or face. The varicella-zoster virus that causes it is a first cousin to HSV-1 and HSV-2 and is the same virus that causes chicken pox.

More than 90 percent of American children get chicken pox. The virus enters through the respiratory tract and disseminates in the bloodstream, causing the itchy rash that heals in a week or two. The virus, however, is not dead. It is just hiding inside your nerve cells.

Decades later, if your immunity starts to flag, the virus descends along the pain and touch nerves that lead to your skin. It triggers inflammation, causing a stabbing or burning pain that shoots up the nerves to your brain. This is the beginning of shingles. As the virus escapes from the nerves into the skin, it causes the painful rash.

Not everyone who has had chicken pox will get shingles. Overall, about 10 to 20 percent of people have a bout of this miserable condition. It occurs four times more often in whites than blacks, presumably for some genetic reason that has yet to be characterized.

For most, the condition is gone within several weeks. For others, unfortunately, the pain persists after the rash is gone, a complication called *postherpetic neuralgia*. For people who get shingles in their sixties, about half will have persistent pain that can take months or even years to go away.

Antiviral drugs, such as acyclovir, are helpful during the acute shingles attack and are generally safe. If they are started early on, they can reduce the pain of the acute attack and may reduce the likelihood that postherpetic neuralgia will occur.

Once postherpetic neuralgia begins, the usual treatment is with antidepressants, not for your mood, but for pain. The ones that work are the older ones, particularly nortriptyline, desipramine, and amitriptyline (Elavil), which boost a brain chemical called noradrenaline.[10] Some experts recommend that they be begun as soon as shingles is diagnosed. Prozac and other antidepressants that affect only serotonin are not helpful for this kind of pain. Some doctors also prescribe codeine or other narcotic painkillers.[11]

There has been little research on the use of lysine for herpes zoster. In a 1983 survey of people using lysine for shingles, 90 percent rated lysine as either "effective" or "very effective," while 10 percent reported no benefit.[8] The dose used is generally the same as for herpes simplex. This study was encouraging, but given that herpes zoster pain eventually remits on its own anyway, a comparison of lysine to a placebo is needed to sort out whether it really helps.

Some people with shingles or postherpetic neuralgia have gotten benefit from capsaicin cream, the unusual pain treatment described in chapter 5, made from the "hot" ingredient in chili peppers. It works by depleting a nerve chemical called *substance P* and dulls the sensitivity to pain.[12]

In a study of patients who had been suffering with postherpetic neuralgia for over a year without relief, the cream yielded improvements in 64 percent of cases. It will not usually make the pain disappear (fewer than 20 percent had a complete remission of pain with capsaicin treatment), but it will usually reduce it.[13] It can safely be used with antidepressants.

You will find capsaicin at drugstores under the brand names Zostrix and Dolorac. It is applied to sore skin four to five times per day. Allow four weeks to assess its benefits, as it sometimes has a delayed action. Wash your hands carefully after applying it, so as not to get any into your eyes. The stinging of the capsaicin cream diminishes after the first week, and you can reduce it further by pretreating your skin with 5 percent Xylocaine ointment or a lidocaine spray such as Solarcaine. I would encourage you to use it in consultation with your doctor to find the best dose and treatment combination possible.

My recommendation for shingles is to pull out all the stops to treat the pain and to try to prevent it from turning into postherpetic neuralgia. This means using antiviral medications, antidepressants, and even narcotic painkillers as soon as it is diagnosed, along with capsaicin. The goal is to keep the attack as short as possible to prevent the onset of persistent pain.

BOOSTING IMMUNITY

The reawakening of the varicella-zoster virus is, in most cases, a sign that your immunity is waning.[14] Foods can help strengthen your immune defenses. As noted in chapter 8, low-fat, vegetarian foods help boost immunity. Partly, this is because avoiding fat and cholesterol helps your immune cells to function better, but vegetables, beans, and fruits also contain nutrients that boost immunity.

Because we tend to be less active as we get older, we work up less of an appetite. If we then eat less vegetables and fruits, we are likely to miss out on the vitamins and minerals we need for a strong immune system. More physical activity and more healthful meals can make up for that. Researchers have also found that even a simple daily multivitamin can correct minor deficiencies and measurably improve your immune strength.[15]

THE EFFECT OF STRESS

Stress can trigger herpes viruses, causing cold sores and genital herpes, and the same appears to be true for shingles attacks. Stress aggravates the pain of postherpetic neuralgia, and relaxation techniques can help relieve it.[10] See chapter 17 for techniques for reducing stress that are easy and quick.

Viruses remain enigmatic, and treatments are not nearly as good as we would like. Nonetheless, the above steps can help reduce the likelihood of viral eruptions and shorten the attacks when they do occur.

CHAPTER 14

Sickle-Cell Anemia

In sickle-cell anemia, healthy round red blood cells collapse into sickle shapes and other irregular configurations that clog tiny blood vessels, blocking the flow of blood and oxygen to body tissues. The result is one painful crisis after another and damage to the spleen, lungs, brain, or other organs. In addition, the abnormal cells have to be replaced, so your bone marrow works overtime to produce new blood cells. Diet and lifestyle cannot eliminate the disease, but they can cut down on the number of painful episodes.

Sickle-cell disease is caused by an inherited change in hemoglobin, the molecule that carries oxygen in red blood cells.* The sickle-cell gene is recessive, meaning that you get the disease only when you get the gene from both of your parents. About three out of every thousand African-Americans are born with sickle-cell anemia.

If you receive the sickle-cell gene from one parent and a normal gene from the other, you have what is called sickle-cell trait. Your red blood cells will retain their normal shape, except in very adverse circumstances—at high altitudes where there is little oxygen, for example. About 80 million people worldwide have sickle-cell trait, including 8 percent of African-Americans.[1,2]

---

*The hemoglobin molecule consists of four chains of amino acids. The two alpha chains have 141 amino acids. The two beta chains have 146. Near one end of the beta chains, the amino acid valine takes the place of another amino acid, called glutamic acid. The substitution of this single amino acid is what causes the cell's tendency to collapse.

THE ORIGIN OF THE SICKLE-CELL GENE

Why should such a gene arise, and why would it persist? The reason is that it protects against malaria. About four thousand years ago in India, and three thousand years ago in Africa, the transition from food gathering to food *producing* led to the cutting down of large sections of forest growth, which in turn resulted in swamps and open pools of water, which are the preferred breeding spots of anopheles mosquitoes.[1] These mosquitoes transmit malaria. At the same time, the growing human population became readily available hosts for the infection.*

The gene for sickling emerged in at least four separate places in Africa and one in India.[1] It has a remarkable property. When the malaria parasite enters a cell that has the sickle gene, the cell collapses. The body spots the abnormal cell and eliminates it. In effect, the malaria parasite commits suicide when it tries to make this kind of cell its home.

Where malaria is endemic, people who have sickle-cell *trait* have a real advantage. Their cells do not go into the sickle shape normally, but will when infected with malaria and can then be rapidly eliminated. Infants with sickle-cell trait are much more likely to survive the rigors of malaria than are children with normal hemoglobin.

PAIN MEDICATIONS

When a sickle-cell crisis occurs, narcotic painkillers are usually necessary to treat the intense pain. Sometimes doctors are hesitant to use narcotics for fear that they will encourage addiction. However, this reticence probably does more harm than good. When pain relief is inadequate, the patient's anxiety increases, and he or she is forced to ask for more medications, setting the stage for power struggles between the patient and the hospital staff.[2] The use of narcotics can be reduced with steps that help prevent crises, and the use of adjuvant nonnarcotic pain medicines and antidepressants for pain control.

---

*Anopheles mosquitoes transmit the protozoan *Plasmodium falciparum* to humans. It enters the red blood cells, causing malaria.

People who have sickle-cell anemia—that is, those who got the gene from both parents—do not have an advantage, because there are simply too many collapsing cells. In countries without adequate medical facilities, nearly all infants with sickle-cell anemia die in the first few years of life.

NUTRITION AND SICKLE-CELL ANEMIA

The role of nutrition in sickle-cell anemia is by no means settled, but certain points are clear. First, keeping alcohol use modest helps. A drink or two every now and then is okay, but overdoing it can easily trigger a sickle-cell crisis. Second, it is important to emphasis plant foods—vegetables, beans, grains, and fruits—in your daily routine. Vegetables and beans, in particular, are rich in the folic acid needed to make blood cells. Also, these foods give you plenty of protein without using animal products. This is important, because sickle cells can clog the kidney's tiny blood vessels, causing it to gradually lose its filtering ability. Animal proteins accelerate the loss of kidney function, as we will see in more detail in chapter 15. Getting your protein from plant sources helps preserve your kidneys.

Third, taking a daily vitamin-mineral supplement is good insurance. In addition to supplying folic acid and zinc, which are low in some people with sickle-cell disease, it also supplies vitamin B_{12}, which is missing from grains, beans, vegetables, and fruits.[3]

Iron supplements should be used only if prescribed by your physician. While some people with sickle-cell disease are low in iron, others are iron-overloaded, particularly if they have had numerous blood transfusions.[3] Guidelines to help you interpret your iron level test are given on page 91.

Some care providers have also suggested the use of vitamin E, 450 IU per day, although the evidence that it helps is only modest at present.[3,4]

MILLET, YAMS, AND CYANATE

In the early 1970s, researchers discovered that a simple molecule, called cyanate, could prevent cells from sickling. Cyanate attaches to the hemoglobin molecule and holds on for the life of the cell. It does not cure the disease, but a report in the *New England Journal of Medicine* showed that it could cut the frequency of crises from an average of 3.6 per year to 2.1, a drop of 40 percent.[5]

Unfortunately, although it looked safe in short-term tests, cyanate caused nerve problems, cataracts, and weight loss in several patients after long-term use, and in spite of its benefits, it had to be abandoned.[6] However, researchers have noted that several foods that are staples in Africa—cassava, yams, sorghum, and millet—are rich in compounds that release cyanate in the body, and these foods have no known side effects. Cassava is also used in Jamaica, where some people with sickle-cell disease live remarkably long lives.[7-9] This raises the question as to whether foods could deliver the benefits of cyanate without its risks. Unfortunately, no one has yet tested this idea.

EXERCISE

Stress, infections, and cold temperatures can trigger sickle crises, and you will want to do what you can to avoid them. It is also important to be careful about exercise, because overexertion can cause a crisis, too.

If you have sickle-cell disease, you are well aware of the risks of overexertion. But people with sickle-cell trait may need to be careful, as well. In 1970, the *New England Journal of Medicine* reported four deaths among Army recruits during strenuous exercise at Fort Bliss, Texas. All had sickle-cell trait, and sickle cells were found in their blood at autopsy. In subsequent reports, thirty people with sickle-cell trait had collapsed after intense exercise, and most died.[10]

Investigators believe that people with sickle-cell trait are vulnerable to the heat of overexertion, and the breakdown of muscle tissue. If this includes you, the following precautions are important while you are exercising:

1. Drink plenty of water, beyond the amount needed to satisfy thirst.
2. Take rest breaks as needed.
3. Wear cool clothing.
4. Limit activity in hot and humid weather, or whenever your medical condition merits it.

CHAPTER 15

Kidney Stones and Urinary Infections

If you've ever had a kidney stone, you know you definitely do not want another. Unlike the pain of childbirth, which, I am told, fades into memory—a phenomenon also found among writers approaching the drafting of another book—a kidney stone leaves an impression like a huge crashing meteorite.

About 12 percent of Americans have a kidney stone at some point in their lives. For some reason, they hit men three times more often than women, and whites more than Asians or blacks. They are especially likely to strike between the ages of forty and sixty.

You are right to be concerned about a recurrence, because that is exactly what happens in 30–50 percent of people within five years of their first stone. The good news is that foods offer a powerful and easy way to shrink those odds.

A kidney stone forms like a salt crystal in a glass of water. If you stir a few grains of salt into water, they easily dissolve. But if you pour in more and more salt, eventually the water cannot hold it in solution, and it begins to form crystals. In the kidneys, crystals form, not from table salt, but from calcium oxalate, which is simply a mixture of the calcium that originally came in foods or supplements, along with oxalate, a part of many plant foods. Less commonly, stones form from uric acid, which is a product of protein breakdown.

To keep a salt crystal from forming in a glass of water, you can either use less salt or add more water. To keep a stone from forming in your kidney, you need less calcium, oxalate, or uric acid flowing through it, or more water to keep them dissolved. Some people have a tendency to quickly lose calcium or oxalate through their kidneys, and they have a greater likelihood of a stone. But there are simple steps that anyone can take to greatly reduce their risk.[1–4]

WHAT'S IN A STONE?[1]

Calcium oxalate	72%
Uric acid	23
Ammoniomagnesium phosphate (struvite)	5
Cystine	<1

To piece together the kind of diet that can help prevent stones, researchers have tracked the diets of large groups of people and watched to see who developed stones and who did not. They have also experimented with different diets, to see which ones slow down the loss of calcium or other stone precursors.

It turns out that putting these findings to work is really quite easy. First, let's look at the protective foods, then at those that encourage stones to form.

PROTECTIVE FOODS

Certain parts of the diet clearly help reduce the risk. The first is no surprise.

Water. Drinking extra water helps. It dilutes the urine and keeps calcium, oxalates, and uric acid from turning into solid crystals. If your fluid intake in a day, including any water, juice, coffee, tea, soup, wine, or anything else you might have, adds up to about two and one-half quarts (or roughly 2.5 liters), your risk of a stone is about one-third less than that of a person drinking only half that much.[1] This is true even if you do nothing to change the rest of your diet. But several other steps let you cut the risk much more.

Your thirst is a fairly good guide to how much water you need over the long run. But it tends to fall behind, letting you become a bit dehydrated before signaling you to have some water. It helps to drink water regularly.

High-potassium, low-sodium foods. A study of 46,000 men done by Harvard University researchers found that a high potassium intake can cut the risk of kidney stones in half. Potassium helps the kidneys keep calcium in the bones and bloodstream, instead of sending it out into the urine. This does not mean taking a potassium supplement or even measuring how much potassium you get every day. It just means having bananas, broccoli, cauliflower, or just about any other fruits, vegetables, or beans in generous amounts daily. Plants are naturally high in potassium.

At the same time, choose foods that keep sodium to a minimum. Sodium increases the loss of calcium through the kidney and adds to the risk of stones.[3] While this effect is not well-known among the lay public, it is well-accepted among researchers, who have found that when people cut their salt (sodium chloride) intake in half, they reduce their daily need for calcium by about 160 mg.[5]

SODIUM AND POTASSIUM IN FOODS (MG)

PLANT PRODUCTS	SODIUM	POTASSIUM	ANIMAL PRODUCTS	SODIUM	POTASSIUM
Apple (1 medium)	1	159	Whole milk (1 cup)	120	370
Banana (1 medium)	1	451	Skim milk (1 cup)	126	406
Black beans (1 cup*)	1	611	Goat's milk (1 cup)	122	499
Broccoli (1 cup*)	44	332	Human milk (1 cup)	40	128
Cauliflower (1 cup*)	8	400	Yogurt (1 cup)	105	351
Cream of wheat (1 cup*)	7	48	Cheddar cheese (2 oz)	352	56
Grapefruit (1 medium)	0	316	Ground beef (4 oz*)	69	253
Navy beans (1 cup*)	2	669	Roast beef (4 oz*)	51	377
Orange (1 medium)	1	250	Chicken breast (no skin) (4 oz*)	82	286
Potato (1 medium*)	16	844	Haddock (4 oz*)	98	447
Rice (1 cup*)	1	60	Swordfish (4 oz*)	130	414

SOURCE: J. A. T. Pennington, *Bowes and Church's Food Values of Portions Commonly Used*, 16th ed. (Philadelphia: J. B. Lippincott, 1994).
*Figures refer to cooked servings.

Plants of any kind—rice, broccoli, chickpeas, apples, potatoes, cauliflower—contain almost no sodium at all in their natural state. Only when they are canned or processed into soups or other commercial products is a substantial amount of salt added. Dairy products and meats contain more salt than plant products, and canned and snack foods contain more still. The table on page 194 gives the potassium and sodium content of common foods. As you can see, plant foods are consistently better choices.

Calcium. Even though most stones contain calcium, calcium in foods is not always a problem. If you take calcium supplements between meals, they may well increase the risk of stones, because about 8 percent of any extra calcium you take in ends up in the urine.[3,6] On the other hand, when you have your calcium *with* a meal, it has the opposite effect. It can actually help prevent stones. The reason, presumably, is that calcium binds to the oxalates in that meal and keeps them in the digestive tract, rather than allowing them to be absorbed. That means less oxalate to filter through the kidneys or to make its way into stones.

By the way, you do not need to have dairy products to get calcium's benefits. As you know, dairy products have many undesirable features, including their animal proteins, lactose sugar, contaminants, and all too often, a serious load of fat. The Harvard study found that plant sources of calcium, such as broccoli and oranges, help reduce the risk of kidney stones.

Coffee and tea. Coffee—caffeinated or decaf—cuts the risk of stones. The same is true of tea. Caffeine is a diuretic, causing extra fluid to pass through the kidney. While it also causes calcium to filter along with it, you lose more water than calcium, so, all things considered, it does reduce the risk of stones.

Also in the not-so-healthy-but-won't-hurt-your-kidneys category, alcoholic beverages are associated with a reduced risk of kidney stones. Their diuretic effect probably gets the credit.

PROBLEM FOODS

Animal protein. Animal protein is the worst enemy of people with a tendency toward kidney stones, or any kidney disease for that matter. It has long been known that animal protein (fish, poultry, "red meat," eggs, or milk) tends to overwork the kidneys and causes their filtering ability to gradually decline. Doctors routinely advise people with kidney disease to keep meat and other animal products to a minimum.

But animal proteins have another effect on the kidney. They cause calcium to be pulled from the bones and excreted in the urine, where it can form stones. They send extra uric acid into the urine as well. In a controlled research study, published in the *American Journal of Clinical Nutrition*, research subjects on a vegetarian diet had less than half the calcium loss that they had on a typical meat-based diet.[7]

The Harvard study found that even a modest increase in animal protein, from less than 50 grams per day to 77 grams, was associated with a 33 percent increased risk of stones in men.[1] The same is true for women. The Nurses' Health Study, a long-term study of various health factors in a large group of women, revealed an even greater risk of stones from animal protein than had been found in men.[3]

The problem with animal products is not just the *amount* of protein they contain. The *type* of protein is a problem, too. A protein molecule is like a string of beads, each "bead" being an amino acid. What makes the proteins in a chicken's thigh or a fish's tail different from those in baked beans or broccoli is the type of amino acids they contain and also the order in which they are joined together in the protein chain.

Animal products are high in amino acids that contain sulfur, which tends to leach calcium from the bones. The calcium passes from the bones into the bloodstream and ends up filtering through the kidneys into the urine, where it can form stones.*

Meats and eggs contain two to five times more of these sulfur-containing amino acids than are found in grains and beans.[8] Needless to say, vegetarians have a tremendous advantage. Since they avoid animal protein, they tend to keep their calcium in their bones where it belongs and end up with both stronger bones and fewer kidney stones, compared to meat-eaters.[6,8]

Between 1958 and the late 1960s, the incidence of kidney stones in Great Britain sharply increased. Obviously, the genetics of the population had not suddenly changed, so a team of researchers in Leeds decided to try to track down whether there were any major changes in eating habits during those years. There was no big difference in the amount of calcium or oxalate-containing foods that people consumed. However, the con-

---

*For those who enjoy technical details, the common sulfur-containing amino acids are cystine and methionine. Their sulfur is converted to sulfate, which tends to acidify the blood. In neutralizing this acid, bone is dissolved, and bone calcium ends up in the urine.

sumption of vegetables decreased, and the use of poultry, fish, and meat increased. The statistics showed a "striking relationship between stone incidence and the consumption of animal protein, particularly that derived from meat, fish, and poultry."[9]

Salt. As we saw earlier, sodium increases the passage of calcium through the kidneys and increases the risk of stones. This is true of sodium that is naturally in foods, as well as salt that is added during cooking. It helps to keep total sodium intake to between one and two grams per day.

Sugar. Sugar's tarnished image comes mainly from its contribution to dental cavities and moodiness. But it also disrupts your calcium balance and increases the risk of kidney stones. Like animal protein and salt, sugar accelerates calcium losses through the kidney.[10] In the Nurses' Health Study, those who consumed, on average, about sixty grams or more of sugar (sucrose) per day had a 50 percent higher risk of stones than those who consumed only about twenty grams.[3]

SUGAR IN COMMON FOODS (GM)

Chocolate bar (2 oz)	22–35	Fruit cocktail (1/2 cup, 124 gm)	14
Cookies (3)	11–14	Grape jam (1 tbsp)	13
Corn flakes (1 cup, 28 gm)	2	Ice cream (1/2 cup, 106 gm)	21
Frosted flakes (1 cup, 41 gm)	17	Soda (12 oz)	40
Crackers (5)	1	White bread (2 slices)	1

Your risk of kidney stones is higher if you live in a warm climate, such as the hot and sunny southern United States. Perspiration can dehydrate you, leading to a more concentrated urine. Also, sunlight increases the amount of vitamin D produced in the skin, which, in turn, increases the absorption of calcium from the digestive tract.[11]

Oddly enough, foods rich in oxalates, such as chocolate, nuts, tea, and spinach, do not seem to be linked to a higher risk of stones.[1] Likewise, vitamin C had been thought by some to increase the risk of kidney stones because it can be converted to oxalate. Its chief advocate, Linus Pauling, consistently maintained it would do no such thing. Pauling was right. A large study of men taking vitamin C supplements found that they had no more kidney stones than men who do not take them.[2]

PUTTING IT ALL TOGETHER

Here are the simple steps for avoiding kidney stones. Keeping calcium out of your urine also helps you keep it in your bones where it belongs.

1. Drink plenty of water or other fluids. It helps to stay ahead of your thirst.
2. Have plenty of vegetables, fruits, and beans. They are rich in potassium and low in sodium.
3. If you use calcium supplements, have them with meals, rather than between meals.
4. Avoid animal products. Their proteins and sodium content increase the risk of stones.
5. To insure complete nutrition, it is important to have a source of vitamin B_{12}, which could include any common multivitamin, fortified soymilk or cereals, or a vitamin B_{12} supplement of 5 mcg or more per day.
6. Keep salt and sugar use modest.

CRANBERRY JUICE AGAINST URINARY INFECTIONS

For many years, cranberry juice has been used to reduce the risk of urinary infections. A 1994 report in the *Journal of the American Medical Association* showed that it works. In a test involving 153 elderly women in Boston, half the subjects drank three hundred milliliters (about one and one-quarter cups) of cranberry juice cocktail each day.[12] This is the same bottled beverage that is sold in grocery stores. The other half consumed a drink that looked and tasted like cranberry juice, but had no real juice in it.

Over the next six months, urine samples were collected and tested for signs of bacteria. The women consuming cranberry juice had fewer than half as many urinary infections as the control group—42 percent, to be exact. The number of cases that had to be treated with antibiotics was also only about half, which is a real advantage, since antibiotics can sometimes lead to yeast infections and other problems. It takes about four to eight weeks for the preventive effect to be seen.

The explanation for the effect of cranberry juice is probably not that it acidifies the urine, because the placebo drink did that just as well. Rather, cranberries contain a substance that stops bacteria from attaching to cells, and this is probably true whether the cranberry juice reaches the bacteria in the digestive tract or the urinary tract. Substances that interfere with bacterial adhesion have also been found in blueberry juice, but not in orange, grapefruit, pineapple, mango, or guava juice.

After the *JAMA* article appeared, Dutch researchers wrote of a similar experience. Cranberries first arrived in Holland when an American ship wrecked on the Dutch coast. Crates of berries washed ashore on a small island called Terschelling. Some of them took root, and cranberries have been cultivated there ever since. The Dutch researchers tested cranberry juice in a group of elderly men and women and found that, indeed, it helps prevent urinary tract infections.[13]

A SIMPLE AMINO ACID FOR INTERSTITIAL CYSTITIS

Interstitial cystitis is a painful condition that feels like a urinary tract infection, with pain, pressure, and burning on urination, but no bacteria show up on urine tests, and antibiotics do not help. About 90 percent of the people affected are women, and it usually hits at around age forty.

Doctors have assumed that this frustrating and chronic condition must be caused by a hidden infection in the wall of the bladder or by some sort of immune system attack on the bladder tissues. But no cause has been nailed down, and available treatments leave much to be desired.

Yale University researchers recently tried a new approach, using a natural amino acid (protein building-block), called L-arginine.[14] In the bladder, L-arginine turns into nitric oxide, a compound that relaxes the muscles that surround the bladder and also seems to help it resist invading bacteria. The Yale researchers gave 500 mg of L-arginine three times a day to ten interstitial cystitis patients. In the first month, most found a significant reduction in their symptoms. By three months, all patients rated L-arginine as the best treatment they had ever had for their problem. By six months, the patients' pain ratings had dropped from an average of 5, on a scale from 0 to 10, to nearly 1. There were no side effects reported. L-arginine is available at health food stores.

PART V

ACTIVITY, REST, AND FOOD

CHAPTER 16

Exercise and Endorphins

A big part of your natural defenses against pain depends on physical activity and rest. Exercise stimulates the release of natural painkillers, called endorphins, improves circulation, limbers up your muscles, and helps you sleep. Rest and sleep allow your body to heal from the traumas of the day and are vital for undoing tension headaches and increasing your general pain resistance.

EXERCISE BLOCKS OUT PAIN

People who exercise frequently (six hours or more per week) have dramatically better resistance to pain than other people.[1] The pain relief comes from endorphins, natural painkillers that are made in the pituitary gland at the base of your brain. They work within the brain and nerves themselves and are also released into your bloodstream.

The kind of exercise that stimulates endorphin release is *aerobic* exercise—that is, walking, bicycling, or other exercises that get your heart beating and your lungs working, as opposed to weight lifting, which works your muscles, but does not increase your heart rate appreciably.

Long-distance runners experience endorphin effects as the "runner's high." Researchers have tested athletes before and after exercise, measuring pain sensitivity by, for example, asking them to immerse their hands in a bucket of ice for as long as they can stand it. The natural analgesic effect of a six-mile run is roughly equivalent to 10 mg of morphine.[2]

Physical activity has other effects, too. When people exercise regularly, their muscles are looser and more compliant, and if you pinch their skin, it is actually less likely to turn red. In other words, they are able, *both physically and mentally,* to ignore painful things a bit more easily than the rest of us. People who rarely get any exercise have a higher sensitivity to pain, and their muscles are more tense.[1]

Physical activity is also a key ingredient in programs for reversing artery blockages, which is critical for people with heart disease and for many people with chronic back pain.

HOW MUCH EXERCISE?

The amount of exercise that is right for you depends on your physical condition, and you should discuss this with your doctor. If you have fibromyalgia or chronic fatigue syndrome, a daily walk lasting between five and fifteen minutes may be plenty for starters. You can increase the duration of the walk by one to two minutes each day until you reach thirty minutes. People with fibromyalgia often find that the more exercise they do, the better they feel.

If you are exercising to open your arteries, the regimen used in Dr. Dean Ornish's program for reversing heart disease was a brisk half-hour walk per day, or an hour three times per week. If you are ready for more, you can gradually increase your activity. Many people find that they feel better and better as they reach new levels of endurance.

The key ingredient in exercise is fun, because, if you enjoy it, you will stick with it. All the exercise equipment in the world is of no value if using it is so tedious that you cannot bear to continue. A little social support goes a long way, too. Walking with a friend, aerobics classes at a health club, or social dancing are fun and help you stick with it.

Exercise has powerful benefits, and it also has potential side effects. The more you work, the faster your heart has to pump to meet your needs. If you have not been active regularly, it is easy to overdo it, particularly if a newfound sense of well-being makes you feel like taking on the world. Resist the urge to reach perfect cardiovascular fitness or burn off ten pounds in one session. Your heart is not up to it yet.

Exercise also puts stress on your muscles, tendons, and ligaments. Within limits, this is beneficial, but joint injuries are common among people who attempt to rebound too quickly from a prolonged period of inactivity.

Let me reiterate a caution that I mentioned in chapter 7. Some people with chronic fatigue syndrome have a condition called neurally mediated hypotension, which causes an unexpected drop in blood pressure while they are exercising. Let your doctor evaluate your ability to exercise safely before you get started.

Exercise is like breathing: doing it regularly is more important than doing it especially vigorously. If you have any medical condition, take medication regularly, or are over forty, you should discuss your exercise plans with your doctor.

CHAPTER 17

Rest and Sleep

Sleep is essential to pain relief. It makes both physical and emotional stresses hurt less. Researchers have found that sleep deprivation can measurably reduce your pain resistance, bringing on pain, tenderness, and fatigue not unlike fibromyalgia.[1,2]

You can do several things to get a good night's sleep.

• Sugar can help you sleep. While sugar is not health food by any stretch of the imagination, it can help you sleep. It causes the brain to produce serotonin, the neurotransmitter that plays a central role in sleep, moods, and pain control, as we saw in chapters 3 and 7. Fruit sugars work as well as table sugar. So have some orange juice and a cookie an hour before bed, and see how it works for you.

• Avoid high-protein foods in the evening. They can block serotonin production. Of course, I never encourage the use of fish, poultry, meats, or eggs at any time, but the same goes for large servings of beans or tofu in the evening if a good night's sleep is your goal.

• You may find that it helps to have your evening meal early, avoiding late-night digestive challenges.

• Physical activity helps you sleep. Sleep rests both the body and the mind. For many of us, our minds are tired out by the challenges of the day, but our bodies have had no exercise at all. You are likely to sleep better if you tire out your muscles in the evening. Try push-ups (on your knees unless you are in good physical shape), squats, or other exercises that work your muscles, in addition to whatever aerobic exercise you are doing.

When people have had surgery, they often sleep deeply, long after the anesthesia has worn off. It is as if the body has shut down temporarily to concentrate on healing. Vigorous exercise does something similar. To the extent that it works your muscles, your body may demand sleep as part of normal recovery.

• Be careful about alcohol. Many people think of alcohol as a sedative. It is, at first. But to get rid of alcohol, your body converts it to another chemical, called acetaldehyde, which is a stimulant.[3] So a drink with dinner might relax you in the evening only to awaken you in the wee hours of the morning. Acetaldehyde tends to build up more in men than women.

• Avoid stimulants. Caffeine is not just in coffee and tea. It is also in colas, chocolate, and many painkillers, and it can keep you awake for hours. Similarly, cold pills containing pseudoephedrine act like stimulants, making it difficult to sleep, unless the effect is counteracted by other ingredients, as in the case of medications designed for nighttime use.

STRESS-REDUCING EXERCISES

Here are some simple exercises that you can use to melt away stress. You will feel the tension leave your muscles and your mind, and the more you do them, the better they work.

DIRECTED BREATHING

This exercise works wonderfully for both relaxation and for inducing sleep.

First, simply relax with your eyes closed for a minute or so. Listen to the sound of your breathing. As you do so, let your breathing become slower and a bit deeper, like a person sleeping. Feel the air come in through your nose and then out again. As you exhale, imagine that your breath carries tension out of your body.

Now, as you breathe in, imagine that the air goes in through your nostrils and then up to your face. As you breathe out, imagine that the exhalation takes the tension from your face and carries it out of your body. Imagine that the inhalation caresses your face like a breeze, and the exhalation carries the tension away. Allow this image to continue in your mind for two or three breaths.

Now, as you breathe in, imagine that the inhalation carries gentle air up over the top of your head. As you exhale, the tension leaves your head and passes out of your body. Then imagine your breath reaching the sides of your head and carrying tension out with it.

Take it slow and easy, and feel the relaxation come over each body part as you let the tension go.

Imagine the inhalation carrying the air to your neck, and as you breathe out, tension leaves with the exhaled air. Then do the same for each part of your body: your shoulders, your upper and lower arms, your hands, and then your chest, stomach, thighs, calves, and feet. Focus your attention on each part, and imagine each breath of air carrying relaxation in, and let the tension leave as you breathe out.

Give yourself several minutes to do this exercise. When you have finished, sit quietly for a minute or two before getting up.

PROGRESSIVE RELAXATION

This exercise is good both for relaxation and for drifting off to sleep. It is very simple. All you do is gently tighten each muscle group of your body for an instant, then release it, letting tension go. We will start at your head and work down to your feet.

Begin by sitting quietly for a minute or so, and allow your breathing to become a bit slower and deeper. Now, gently raise your eyebrows, tensing the muscles of your forehead. Hold this tension for just a second, then relax. Let any tension in your brow drift away. Continue to breathe slowly in and out. Now gently tighten the muscles of your cheeks for a second, then let them relax as completely as you can. Then gently clench your jaw for just an instant and release it.

Continue to tighten and then release your muscles, focusing on one part at a time: neck, shoulders, upper arms, lower arms, hands, chest, abdomen, thighs, calves, and feet. Take your time, and relax each muscle group completely. When you are finished, sit quietly for a minute or two before getting up.

NECK CIRCLES

Golfer Greg Norman describes a simple stress-reducer: Simply lower your head to the front and then slowly turn it in a circle over your right ear, to the back, over your left ear and back to the front. Repeat this, then do it twice in the opposite direction.

These muscle-loosening exercises work on the theory that stress is always both physical and emotional. If your muscles are deeply relaxed, it is all but impossible for your mind to feel tension.

FOUR-SEVEN-EIGHT BREATHING

This is a quick de-stressor that I learned from Andrew Weil, M.D. It takes only about a minute, and you can do it while you are walking, driving, or anywhere else.

Start by placing your tongue on the ridge behind your front teeth, and keep it there for the entire exercise. Breathe in slowly and easily through your nose for a count of four. Then hold your breath for seven counts, then let the breath out through your mouth over eight counts, listening to the whooshing sound as the air goes past your tongue. Do this sequence a total of four times at whatever rate is comfortable for you. Something about this pacing of your breathing and attention to your body processes helps stress melt away.

An equally quick breathing exercise is to take a deep breath in, as deep as you can. Then, without exhaling, take in even a bit more air, really feeling it in your lungs. Then take in even a bit more. Hold it for several counts and then let it all go. Feel your muscles relax as you do so, and you may notice a little involuntary smile arriving. Do this twice.

REST YOUR EYES

When your eyes are tired, a feeling of fatigue comes over your whole body. Practitioners of hypnosis have exploited this phenomenon for many years, asking subjects to stare at an object positioned so as to strain the eyes. You are doing much the same thing every day as your eyes move back and forth across a book or a computer screen. The eye strain triggers an overall sense of fatigue.

You can rest your eyes by draping a cool, damp cloth over them for a few minutes. If you can, put your feet up at the same time. The combination of rest for your eyes and blood returning from your feet is wonderfully restorative. If you are not in a position to close both eyes, try covering one eye at a time for several seconds.

VISUALIZATION

Visualization has many applications. Perhaps best known is its use in cancer treatment programs, where, for example, cancer patients are asked to picture white blood cells swallowing up cancer cells, resulting in a broad range of physical and psychological benefits.

Visualization is a great relaxation tool. A basic technique is simply to guide your thoughts in a story that you imagine and that leaves room for one or two unexpected scenes.

I will give you a generic visualization exercise designed for relaxation. If you have a particular health scenario you would like to visualize, however, feel free.

Start by picturing an outdoor setting, one that is appealing and restful. The setting is up to you. The temperature is perfect. A light breeze is blowing. Take a minute and just picture this scene, allowing it to become clear in your mind. Imagine the sights, sounds, and smells around you.

After a minute or two, you notice a path that leads into a sunny meadow. You decide to follow the path for a bit to see where it might go. Along the way, there are pretty flowers with lovely scents. Take a minute or two and imagine what you see and hear as you go.

Eventually, you come to a shallow brook that is bubbling along. And next to the brook is a friendly looking person who has walked up and has something to show you, something you will like.

Take a look. What is it? How do you feel as you look at it?

You can take it with you or not, as you like, and return along the path to where we started. The air feels perfect, and your body feels comfortable.

Take your time, and let yourself enter the story. After you are done, you might reflect on the scene you imagined, and how your internal movie director made the choices you saw.

CHAPTER 18

Yogurt and Corn Dogs: Why Our Bodies Rebel Against Certain Foods

W hen we look at the foods that cause painful symptoms—migraines, arthritis, or digestive problems—clear patterns emerge. The foods that trigger migraines are strikingly similar to the list of culprits for arthritis. These same problem foods show up again in irritable bowel symptoms, Crohn's disease, and fibromyalgia and are compiled in the chart below

MULTI-SYMPTOM TRIGGERS

The following list includes the foods most often identified in research studies as triggers for migraines, arthritis, irritable bowel syndrome, Crohn's disease, and fibromyalgia.[1-21]

dairy products	corn	nuts
wheat	caffeine	tomatoes
citrus fruits	meat	eggs

These foods are popular, yet for many of us they are like a subtle form of poison ivy. It is as if the proteins in cow's milk, wheat, citrus fruits, tomatoes, and other common trigger foods are biological strangers, sparking inflammation and pain in sensitive people.

What is it about these innocent-seeming foods that makes them such a problem? The answer becomes clearer when we look at their origins. We can gain further insights from the reactions of babies encountering them for the first time and from the food choices of our closest biological relatives, the other primates.

ANTHROPOLOGY IN THE KITCHEN

For the most part, these culinary troublemakers were not part of human experience when our species first appeared. In the grand scheme of human history, stretching back millions of years, many of these foods are new arrivals, never having passed human lips until a few thousand—or even a few hundred—years ago.

Most anthropologists, having studied the roughly one thousand existing human skeletons dating from 1 to 4 million years ago, put the origins of modern humans in South and East Africa, and some might argue for the Middle East. But migration to Asia did not occur until well after humans existed in modern form. We did not make our way to Australia until about fifty-five thousand years ago or to the Americas until twenty thousand years ago—a mere blink of the eye in our species' history.[22]

At the time when our digestive tracts, arteries, and nervous systems were taking human form, there were no grapefruit trees, dairies, or bakeries on the surface of the earth, and tomato plants, cornstalks, and orange groves were nowhere in sight. All of these are as new and alien to us as an oil slick is to seagulls or power lines are to migrating birds.

Of course, our species does have some ability to adapt. We might imagine that, even if these foods were not part of early human experience and some of us had sensitivities to them, we should have adapted after all these years.

The fact is, however, there is little evolutionary pressure to adapt to anything unless our ability to reproduce hangs in the balance. Let's take tobacco as an example. In spite of centuries of tobacco use, we still have not developed any resistance to its dangers.

Now, if tobacco killed or sterilized its users in early life, only those smokers who had a natural resistance to its ill effects could reproduce. They could pass their natural resistance on to their children, while users who could not adapt would gradually die out. The human species would adapt to tobacco, and it would cease to be a problem. But, of course, tobacco nearly always waits until long after the age of reproduction to take its victims, so there is no pressure to adapt to it. For each generation, it is as dangerous as for the first man or woman who ever used it.

Similarly, if dairy products or wheat cause arthritis or migraines that do not affect the ability to reproduce, this will have no influence whatsoever on future generations. No adaptation will occur. Meat-eating clearly contributes to heart disease and several forms of cancer. However, these diseases are rarely symptomatic until well after the age of reproduction.

Let us take another look at the problem foods. Although human migration and inventions from milling to microwaves have obscured our culinary roots, it is clear that many of our most common foods are no more natural for us than a pineapple is for a penguin.

Cow's milk. The peculiar practice of drinking the milk of another species did not begin until after animals were domesticated. Sheep came under human control about 11,000 years ago, and goats followed, about 9,500 years ago. Cows, being larger and more difficult to manage, were not domesticated for another thousand years or so. The first evidence of milk production comes from about 4,000 B.C.[23]

As we saw in chapter 6, the vast majority of humans, other than Caucasians, do not retain the enzymes for digesting milk sugars after weaning. If they drink more than a modest amount, they have digestive symptoms, unless the milk is in some way modified (e.g., with added enzymes).

About 85 percent of Caucasians have a genetic adaptation to the immediate digestive effects of milk consumption, although there is no evidence that they have adapted to the apparent long-term problems caused by dairy products: cataracts and ovarian problems due to breakdown products of lactose sugar;[24] insulin-dependent diabetes and some cases of arthritis, migraines, and other sensitivities to milk proteins; coronary artery disease and obesity from milk fat and cholesterol; and possibly breast cancer from the fat, hormones, and growth factors in milk.[25] Although all of these problems are still under investigation, evidence of their links with dairy products is already far beyond the point where it can easily be dismissed.

While most North Americans and Europeans accept animal milk consumption as natural, it is a biologically recent phenomenon that remains alien to much of the rest of the world.

Wheat. Wheat consumption was impossible until the advent of fire and cooking, by which time modern human biology had long been established. Once consumed, however, wheat grew in popularity quickly. In 2700 B.C., Chinese emperor Shen Nung included it as one of the five principal and sacred crops, along with barley, millet, rice, and soybeans.[26]

Wheat's attraction comes from physical properties that set it apart from other grains. It has less natural oil than oats so it resists rancidity, and its gluten proteins make a flexible, yet adherent dough that can be formed into loaves and set to rise.

Citrus fruits. Citrus trees are native not to Africa but to Southeast Asia. They were cultivated in India, where the word *orange* came from the Hindi language. The grapefruit was born in the West Indies in the eighteenth century as a cross between the orange and the pummelo, a large citrus fruit. Ruby red grapefruits were a mutation discovered in McAllen, Texas, in 1929.

Tomatoes. Tomatoes are indigenous to South America. While they made their way to Europe in the 1500s, they were not widely consumed in Europe, except in Italy, or in America until the mid-1800s. The major use for the tomato was as an ornamental plant, rather than a food, owing to its once being viewed as potentially poisonous. While this concern seems ludicrous today, the frequent appearance of tomatoes as a trigger for migraines, arthritis, and digestive problems suggests that the ancient concern may have had merit.

Corn. Like tomatoes (and chocolate), corn is one of the New World's additions to the human menu, and one with nutritional advantages and disadvantages. It is low in fat and, like all plant products, has no cholesterol. Small wonder that the Incas of Peru, the Aztecs of Mexico, and the Native Americans of the American Southwest who made it their dietary staple had virtually no coronary heart disease.

Unfortunately, corn is extremely low in the amino acid tryptophan, which, as we saw in chapter 7, we need to make the brain chemical serotonin, which reduces our sensitivity to pain. In fact, corn is so low in tryptophan that it has been administered to animals in gruesome experiments to reduce serotonin in their brains and lower their resistance to experimentally induced pain. Corn is also low in virus-fighting lysine, and its oils are nearly devoid of the alpha-linolenic acid needed to keep inflammation at bay. All of these faults can be made up for by combining corn with other plant foods. However, it remains a common trigger for migraines, arthritis, and digestive problems.

Caffeine. Caffeine's history began in Africa, where the coffee tree is indigenous. Its berries were occasionally eaten or used to make wine. It was not until around A.D. 1,000, however, when Ethiopian Arabs invented coffee as a beverage, that its use became at all common, and not until the early 1600s that it became common in Europe. English adventurer George Sandys wrote in 1601 that this novel concoction was "black as soote and tasting not much unlike it."[27]

There is caffeine in tea, too, and while we think of tea as being as old as time, the fact is, no Cro-Magnon man or woman ever dipped a tea bag into hot water. Tea cultivation probably began in China in the third or fourth century A.D. and did not gain popularity until the eighth century. The following century saw its introduction to Japan. It was not popular in England until the 1700s.

The caffeine in cocoa beans was first cultivated by Mayas, Aztecs, and Toltecs. The Aztecs taught the Spanish how to make it into a beverage, which became popular in Europe. Modern chocolate candy was not produced until the mid-1800s.

Meat. Meat-eating was a challenge for humans until the advent of the Stone Age. Without the speed or claws that true carnivores use to catch prey, and with canine teeth that shrank away to be no longer than our incisors at least 3.5 million years ago, early humans lived on fruits, leaves, nuts, berries, and other plant foods, as do other primates for the most part (although chimpanzees' long canines and enormous strength do permit them to dispatch rare prey with less effort than we would require).

Only when we started making stone arrowheads and cutting implements could we capture prey and remove its hide. The few existing groups of modern-day hunter-gatherers do not reflect the beginnings of human existence. In fact, they use fire, cooking, and tools that were not available to our pre–Stone Age ancestors.

Most anthropologists believe that meat-eating probably began by scavenging from the remains of kills left behind by true carnivores.[28] In spite of a fairly long exposure to at least limited amounts of meat, and as seductive as it has been, particularly to Western cultures, we have yet to adapt to meat's risks, none of which are fatal before the age of reproduction.

Eggs. Eggs have existed for as long as there have been birds or other animals to lay them. However, given the remoteness of birds' nests, it is unlikely that early humans had more than an occasional egg, and none at all from chickens, who are of Asian ancestry. Birds resembling modern chickens were first domesticated four to five thousand years ago.

Nuts. Nuts are the one food group on the triggers list that early humans did undoubtedly have access to. Unfortunately, most migraine and arthritis researchers have not listed *which* nuts are the problem. This would be interesting to know, because some nuts, such as acorns, chestnuts, coconuts, and pine nuts, have grown in a wide geographic pattern since time immemorial.

Walnuts are native to Asia, Europe, and North America. Almonds are from western India, pistachios are from central Asia, and macadamias come from northeastern Australia. Brazil nuts really do come from Brazil, and cashews are also native to the Amazon.

Peanuts are from South America. The peanut, by the way, is more pea than nut. A true nut is defined as a one-seeded, dry-fleshed fruit. Peanuts come in a pod like peas and beans, so they qualify as a legume.

As our species began, we did not have the technology for consuming dairy products, meat, or wheat. Citrus fruits awaited our arrival in Asia, and corn, tomatoes, and peanuts were in the faraway New World. The proteins in these foods can elicit reactions today as readily as they did when adventurous taste buds first tried them out.

WHEN BABIES WRINKLE THEIR NOSES

In trying to come to grips with food triggers, we might gain another perspective from the reactions of infants as they try foods for the first time. Babies give us clues, rather like the canaries who once involuntarily served as gas detectors for old-time miners. As parents and pediatricians can attest, babies tolerate certain foods well and have problems with others.

Rice cereal generally goes well, while wheat is a more common allergen. Babies love fruit. Apples, peaches, pears, apricots, and prunes are usually the first fruits for babies, followed by bananas and avocados.

Among the vegetables, string beans, peas, squash, carrots, beets, and sweet potatoes are the first ones parents usually offer, and babies do well with them. Babies have trouble with the toughness of corn and often do not care for the bitterness of broccoli, cauliflower, cabbage, turnips, kale, and onions. Their intuition has a good basis, as cruciferous vegetables and onions are common triggers for colic.

Cow's milk proteins are an even more common cause of colic, which makes life miserable for one baby in five. Milk proteins are also under investigation for their role in juvenile-onset diabetes. While human milk is perfect for newborns, cow's milk is not at all suitable for infants, unless it is modified in several ways. To support human growth, its butter fat has to be replaced with vegetable oils, its protein content is reduced, and carbohydrates, vitamins, and minerals are added.

WHAT DO OUR COUSINS EAT?

One final line of evidence: What do the other great apes eat? Gorillas and orangutans are vegetarians. Neither they nor chimpanzees consume milk of any kind, except as nursing infants, nor do they have corn, wheat, tomatoes, or any of the other major diet triggers, except for certain nuts. Chimps eat mainly fruits, followed by leaves, blossoms, seeds, and occasional insects. Obviously these primates never eat beef, pork, or fish. Although chimps will occasionally use their long canines to kill and eat monkeys, this never constitutes more than a small percentage of their diet. They cook nothing. While we may imagine that chimps love bananas, these fruits are not native to Africa at all. They began in India and Malaya and arrived in Africa around A.D. 500.

OVERLOOKING FOODS' EFFECTS

If a food causes symptoms in only a minority of people within a given culture, its role in causing these symptoms may remain unknown, particularly if the problem is subtle, such as gradually stiffening joints, as opposed to a sudden rash or anaphylactic shock. It is common for people with joint symptoms or migraines to have no idea at all that specific foods have triggered them until, for whatever reason, they happen to avoid those foods for a while.

Of course, sometimes we put up with certain foods' disadvantages in order to have their special effects. Caffeine and alcohol are obvious examples. Similarly, hot peppers are habituating, at least to a degree. The ability of their active ingredient, capsaicin, to deplete the pain neurotransmitter substance P is only gradually becoming understood. Chocolate and cheese contain phenylethylamine, a compound with mild amphetamine-like effects that may partially account for these foods' near druglike appeal for some people.

It may also be that, given an absence of high-protein, high-fat foods in the diet of early humans, a tendency to be drawn toward those foods that were slightly higher in protein or fat would be understandable and even advantageous. However, that tendency becomes potentially devastating if high-protein or high-fat foods become widely available. Just as the Pima Indians developed an epidemic of weight problems and diabetes when high-fat foods arrived in southwestern North America, our built-in nutritional sensors end up misleading us when we gain access to new foods through modern agriculture and shipping.

Of course, nothing says that a food has to be "natural." If wheat or citrus fruits cause no symptoms for you, there is no reason to avoid them, since they are not linked to any risk of serious diseases. That is also true for corn, tomatoes, and probably caffeine, as well, within limits.

The origin of the foods that make up modern diets is a fascinating area for exploration. Detailed works on this subject are listed in the references for this chapter.

CHAPTER 19

From Laboratory to Kitchen

Thank you for coming along with me in an exploration of foods that fight pain. Let's set the research studies aside for the moment and step into the kitchen. It is time to start feeling better.

If you have been looking only for pain relief, changing the foods you eat may bring unexpected benefits. When Dr. Dean Ornish's research subjects used diet and lifestyle changes to dissolve artery blockages and melt away chest pain, they also burned off a considerable amount of weight—more than twenty pounds on average. We found the same result in our research on diabetes and menstrual pain. In fact, our research subjects appreciated their weight loss, among other diet benefits, so much that it was hard to convince them to *stop* using our experimental food program when the research called for a return to their previous eating habits. Their energy levels improved dramatically, and they had no desire to return to the weight problems and fatigue—not to mention pain—their old diets had caused.

The diet that eliminates sensitizing proteins and brings your hormones into balance to ease your joints may also help your digestion and even give your skin a healthy glow. Likewise, foods that protect against kidney stones also keep calcium in your bones where it belongs, protecting against osteoporosis and back pain. As you experiment with new foods, you can enjoy the surprising benefits they bring.

FEELING GOOD AT LAST

For many of us, finding the right foods is like putting the right fuel in your car. It makes everything work better. If you had accidentally filled your tank with outboard-motor fuel instead of normal gasoline, your car would run, more or less. But it would idle roughly, it would not accelerate well, the ride would be terrible, and its exhaust would look like Pittsburgh's bitter memories. It would bear no resemblance to a normal drive. When you discover the error and put in the right fuel, the engine gradually cleans out the old fuel and starts to purr. It accelerates with real power, and the ride is smoother and quieter than you could have imagined.

Many people put the wrong fuel in their bodies, day after day—foods that clog their arteries, push hormones out of balance, irritate their tissues, and cause gradually worsening pain. They will never know how good their bodies can feel until they find the right foods and their healing begins. It can be like having a brand-new body.

RECIPES FOR YOUR OWN NEEDS

The following section includes recipes for people with different needs. All the recipes are suitable if you have back pain, heart disease, diabetes, menstrual pain, breast pain, cancer, kidney stones, osteoporosis, or sickle-cell anemia, unless you have a specific food allergy or medical limitation. All are low in fat, with no cholesterol or animal ingredients, and are perfect for cholesterol-lowering and hormone-balancing. Their protein comes from plants, and most are high in potassium and low in sodium, so they help protect your bones and prevent kidney stones. They are rich in folic acid and moderate in iron, which are important features for sickle-cell anemia.

If you have migraines, arthritis, digestive problems, or fibromyalgia, you will want to go one step further and note the ingredients marked with an asterisk (*). These could be pain triggers for some people, and you will want to leave them out until you have tested your sensitivities.

The special elimination menu avoids virtually all triggers and lets you track down your food sensitivities. Use this program following the instructions on pages 48–49.

I would encourage you to be guided by your doctor as you plan your menu in order to meet any special dietary needs.

ENSURING COMPLETE NUTRITION

Whatever your health, I would encourage you to build your diet from these four food groups: vegetables, legumes (beans, peas, and lentils), grains, and fruits. Avoiding animal products and added vegetable oils allows you to avoid the hazards of cholesterol, excess fat, and animal proteins.

A varied diet drawn from these four groups provides plenty of protein without any careful planning or combining of foods in any particular way. The old idea of "protein complementing," which required various food combinations for adequate protein, has been discarded both by dietitians and the U.S. government. Green vegetables and legumes easily meet the body's calcium needs, too, as we saw in chapter 1.

There are, however, two nutrients that deserve attention. Vitamin D controls your ability to absorb and retain calcium, so it is important for healthy bones. It is made by the action of the sun on the skin. If, however, you get little sun, you should take a vitamin D supplement. The recommended dietary allowance is 200 IU (5 mcg) per day and can be doubled for those who get no sun at all.

Vitamin B_{12} is needed for healthy nerves and healthy blood cells. The recommended dietary allowance is tiny, only 2 mcg per day, and most people have a three-year supply stored in their livers. Nonetheless, you do need B_{12} in your diet.

Vitamin B_{12} is not made by plants or animals but, rather, by bacteria and other one-celled organisms. The bacteria on plants, in the soil, or even in our mouths may provide occasional traces of B_{12}, but modern hygiene has essentially eliminated them as reliable sources.

Animal products contain vitamin B_{12} because bacteria in animals' intestines produce it, and it is then absorbed into their tissues. However, these products do much more harm than good and are not recommended.

You will find B_{12} in enriched breakfast cereals and many soymilk products. It may be listed by its chemical name, *cobalamin* or *cyanocobalamin*. Red Star nutritional yeast, which is sometimes used to add a cheeselike flavor to foods, is naturally enriched in B_{12}.

If these products are not part of your routine, the most convenient B$_{12}$ source is any common multivitamin, which will also give you the vitamin D you may need.

GIVE IT 100 PERCENT

As you put these principles to work, let me encourage you to follow the guidelines in each chapter exactly. Research on cholesterol-lowering, heart-disease reversal, diabetes, and menstrual pain has shown that even minor deviations from the prescribed regimen can greatly reduce your benefits.

Even so, there is no need for a long-term commitment to any diet change. Rather, I would suggest that you focus on the short term. If you explore and enjoy new foods for just three weeks or so, your benefits will begin, and if you like how you feel, you can continue for as long as you like.

If you have found the information in this book helpful, I hope you will share it with others. You may also wish to join the Physicians Committee for Responsible Medicine (PCRM), a nonprofit organization I founded in 1985 to promote preventive medicine, good nutrition, and higher standards in research. PCRM's magazine, *Good Medicine,* is available for both doctors and laypersons. You can write to PCRM at 5100 Wisconsin Avenue, Suite 404, Washington, D.C. 20016.

I wish you the very best of health!

PART VI

MENUS AND RECIPES

BY JENNIFER RAYMOND

A WORD FROM THE COOK

When Neal Barnard described this book and asked me to do the recipes, I must admit I had some misgivings. The low-fat, no-cholesterol recipes were no problem. We have been using them for years to help people open up arteries, balance their hormones, and get diabetes under control. What I found challenging was cooking without the foods that can trigger migraines and arthritis.

The list of trigger foods included many of my dietary staples. Then, as Dr. Barnard went on to outline the ground rules for the Elimination Diet, I thought to myself, "How on earth can anyone make foods as simple as brown rice, cooked vegetables, and cooked fruits seem interesting, varied, and tasty?"

But I was intrigued by the challenge, and I had a personal reason for wanting to try the approach that Dr. Barnard was advocating. As I reached my midforties, I'd begun noticing increasing stiffness and pain in my joints, especially my fingers and toes. When I asked my doctor about this, his response was "Welcome to middle age!" He suggested that I begin taking nonsteroidal anti-inflammatory drugs to ease the pain. "But that doesn't get to the root of the problem, it just masks the symptoms," I objected. "Isn't there anything I can do about the cause?" He just shrugged and shook his head.

When Dr. Barnard began explaining that certain foods could trigger the inflammation that causes arthritis, as well as other conditions, my ears perked up. Avoiding those foods on a trial basis would certainly be worth a try. After all, I could stick with just about any diet for a few weeks. So with a dual mission, one professional and one personal, I embarked on the challenging task of developing the recipes for this book.

In addition to meeting the guidelines laid out by Dr. Barnard, I wanted the recipes to be quick, easy, and appealing to a variety of tastes. I also wanted, as much as possible, to use familiar ingredients that could be purchased in most supermarkets and grocery stores. As I began developing the recipes, I was pleasantly surprised by how delicious simple foods can be, and as I served them to friends and family, it was clear that other people really enjoyed them as well. I also discovered that limiting the number of ingredients was actually a blessing in disguise, because it made the recipes truly quick and easy to prepare. Most of the recipes in this section take fifteen minutes or less to assemble.

But my greatest surprise, by far, was that I began to feel better. As I followed the diet, the stiffness in my joints disappeared, allowing me to move freely without pain (and without pain medications!). I also had significantly fewer tension headaches, and indigestion, which had been a lifelong problem, disappeared altogether.

The recipes are given in two groups. First are those that meet the guidelines for the Elimination Diet. Then there are recipes that may contain trigger foods. The trigger foods are indicated with an asterisk (*).

As you look through the recipes, you may notice some ingredients that are unfamiliar to you. This is especially true of some of the flours used to replace wheat flour in baked goods. For a description of these and suggestions for where to find them, turn to the section "Ingredients That May Be New to You," beginning on page 301, and look under the name of the flour that interests you.

IDENTIFYING HIDDEN TRIGGERS

Processed foods often contain ingredients that are triggers for migraines, arthritis, and other conditions, so it is important to read all food labels carefully. Even labels you have checked before should be checked periodically, since manufacturers sometimes change the formulation of their products. Some trigger ingredients, such as milk and eggs, are easily recognizable. Others, like whey (a milk derivative) and albumen (a protein derived from eggs), may be less obvious. A list of ingredients derived from trigger foods follows.

Meat, Poultry, Fish

beef broth	gelatin
beef stock	lamb broth
chicken broth	lamb stock
chicken stock	lard

Milk and Dairy Products

As you begin reading labels, you will be amazed at the widespread use of milk and its derivatives. Some are obvious, such as cheese, yogurt, cream, and butter. Less obvious milk-containing foods include everything from breads, pastries, and muffins to "nondairy" creamers and margarine. The following ingredients are all derived from milk:

casein, caseinate, sodium	lactose
caseinate, potassium	milk solids
caseinate	nonfat milk solids
lactalbumin	whey
lactoglobulin	

Corn

Corn and corn-based ingredients are used in everything from chewing gum and carbonated beverages to envelope and stamp adhesive. And don't forget popcorn and tortilla chips! Common corn ingredients include:

caramel color	hominy
corn flour, cornmeal	lactic acid
corn oil	maltodextrins
corn starch	mannitol
corn syrup	masa harina
dextrin, dextrose	modified food starch
fructose	sorbitol
grits	zein

Wheat

In addition to being the main ingredient in breads, muffins, and pastries, wheat and its derivatives are found in a wide variety of foods, including prepared soups and soup mixes, some brands of soy sauce, some instant and flavored coffees, gravy mixes, instant puddings, and prepared frosting. The following indicate the presence of wheat:

all-purpose flour
bran
bread crumbs
bread flour
bromated flour
bulgur
cake flour
couscous
cracked wheat
cracker crumbs
durum
enriched flour
farina
flour

gluten, gluten flour
graham flour
hydrolyzed vegetable
    protein (TVP)
malt, malt syrup
modified food starch
monosodium glutamate
pastry flour
semolina
unbleached flour
wheat flour, whole wheat flour
wheat germ
white flour

Soy

Soy finds its way into hundreds of foods, from vegetarian burgers and meat analogs to salad dressings, margarine, and nonstick cooking sprays. Common soy-derived ingredients include:

hydrolyzed vegetable
    protein (HVP)
lecithin
miso
natto
okara
soybeans
soy flour, soy meal

soy milk
soy oil
soy protein concentrate
soy protein isolate
soy sauce
tempeh
textured vegetable protein (TVP)
tofu

THE ELIMINATION DIET

For a brief time your diet will be based on simple, tasty foods that are free of all common pain triggers. The Elimination Diet includes brown rice; green, yellow, and orange vegetables; and noncitrus fruits. All foods must be cooked. Seasonings may include minimal amounts of salt, vinegar, maple syrup, and vanilla extract.

After your initial test period, you will systematically add other foods to this simple diet as described on pages 48–49.

Getting Started. Before beginning the Elimination Diet, stock up on a selection of the foods that you will be eating. These can include any of the following:

Starches
Many of the following products are available in natural food stores.

arrowroot powder	rice crackers
brown rice, short- and long-grain	rice flour
	rice milk
mochi	rice pasta
rice cakes (plain or salted only)	tapioca flour
	taro root
rice cereals, hot and cold	

Vegetables (may be fresh, canned, or frozen)

artichokes	mushrooms
asparagus	New Zealand spinach
beets	parsnips
bok choy	radishes
broccoli	rutabagas
brussels sprouts	snow peas, sugar snap peas
cabbage (including napa cabbage)	spinach
carrots	summer squash (zucchini, crookneck, and scalloped varieties)
celery	
collard greens	sweet potatoes
cucumber	Swiss chard
daikon	turnips
endive	white potatoes
fennel	winter squash (acorn, banana, butternut, delicata, kabocha, and others)
green beans	
jicama	
kale	yams
kohlrabi	
lettuce (butter lettuce, romaine, and green leaf varieties are the most nutritious)	

Fruit
The fruit you select may be fresh, dried, frozen, or canned in its own juice. Avoid canned fruit in syrup.

berries (including
   raspberries,
   blackberries,
   blueberries,
   boysenberries)
cherries
cranberries
grapes
kiwifruit
mangoes

melon (including
   watermelon, cantaloupe,
   honeydew, and others)
nectarines
papayas
pears
persimmons
pineapple
plums
pomegranates

ELIMINATION MENUS

DAY 1

BREAKFAST
Breakfast Rice Pudding (page 235)
Rice bread toast with natural fruit preserves
Summer Fruit Compote (page 237)

LUNCH
Creamy Carrot Soup (page 239)
Always Great Brown Rice (page 238)
Steamed broccoli
Melon slice

DINNER
Cabbage Rolls (page 248)
Beet Soup (page 240)
Steamed Yams (page 247)
Prune Whip (page 250)

DAY 2

BREAKFAST

*Always Great Brown Rice (page 238) with rice milk and maple
   syrup*
Chunky Applesauce (page 236)
Papaya half

LUNCH

Beet Soup (page 240)
French Vegetable Salad (page 243)
Poached Apples (page 253)

DINNER

Rice Pasta with Creamy Zucchini Pesto (page 247)
Creamy Carrot Soup (page 239)
Braised Kale or Collard Greens (page 245)
Fruit Gel (page 249)

DAY 3

BREAKFAST

Rice bread toast
Natural fruit preserves
Stewed Prunes (page 237)

LUNCH

Potato Vegetable Soup (page 242)
Basil-Lover's Green Beans (page 244)
Always Great Brown Rice (page 238) or rice bread
Strawberry Applesauce (page 236)

DINNER

Green Pea and Cauliflower Soup (page 241)
Wild Brown Rice (page 239)
Steamed broccoli
Poached Pears (page 252)

DAY 4

BREAKFAST
Peachy Sweet Potatoes (page 238)
Rice bread toast with natural fruit preserves
Date Cooler (page 250)

LUNCH
Vegetable Soup (page 242)
Steamed green beans
Rice crackers or rice cakes
Fruit salad

DINNER
Steamed white potatoes with Creamy Zucchini Pesto (page 247)
Beet Soup (page 240)
Steamed carrots
Summer Fruit Compote (page 237)

DAY 5

BREAKFAST
French Toast (page 234)
Chunky Applesauce (page 236)
Prune Whip (page 250)

LUNCH
Cream of Asparagus Soup (page 240)
Rice bread or rice crackers
Yams with Pineapple (page 246)
Steamed zucchini

DINNER
Cabbage Rolls (page 248)
Oven Fries (page 246)
Basil-Lover's Green Beans (page 244)
Carrot Pudding (page 251)

DAY 6

BREAKFAST

Always Great Brown Rice (page 238) or cream of rice cereal
Rice bread toast with natural fruit preserves
Chunky Applesauce (page 236)

LUNCH

Green-Pea and Cauliflower Soup (page 241)
Always Great Brown Rice (page 238)
Braised Collards (page 245)
Poached Apple (page 253)

DINNER

French Vegetable Salad (page 243)
Wild Brown Rice (page 239)
Braised Cabbage (page 244)
Fruit Gel (page 249)

DAY 7

BREAKFAST

Puffed Rice or other cold cereal
Rice bread toast with Strawberry Applesauce (page 236)
Poached Pears (page 252)

LUNCH

Beet Soup (page 240)
Always Great Brown Rice (page 238)
Steamed broccoli

DINNER

Cream of Asparagus Soup (page 240)
Always Great Brown Rice (page 238)
French Vegetable Salad (page 243)
Apricot-Pineapple Gel (page 249)

RECIPES SUITABLE FOR
THE ELIMINATION DIET

NOTE: A few of the recipes in this section contain ingredients that should be omitted while you are following the Elimination Diet. These are noted in parentheses, and may be replaced when you return to a regular diet.

FRENCH TOAST
Makes four to six slices

This French toast is suitable for the Elimination Diet if you use rice bread and rice milk.

> ½ cup soymilk or rice milk
> 3 tablespoons arrowroot powder
> 1 teaspoon vanilla extract
> ¼ teaspoon cinnamon (omit during Elimination Diet)
> 4–6 slices rice bread
> Vegetable-oil spray, for cooking surface
> Fresh fruit, fruit preserves, or maple syrup, for topping

In a medium-size bowl whisk together soymilk, arrowroot, vanilla, and cinnamon. Pour batter into a flat container, and dip the bread into the batter, turning it to coat both sides.

Heat a nonstick griddle or large skillet, then lightly coat it with vegetable-oil spray. Cook each side of the coated slices over medium-high heat for 2 to 3 minutes, or until golden brown. Serve with fresh fruit, fruit preserves, or syrup. PER SLICE (WITHOUT TOPPING): 117 CALORIES, 2 G PROTEIN, 24 G CARBOHYDRATE, 1 G FAT, 118 MG SODIUM

BREAKFAST RICE PUDDING
Makes six ¹/₂-cup servings

2 cups cooked Always Great Brown Rice (page 238)
1½ cups vanilla rice milk
3 tablespoons raisins
2 tablespoons maple syrup
1 teaspoon vanilla extract
¼ teaspoon cinnamon (omit during Elimination Diet)

In a medium-size saucepan combine all ingredients and bring to a slow simmer. Cook, uncovered—stirring occasionally—for about 20 minutes, or until thick. Serve hot or cold. PER ½-CUP SERVING: 205 CALORIES, 3 G PROTEIN, 45 G CARBOHYDRATE, 1 G FAT, 169 MG SODIUM

RICE PANCAKES
Makes about sixteen 3-inch pancakes

1 cup Ener-G Rice Mix
1 cup rice milk
1 tablespoon maple syrup
1 tablespoon canola oil (omit during Elimination Diet)
Vegetable-oil spray, for cooking surface
Fresh fruit, fruit preserves, or maple syrup, for serving

In a medium-size bowl combine all ingredients and stir until smooth.

Heat a nonstick griddle or large skillet and lightly coat it with vegetable-oil spray. Pour small amounts of batter onto the heated surface and cook for 2 to 3 minutes, or until the edges are dry and the tops bubble. Turn pancakes and cook the second sides for about 1 minute, or until golden brown. Serve with fresh fruit, fruit preserves, or syrup. PER PANCAKE (WITHOUT TOPPING): 65 CALORIES, 1 G PROTEIN, 12 G CARBOHYDRATE, 1.5 G FAT; 43 MG SODIUM

CHUNKY APPLESAUCE

Makes 2 1/2 cups

Serve this applesauce hot or cold.

    4 large green apples
    ½ cup frozen apple juice concentrate
    ½ teaspoon cinnamon (omit during Elimination Diet)

Peel, core, and dice apples. Put apples into a medium-size saucepan. Add apple juice concentrate, then cover and cook over very low heat for about twenty minutes, or until apples are tender when pierced with a fork. Mash slightly and stir in the cinnamon, if used. PER ½ CUP: 112 CALORIES, 0 G PROTEIN, 27 G CARBOHYDRATE, 0 G FAT, 8 MG SODIUM

STRAWBERRY APPLESAUCE

Makes 2 cups

Serve this applesauce hot or cold.

    2 cups peeled, cored, and coarse-chopped apples
    2 cups hulled strawberries, fresh or frozen
    ½ cup frozen apple juice concentrate

In a medium-size saucepan combine all ingredients. Bring to a simmer, then cover and cook over very low heat for about 25 minutes, or until apples are tender when pierced with a fork. Mash slightly or puree in a food processor, if desired. PER ½ CUP: 112 CALORIES, 1 G PROTEIN, 26 G CARBOHYDRATE, 0 G FAT, 10 MG SODIUM

SUMMER FRUIT COMPOTE
Makes 2 cups

2 cups peeled and sliced fresh peaches (peeling is optional)
2 cups hulled fresh strawberries
½ cup white grape juice concentrate or apple juice concentrate

In a large saucepan combine all ingredients. Bring to a simmer and cook for about 5 minutes, or until fruit just becomes soft. Serve warm or cold.
PER ½ CUP: 78 CALORIES, 1 G PROTEIN, 18 G CARBOHYDRATE, 0 G FAT, 7 MG SODIUM

STEWED PRUNES
Makes 2 cups

2 cups pitted prunes
1½ cups water

In a medium-size saucepan combine prunes and the water. Bring water to a simmer and cook, loosely covered, for about 15 minutes, or until prunes are soft. (Cook longer if softer prunes are desired.) PER ½ CUP: 193 CALORIES, 2 G PROTEIN, 45 G CARBOHYDRATE, 0 G FAT, 3 MG SODIUM

DRIED FRUIT COMPOTE
Makes 2 cups

½ cup raisins
½ cup pitted prunes
½ cup dried figs, halved
½ cup dried peach or apricot slices
½ cup white grape juice concentrate or apple juice concentrate

In a large saucepan combine the fruits. Add white grape juice concentrate and enough water to just cover the fruits. Bring liquid to a simmer, then cover and cook for about 15 minutes or until fruit is tender. Serve warm or cold. PER ½ CUP: 319 CALORIES, 3 G PROTEIN, 75 G CARBOHYDRATE, 1 G FAT, 18 MG SODIUM

PEACHY SWEET POTATOES
Makes 2 cups

This simple breakfast pudding is a rich source of beta-carotene and other important nutrients.

>1 medium-size sweet potato or yam (1 cup cooked)
>2 small peaches or nectarines

Scrub sweet potato, then steam or microwave until it is tender when pierced with a fork. Set aside to cool.

Cut peaches in half and remove the pits. Cut each half into 2 or 3 slices. Place slices into a food processor. Chop into pieces, using a few quick pulses.

Peel sweet potato and add flesh to the food processor. Using quick pulses, chop sweet potato and blend it with peaches. There should still be some chunks.

Transfer the mixture to a small microwavable container and heat in the microwave for 2 to 3 minutes, or until hot throughout. PER ½ CUP: 98 CALORIES, 1 G PROTEIN, 23 G CARBOHYDRATE, 0 G FAT, 6 MG SODIUM

ALWAYS GREAT BROWN RICE
Makes 3 cups

Brown rice supplies more vitamins, minerals, protein, and fiber than does white rice, and this cooking method ensures perfect rice and actually reduces the cooking time. Short-grain brown rice tends to be a bit chewy; long-grain brown rice is slightly more tender and fluffy. If brown rice is new to you, I recommend starting with the long-grain variety.

>1 cup short- or long-grain brown rice
>3 cups water
>½ teaspoon salt (optional)

In a medium-size saucepan of cool water, rinse rice; drain off water as thoroughly as possible. Put the saucepan on medium heat—stirring constantly—for about 2 minutes, or until rice dries. Add the 3 cups water and salt (if used). Bring to a boil, then lower heat slightly; cover and simmer for about 40 minutes, or until rice is soft but still retains a hint of crunchiness. Drain excess liquid (this can be saved and used as a broth for soups and stews). PER ½ CUP: 115 CALORIES, 2.5 G PROTEIN, 25 G CARBOHYDRATE, 1 G FAT; 178 MG SODIUM

WILD BROWN RICE
Makes 3 cups

½ cup long-grain brown rice
½ cup wild rice
¼ teaspoon salt
4 cups water

In a medium-size saucepan combine all ingredients. Bring to a simmer. Cover loosely and cook about 50 minutes, or until both rices are tender. Drain excess liquid (this may be saved for later use as a soup stock). PER ½ CUP: 104 CALORIES, 3 G PROTEIN, 23 G CARBOHYDRATE, 0 G FAT, 99 MG SODIUM

CREAMY CARROT SOUP
Makes about 6 cups

So simple and so good!

4 large carrots
1½ cups water
1½ cups plain rice milk
⅛ teaspoon salt

Scrub carrots, cut them into chunks, and place them in a medium-size saucepan with the water. Cover and simmer for about 20 minutes, or until tender when pierced with a fork. Pour rice milk into a blender and add cooked carrots, cooking liquid, and salt. Puree until completely smooth, adding a bit more rice milk if the soup is too thick. Serve hot or chilled. PER 1-CUP SERVING: 76 CALORIES, 1 G PROTEIN, 16 G CARBOHYDRATE, 1 G FAT, 125 MG SODIUM

BEET SOUP
Makes about 6 cups

3 medium-size beets
1½ cups water
1½ cups plain rice milk
2 tablespoons white grape juice concentrate or apple juice
    concentrate
2 teaspoons balsamic vinegar
1 teaspoon dried dill weed

Cut the tops and roots off beets, then scrub and peel them. Cut beets into ½-inch chunks (you should have about 4 cups). Place chunks into a large saucepan with the water. Bring to a simmer, then cover and cook for about 15 minutes, or until tender when pierced with a sharp knife.

Transfer beets to a blender, leaving the cooking liquid in the pan. Add remaining ingredients to the blender and puree at least 1 minute, until completely smooth. Pour beet mixture back into the pan; stir. Heat gently if desired. PER 1-CUP SERVING: 90 CALORIES, 1 G PROTEIN, 20 G CARBOHYDRATE, 1 G FAT, 96 MG SODIUM

CREAM OF ASPARAGUS SOUP
Makes about 7 cups

2 medium-size white potatoes, diced
2 cups water
1 medium-size bunch asparagus (about 4 cups chopped)
2 cups shredded cabbage
1 cup (loosely packed) chopped fresh parsley
¼ cup chopped fresh basil (omit during Elimination Diet)
1–2 cups plain rice milk
¾–1 teaspoon salt

Scrub and dice potatoes (no need to peel them); place them into a large pot with the water. Bring to a simmer, then cover and cook for about 10 minutes, or until tender when pierced with a fork.

Remove the tough ends from asparagus, then cut or break stalks into 1- to 2-inch lengths.

When potatoes are tender when pierced with a fork, add asparagus along with cabbage, parsley, and basil (if used). Cover and simmer for about 5 minutes, or until asparagus is just tender when pierced with a fork.

In a blender puree the vegetables with cooking liquid, in 2 or 3 batches. Add enough of the rice milk to each batch to facilitate blending. (Be sure to start the blender on a low speed.) After pureeing all vegetables, pour soup into the pan. Add salt, then heat gently until steamy. PER 1-CUP SERVING: 100 CALORIES, 3 G PROTEIN, 21 G CARBOHYDRATE, 1 G FAT, 224 MG SODIUM

GREEN-PEA AND CAULIFLOWER SOUP

Makes about 8 cups

2 medium-size white potatoes, scrubbed and diced
2 medium-size stalks celery, sliced
1 medium-size cauliflower
1 cup fine-chopped fresh parsley
2 cups water
2½ cups plain rice milk
2½ cups frozen peas
1 tablespoon balsamic vinegar
¾ teaspoon salt

In a large pot combine potatoes and celery. Cut or break cauliflower into bite-size pieces; add pieces to the pot, along with parsley and the water. Bring to a simmer, then cover and cook for about 15 minutes, or until potatoes are tender when pierced with a fork.

Transfer about half the vegetable mixture and cooking liquid to a blender. Add remaining ingredients and blend until smooth. Return blended mixture to the pot; stir to mix. Heat gently until steamy. PER 1-CUP SERVING: 162 CALORIES, 5 G PROTEIN, 33 G CARBOHYDRATE, 1 G FAT, 307 MG SODIUM

POTATO-VEGETABLE SOUP

Makes about 8 cups

3 medium-size white potatoes, scrubbed and cut into ½-inch cubes
2 medium-size stalks celery, sliced thin
1 large carrot, scrubbed and diced or sliced thin
3 cups water
2 cups shredded green cabbage
1 cup plain rice milk
¾ teaspoon salt

In a large pot combine potatoes, celery, carrot, cabbage and the water. Bring to a simmer, then cover and cook for about 15 minutes, or until potatoes and carrots are tender when pierced with a fork. Transfer about 3 cups of the mixture into a blender; add rice milk and salt. Blend for about 30 seconds, or until completely smooth. Return blended mixture to the pot and stir to mix. Heat gently if desired. PER 1-CUP SERVING: 144 CALORIES, 2 G PROTEIN, 33 G CARBOHYDRATE, 0.5 G FAT, 308 MG SODIUM

VEGETABLE SOUP

Makes about 10 cups

½ cup water
4 medium-size cloves garlic, minced
3 medium-size carrots, cut into 1-inch chunks
2 cups coarse-chopped cabbage
2 medium-size white potatoes, cut into 1-inch chunks
2 cups water
4 cups zucchini slices
2 cups chopped cauliflower
2 cups plain rice milk
¾ teaspoon salt

In a large pot heat the ½ cup water to a simmer. Add garlic and cook about 30 seconds. Add carrots, cabbage, potatoes, and the 2 cups water. Bring liquid to a simmer. Cover and cook for about 15 minutes, or until the vegetables are tender when pierced with a sharp knife.

Add zucchini and cauliflower, then cover and cook over medium heat for another 10 minutes, or until newly added vegetables are tender.

Transfer 3 to 4 cups of the vegetable mixture and cooking liquid to a blender; add some rice milk. Blend until completely smooth. Pour blended mixture into a clean large pot. Blend the rest of the soup with remaining rice milk—blend just enough so vegetables are coarse. Combine with the first batch. Add salt, stir, and heat gently until steamy. PER 1-CUP SERVING: 94 CALORIES, 2 G PROTEIN, 21 G CARBOHYDRATE, 0 G FAT, 196 MG SODIUM

FRENCH VEGETABLE SALAD
Serves 6

This salad contains some optional ingredients—garbanzo beans, mustard, and garlic. These can be omitted to make it suitable during the Elimination Diet.

> 1 16-ounce bag frozen mixed vegetables (green beans, Italian
>   green beans, sliced carrots, cauliflower, zucchini, etc.)
> 1 15-ounce can garbanzo beans, drained (omit during Elimination
>   Diet)
> ¼ cup apple cider vinegar
> ¼ cup white grape juice concentrate or apple juice concentrate
> 1 teaspoon stone-ground mustard (omit during Elimination Diet)
> 2 medium-size cloves garlic, crushed (omit during Elimination Diet)
> ½ teaspoon salt

Place frozen vegetables on a steamer rack and steam over boiling water for about 10 minutes, or until just tender. Transfer to a large bowl and add remaining ingredients. Stir to mix. Serve immediately or chill if desired. PER SERVING: 106 CALORIES, 4 G PROTEIN, 20 G CARBOHYDRATE, 1 G FAT, 305 MG SODIUM

BRAISED CABBAGE

Makes about 2 cups

Braised cabbage is delicious and mildly sweet—a great addition to any meal.

    ½ cup water
    2–3 cups green cabbage, chopped coarse
    ½ teaspoon caraway seeds (omit during Elimination Diet)
    Salt and black pepper, to taste (omit pepper during Elimination
        Diet)

In a medium-size skillet or saucepan, bring the water to a boil. Stir in cabbage and caraway seeds, if used. Cover and cook for about 5 minutes, or until cabbage is just tender when pierced with a fork. Sprinkle with salt and pepper if used. PER ½-CUP SERVING: 16 CALORIES, 0.5 G PROTEIN, 4 G CARBOHYDRATE, 0 G FAT, 80 MG SODIUM

BASIL-LOVER'S GREEN BEANS

Makes about 6 cups

    1 pound green beans
    1 small zucchini or other summer squash (about 1 cup of chunks)
    1 cup fresh basil leaves
    ½ teaspoon salt
    1 medium-size clove garlic (omit during Elimination Diet)
    1 tablespoon olive oil (omit during Elimination Diet)

Trim ends from beans. Break beans into 1-inch pieces. Steam over boiling water for 7 to 10 minutes, or until tender when pierced with a fork.

While beans are cooking, cut zucchini into chunks. Place into a food processor, along with basil and salt. Add garlic and olive oil, if used. Process until smooth.

Transfer beans to a serving dish and toss with the basil mixture. PER 1-CUP SERVING: 40 CALORIES, 1 G PROTEIN, 6 G CARBOHYDRATE, 1 G FAT, 186 MG SODIUM

BRAISED KALE OR COLLARD GREENS
Makes about 4 cups

Kale and collard greens are excellent sources of calcium and beta-carotene. Their flavor is robust and delicious, especially with garlic. Young tender greens have the best flavor and texture.

> 1 medium-size bunch kale or collard greens
> (about 8 cups chopped)
> ½ cup water
> ¼ teaspoon salt
> 2–3 medium-size cloves garlic, minced

Rinse greens and remove stems. Chop leaves into bite-size pieces. In a large pot or skillet, heat the water and salt to a simmer. Add garlic. Cook 30 seconds, then add greens. Toss to mix, then cover and cook over medium heat—stirring occasionally—for about 5 minutes, or until greens are tender. PER ½ CUP: 27 CALORIES, 2 G PROTEIN, 5 G CARBOHYDRATE, 0 G FAT, 106 MG SODIUM

BRAISED SUMMER SQUASH
Makes about 6 cups

> ¼ cup water
> 4 medium-size summer squash (zucchini, crookneck, scallop),
> sliced
> ½ cup chopped fresh basil
> Salt, to taste

In a large skillet or pot, heat the water. Add squash; cover and cook over medium heat for about 3 minutes, or until barely tender when pierced with a fork. Add basil, then cover and cook for another 2 to 3 minutes until basil just begins to wilt. Sprinkle with salt. PER ½-CUP SERVING: 30 CALORIES, 2 G PROTEIN, 6 G CARBOHYDRATE, 0 G FAT, 142 MG SODIUM

OVEN FRIES

Makes about 6 cups

Be sure to try these tasty fat-free fries!

>   4 medium-size or large white potatoes
>   1 teaspoon garlic granules or powder (omit during Elimination Diet)
>   1 teaspoon dried Italian seasoning
>   ½ teaspoon paprika or chili powder (omit during Elimination Diet)
>   ¼ teaspoon salt
>   ¼ teaspoon black pepper (omit during Elimination Diet)

Preheat the oven to 450° F.

Scrub potatoes and cut into "fries." Place into a large bowl and sprinkle with garlic (if used), Italian seasoning, paprika (if used), salt, and pepper (if used). Toss to mix.

Line two 9- × 13-inch baking dishes with baking parchment or foil (lining makes cleanup much easier). Arrange potatoes in a single layer in the baking dishes. Bake for about 30 minutes, or until tender when pierced with a fork. PER 1-CUP SERVING: 147 CALORIES, 2 G PROTEIN, 34 G CARBOHYDRATE, 0 G FAT, 100 MG SODIUM

YAMS WITH PINEAPPLE

Makes about 8 cups

This is absolutely one of the easiest and most delicious ways to prepare yams!

>   5 medium-size yams or sweet potatoes, unpeeled
>   1 15-ounce can juice-packed crushed pineapple

Scrub yams. Steam them over boiling water for about 25 minutes, or until tender when pierced with a fork. Set aside to cool slightly.

When cool enough to handle, cut a lengthwise slit in each yam. Squeeze the ends to open it. Leaving the flesh in the skin, use a fork to mash flesh slightly. Into each yam place 2 to 3 tablespoons undrained crushed pineapple, then mix. Fill each of the cavities with remaining pineapple.

Variation. Peel cooked yams when they are cool enough to handle. In a large bowl mash the flesh, then mix in all the pineapple, with its juice. PER ½-CUP SERVING: 97 CALORIES, 1 G PROTEIN, 23 G CARBOHYDRATE, 0 G FAT, 6 MG SODIUM

STEAMED YAMS
Makes 4 yams

Keep a few cooked yams on hand for a tasty, nutritious snack or addition to a meal. The easiest way to cook a quantity of yams is to steam them.

    4 medium-size yams

Scrub yams and cut out any rough spots. Leave whole or cut into large chunks. Place them on a vegetable steamer over boiling water; cover and steam for about 25 minutes, or until tender when pierced with a fork. PER YAM: 237 CALORIES, 2 G PROTEIN, 57 G CARBOHYDRATE, 0 G FAT, 16 MG SODIUM

RICE PASTA WITH
CREAMY ZUCCHINI PESTO
Makes about 6 cups

    8 ounces rice pasta (or other pasta if not on Elimination Diet)
    2 small zucchini or other summer squash
    2 cups fresh basil
    ½ teaspoon salt
    ½ teaspoon garlic granules
    1 tablespoon tahini (omit during Elimination Diet)

Cook pasta according to package directions until tender. Rinse and drain.

Cut zucchini into 1-inch chunks (you should have about 2 cups). Steam chunks over boiling water for about 5 minutes, or until just tender when pierced with a sharp knife.

Place basil in a food processor fitted with a metal blade; chop fine. Add zucchini, salt, garlic, and tahini (if used). Process in short on-off bursts until everything is chopped fine. Combine with pasta and toss to mix. PER 1-CUP SERVING: 171 CALORIES, 7 G PROTEIN, 32 G CARBOHYDRATE, 2 G FAT, 192 MG SODIUM

CABBAGE ROLLS
Makes 8 generous rolls

1 medium-size green cabbage
1 medium-size beet, peeled and diced (about 1½ cups)
1 medium-size stalk celery, chopped
1 medium-size carrot, cut into chunks
1 medium-size onion, chopped coarse (omit during Elimination
    Diet or if this is a trigger for you)
½ teaspoon dried dill weed
3 cups water
1 cup canned sauerkraut (choose a brand without preservatives)
3 cups Wild Brown Rice (page 239)
3 tablespoons Sesame Seasoning (page 299) (omit during
    Elimination Diet)
¼ cup pumpkin seed (omit during Elimination Diet)
¼ cup raisins

Remove any wilted cabbage leaves; cut out the core with a sharp knife. In a large covered pot steam cabbage for about 20 minutes, or until quite soft when pierced with a fork. Remove cabbage from the pot. When cabbage is cool enough to handle, carefully remove 8 large outside leaves and set aside. Chop enough of the remaining cabbage to make 1 cup.

To make the sauce: In a large saucepan, combine beet, celery, carrot, onion (if used), dill, and 2 cups of the water. Cover and simmer for about 15 minutes, or until beet and carrot pieces are tender when pierced with a sharp knife. Transfer vegetables and cooking liquid to a blender and add 1 more cup of the water. Blend on low speed until smooth. Return blended mixture to the pot. Add sauerkraut and stir.

To make the filling: Combine Wild Brown Rice, Sesame Seasoning and pumpkin seed (if used), raisins, and reserved chopped cabbage.

Preheat the oven to 350° F.

Spread about 2 cups of the beet sauce in a 9- × 12-inch baking dish. Place one eighth of the filling on each cabbage leaf. Roll up each leaf, starting at the core end and tucking in the edges. Arrange leaves in the baking dish; pour the remaining sauce evenly over the leaves. Bake for about 25 minutes, or until sauce bubbles. PER CABBAGE ROLL: 158 CALORIES, 5 G PROTEIN, 26 G CARBOHYDRATE, 3.5 G FAT, 521 MG SODIUM

FRUIT GEL
Makes 4 cups

This is an all-natural alternative to Jell-O! It is made with agar, a sea vegetable that acts as a thickener, and arrowroot powder, which is an excellent substitute for cornstarch.

> 1 quart natural fruit juice (apple-boysenberry and apple-
> strawberry are two delicious choices)
> 1½ teaspoons agar powder
> 2 tablespoons arrowroot powder

In a large saucepan stir all ingredients together until completely smooth. Bring to a simmer. Simmer, uncovered—stirring constantly—for about 3 minutes, until slightly thickened. Pour into serving dishes and chill completely. PER 1-CUP SERVING: 120 CALORIES, 0 G PROTEIN, 30 G CARBOHYDRATE, 0 G FAT, 10 MG SODIUM

APRICOT-PINEAPPLE GEL
Makes about 2¹/₂ cups

Like Fruit Gel, this is an all-natural alternative to Jell-O.

> 2 cups natural apricot juice
> ½ cup crushed pineapple
> 3 tablespoons apple juice concentrate
> 1 tablespoon arrowroot powder
> 1½ teaspoons agar powder

In a large saucepan stir all ingredients together until completely smooth. Bring to a simmer. Simmer uncovered—stirring constantly—for about 3 minutes, until slightly thickened. Pour into serving dishes and chill completely. PER 1-CUP SERVING: 112 CALORIES, 0 G PROTEIN, 27 G CARBOHYDRATE, 0 G FAT, 4 MG SODIUM

PRUNE WHIP
Makes about 1 cup

1 cup stewed prunes (save the cooking liquid)
2 tablespoons carob powder
2 tablespoons maple syrup

In a food processor or blender, puree all ingredients. Use the stewing liquid as needed to ensure a smooth mixture. PER SERVING: 191 CALORIES, 1 G PROTEIN, 46 G CARBOHYDRATE, 0 G FAT, 5 MG SODIUM

DATE COOLER
Makes about 1 1/2 cups

1 cup vanilla rice milk
3 pitted dates
2–3 ice cubes

Place rice milk and dates in a blender; blend until smooth. Add ice cubes and blend until they are chopped fine. PER 1-CUP SERVING: 140 CALORIES, 1 G PROTEIN, 30 G CARBOHYDRATE, 1 G FAT, 45 MG SODIUM

TAPIOCA PUDDING
Makes about 2 cups

2 cups vanilla rice milk
½ cup tapioca
¼ cup maple syrup
⅛ teaspoon salt
1 teaspoon vanilla extract

In a medium saucepan combine rice milk, tapioca, syrup, and salt. Let stand 5 minutes, then bring to a full boil over medium heat, stirring constantly. Remove from heat and stir in vanilla. Pour an equal amount of pudding into 4 serving dishes. Serve warm or chilled. PER ½-CUP SERVING: 170 CALORIES, 0.5 G PROTEIN, 28 G CARBOHYDRATE, 1 G FAT, 114 MG SODIUM

CARROT PUDDING
Serves 2

Whenen I told my friend Kerstin, an aspiring chef, about the recipes I was developing for this book, she promptly shared this one with me.

3 medium-size carrots, grated
⅛ cup raisins
1½ cups plain or vanilla rice milk
¼ teaspoon minced fresh ginger
3 tablespoons tapioca

In a medium-size saucepan combine all ingredients. Cook over low heat—stirring often—for about 15 minutes, or until carrots are soft and most of the liquid has evaporated.

Transfer about half the mixture to a blender; blend until smooth. Return the blended mixture to the pot, and stir to mix. Serve warm or chilled. PER ½-CUP SERVING: 127 CALORIES, 1 G PROTEIN, 29 G CARBOHYDRATE, 1 G FAT, 54 MG SODIUM

PEACH SORBET
Makes about 2 cups

This recipe is suitable for the Elimination Diet if you use canned peaches. To freeze peaches, simply drain off all the liquid and lay slices on a baking sheet in a single layer. Place the sheet in the freezer. Once peaches are frozen, they can be transferred to an airtight container.

2 cups frozen peach slices
1–2 tablespoons frozen apple juice concentrate or white grape
    juice concentrate
½ cup vanilla rice milk

In a blender combine all ingredients. Blend on high speed until thick and smooth. You'll need to stop the blender occasionally and use a spoon or rubber spatula to move the unblended fruit to the center. Serve immediately. PER 1-CUP SERVING: 96 CALORIES, 1 G PROTEIN, 22 G CARBOHYDRATE, 1 G FAT, 28 MG SODIUM

RICE MILK

Makes 2 cups

Commercially prepared rice milk is widely available in natural food stores and many supermarkets. You can also make your own with the following recipe. This rice milk is suitable as a beverage or for cooking. The solids will settle as the milk stands, so shake before using.

> 1 cup Always Great Brown Rice (page 238)
> 2 cups water
> ⅛ teaspoon salt
> 1 tablespoon Date Spread (page 254)

Into a blender place Always Great Brown Rice, the water, salt, and Date Spread. Blend for at least 30 seconds, or until completely smooth. PER ½-CUP SERVING: 65 CALORIES, 1 G PROTEIN, 14 G CARBOHYDRATE, 0 G FAT, 69 MG SODIUM

POACHED PEARS

Serves 2

I like to use Bosc pears for this recipe.

> 2 ripe medium-size pears
> 2 cups boysenberry-apple juice or similar fruit juice
> ½ teaspoon vanilla extract (if sauce is desired)

Peel pears, then cut them in half lengthwise and remove the cores. Place in a medium-size saucepan with boysenberry-apple juice, and bring to a slow simmer. Cook, uncovered, for about 10 minutes, or until pears are tender when pierced with a fork. Transfer pears to 2 small plates or flat dishes.

Increase heat and boil juice, uncovered, until it is reduced to ½ cup. Stir in vanilla, then pour the sauce over pears. Serve warm or chilled. PER PEAR: 107 CALORIES, 0 G PROTEIN, 25 G CARBOHYDRATE, 0 G FAT, 10 MG SODIUM

POACHED APPLES
Makes 2 apples

2 medium-size apples
3–5 large dates, pitted
¼ cup apple juice concentrate
¼ cup water

Remove apple cores to within ¼ inch of the bottom of each apple. Stuff each apple with the dates, then place apples into a medium-size saucepan. Add apple juice concentrate and the water. Bring to a slow simmer. Cover and cook for 20 to 25 minutes, or until tender. Serve hot or chilled. PER APPLE: 124 CALORIES, 0.5 G PROTEIN, 29 G CARBOHYDRATE, 0 G FAT, 0 MG SODIUM

PRUNE PUREE
Makes 1¹/₂ cups

Prune Puree is simple to make and may be used in baking as a substitute for eggs and to replace part or all of the oil. For each egg, use ¼ cup Prune Puree.

2 cups pitted prunes
2 cups water

Place prunes and the water in a medium-size saucepan. Cover and simmer for about 25 minutes, or until prunes are very soft. Puree prunes and cooking liquid in a food processor or blender until completely smooth. Store in an airtight container in the refrigerator. PER ¼-CUP SERVING: 129 CALORIES, 1 G PROTEIN, 30 G CARBOHYDRATE, 0 G FAT, 2 MG SODIUM

DATE SPREAD
Makes 1 cup

Use as a spread on bread, a dessert topping, or a sweetener on cereal.

>1 cup pitted dates
>1 cup water

Into a medium saucepan place dates and the water. Cook over medium heat—stirring constantly—for about 5 minutes, or until smooth and thick.

PER TABLESPOON: 31 CALORIES, 0 G PROTEIN, 7 G CARBOHYDRATE, 0 G FAT, 0 MG SODIUM

LOW-FAT RECIPES WITHOUT
CHOLESTEROL OR ANIMAL PROTEIN

The following recipes are low in fat, with no cholesterol or animal proteins. Like those in the Elimination Diet, they are perfect for people seeking to open their arteries, balance hormones, prevent kidney stones or osteoporosis, or bring diabetes under better control. However, some contain one or more ingredients that may act as triggers for migraines, arthritis, digestive symptoms, or fibromyalgia in some people. These are indicated with an asterisk (*). Omit these ingredients or recipes if you are sensitive to them or have not yet tested your sensitivities.

BREAKFAST BARLEY
Makes about 1 1/2 cups

>1 cup cooked barley (page 263)*
>½ cup vanilla rice milk
>¼ cup chopped pitted dates

In a medium-size saucepan or microwavable dish, combine all ingredients. Heat on the stove or in a microwave until hot. PER ½-CUP SERVING: 117 CALORIES, 2 G PROTEIN, 26 G CARBOHYDRATE, 0.5 G FAT, 17 MG SODIUM

Contains gluten, which may be a trigger food for some individuals.

CREAMY OATMEAL
Makes 3 cups

You'll love this delicious, creamy oatmeal. The vanilla rice milk adds a bit of sweetness as well as creaminess.

> 1 cup quick rolled oats*
> 2 cups vanilla rice milk

In an uncovered medium-size saucepan, combine rolled oats and milk. Bring to a simmer and cook for about 1 minute, or until slightly thickened. Cover pan, remove from heat. Before serving let stand for about 3 minutes. PER ½-CUP SERVING: 90 CALORIES, 4 G PROTEIN, 16 G CARBOHYDRATE, 2 G FAT, 38 MG SODIUM

Contains gluten, which may be a trigger food for some individuals.

FRUITED BREAKFAST QUINOA
Makes about 3 cups

Quinoa (pronounced "keen-wah") is a highly nutritious grain that was a staple in the diet of the ancient Incas. It has a delicious flavor and a light, fluffy texture. It is important to rinse the grain thoroughly prior to cooking. Do this by covering it with water in a mixing bowl, then rubbing it between the palms of your hands. Pour off the cloudy liquid through a strainer, then repeat the process, two or three more times, until the rinse liquid remains clear.

> ½ cup rinsed quinoa
> 1½ cups vanilla rice milk
> 2 tablespoons raisins
> 1 cup chopped fresh or canned apricots
> ¼ teaspoon vanilla extract

Be sure quinoa is well rinsed. In a medium-size saucepan, combine it with rice milk. Bring to a slow simmer, then cover and cook for about 15 minutes until the quinoa is tender. Stir in remaining ingredients, then transfer about 1½ cups to a blender; puree. Return pureed mixture to the pan and stir to mix. Serve warm or chilled. PER ½-CUP SERVING: 102 CALORIES, 3 G PROTEIN, 20 G CARBOHYDRATE, 1 G FAT, 24 MG SODIUM

QUICK BREAKFAST PUDDING
Makes 3 cups

8–10 dried apricot halves
2–3 medium-size dried figs (optional)
¼ cup raisins
1 medium-size apple*
1 cup quick rolled oats*
3 cups vanilla rice milk
¼ teaspoon cinnamon*

In a food processor chop apricot halves, figs (if used), and raisins. Cut and core apple, if used, then add it to the dried fruit in the food processor. Chop fine. Transfer the fruit mixture to a medium-size saucepan and add the remaining ingredients. Simmer slowly—stirring occasionally—for about 5 minutes, or until thickened. PER ½ CUP: 160 CALORIES, 5 G PROTEIN, 31 G CARBOHYDRATE, 2 G FAT, 47 MG SODIUM

May be a trigger food for some individuals.

BARLEY PANCAKES
Makes about sixteen 3-inch pancakes

1 cup barley flour*
½ teaspoon baking soda
¼ teaspoon salt
1¼ cups rice milk or soymilk (use rice milk if soy is a trigger food
    for you)
1 tablespoon maple syrup
1 tablespoon vinegar
1½ teaspoons canola oil*
Maple syrup or fruit preserves, for serving
Vegetable-oil spray, for cooking surface

In a medium-size bowl, stir barley flour, baking soda, and salt. In another medium-size bowl, stir milk, syrup, vinegar, and canola oil. Combine the two mixtures and stir to mix.

Heat a nonstick skillet or griddle. Lightly coat cooking surface with vegetable-oil spray. Pour small amounts of batter onto the heated surface and cook for 1 to 2 minutes, or until the edges are dry and the tops bubble. Turn carefully with a spatula and cook the second side for about 1 minute, or until golden brown. PER PANCAKE: 42 CALORIES, 1 G PROTEIN, 8 G CARBOHYDRATE, 1 G FAT, 66 MG SODIUM

May be a trigger food for some individuals.

BUCKWHEAT PANCAKES
Makes sixteen 3-inch pancakes

1 cup buckwheat flour
1 teaspoon baking powder
⅛ teaspoon salt
¾ cup vanilla rice milk
2 tablespoons maple syrup
1 tablespoon vinegar
Vegetable-oil spray, for cooking surface
Maple syrup or fruit preserves, for serving

In a medium-size bowl stir buckwheat flour, baking powder, and salt. In another medium-size bowl stir rice milk, syrup, and vinegar. Combine the two mixtures and stir to mix.

Heat a nonstick skillet or griddle. Lightly coat cooking surface with vegetable-oil spray. Pour small amounts of batter onto the heated surface and cook for 1 to 2 minutes, or until the tops bubble. Turn carefully with a spatula and cook for about 1 minute, or until the second side is golden brown. Serve immediately. PER PANCAKE: 33 CALORIES, 1 G PROTEIN, 7 G CARBOHYDRATE, 0 G FAT, 21 MG SODIUM

BARLEY WAFFLES
Makes four 6-inch waffles

2 cups barley flour*
1 teaspoon baking soda
½ teaspoon salt
2½ cups rice milk or soymilk (use rice milk if soy is a trigger food
    for you)
2 tablespoons maple syrup
2 tablespoons vinegar
1 tablespoon canola oil*
Maple syrup or fruit preserves, for serving
Vegetable-oil spray, for waffle iron

Preheat waffle iron.

In a medium-size bowl, stir barley flour, baking soda, and salt. In another medium-size bowl, stir milk, syrup, vinegar, and canola oil. Combine the two mixtures and stir to mix.

Lightly coat the waffle iron with vegetable-oil spray, then pour in some of the batter and cook for 3 to 5 minutes, or until golden brown. Serve with syrup or fruit preserves. PER WAFFLE: 166 CALORIES, 3 G PROTEIN, 32 G CARBOHYDRATE, 3 G FAT, 265 MG SODIUM

May be a trigger food for some individuals.

BARLEY SCONES
Makes 6 scones

¼ cup vanilla rice milk
2 tablespoons maple syrup
1 tablespoon sunflower or canola oil*
2 teaspoons vinegar
1 cup plus 3 tablespoons barley flour*
¼ teaspoon baking soda
1 teaspoon baking powder
¼ teaspoon salt
3 tablespoons raisins
Additional barley flour, for dusting

Preheat oven to 350° F.

In a small bowl mix rice milk, syrup, oil, and vinegar. Set aside. In a food processor fitted with a metal blade, combine barley flour, baking soda, baking powder, salt, and raisins. Blend until well mixed and raisins are chopped.

Add the liquid mixture. Process until a ball of dough forms. Dust a flat surface with barley flour. Transfer the dough to the dusted surface. Flatten it into a circle approximately 6 inches in diameter and ¾ inch thick. Use a sharp knife to score the dough into 6 wedges (do not separate), then transfer it to a baking sheet. Bake for about 30 minutes, or until lightly browned. PER SCONE: 221 CALORIES, 4 G PROTEIN, 43 G CARBOHYDRATE, 4 G FAT, 354 MG SODIUM

May be a trigger food for some individuals.

DATE MUFFINS
Makes 12 muffins

1 cup whole wheat pastry flour*
1 cup barley flour
1 teaspoon baking soda
½ teaspoon salt
1½ cups Date spread (page 254)
1 cup water
2 tablespoons apple cider vinegar
2 tablespoons canola or sunflower oil*
Vegetable-oil spray, for muffin pan

Preheat the oven to 375° F.

In a large bowl mix flours, baking soda, and salt. Add Date Spread, the water, vinegar, and oil. Stir until just mixed.

Lightly coat the muffin pan with vegetable-oil spray. Fill cups to the top with batter. Bake for about 30 minutes, or until the top of a muffin bounces back when pressed lightly. Let stand 1 to 2 minutes before removing from the pan. When cool, store in an airtight container in the refrigerator. PER MUFFIN: 148 CALORIES, 3 G PROTEIN, 28 G CARBOHYDRATE, 2 G FAT, 159 MG SODIUM

May be a trigger food for some individuals.

YAM SPICE MUFFINS
Makes 10 to 12 muffins

2 cups whole wheat or whole wheat pastry flour*
½ cup sugar*
1 tablespoon baking powder
½ teaspoon baking soda
½ teaspoon salt
½ teaspoon cinnamon
¼ teaspoon nutmeg
1½ cups cooked, mashed yams
½ cup water
½ cup raisins
Vegetable-oil spray, for muffin pan

Preheat the oven to 375° F.

In a large bowl mix whole wheat flour, sugar, baking powder, baking soda, salt, cinnamon, and nutmeg. Add yams, the water, and raisins; stir until just mixed.

Lightly coat a muffin pan with vegetable-oil spray. Fill cups to the top. Bake for 25 to 30 minutes, or until the top of a muffin bounces back when pressed lightly. Let stand for 1 to 2 minutes before removing from the pan. When cool, store in an airtight container. PER MUFFIN: 137 CALORIES, 3 G PROTEIN, 31 G CARBOHYDRATE, 0 G FAT, 128 MG SODIUM

MIXED FRUIT MUFFINS
Makes 12 muffins

1 cup whole wheat pastry flour*
1 cup barley flour*
1 teaspoon baking soda
½ teaspoon salt
2 cups Summer Fruit Compote, including some of the liquid
    (page 237)
1 cup water
3 tablespoons apple cider vinegar
2 tablespoons canola or sunflower oil*
Vegetable-oil spray, for muffin pan

Preheat the oven to 375° F.

In a large bowl mix flours, baking soda, and salt. In a food processor or blender, puree Summer Fruit Compote until it is quite smooth, then add it to the flour mixture along with the water, vinegar, and oil. Stir until just mixed.

Lightly coat a muffin pan with vegetable-oil spray. Fill cups to the top with batter. Bake for about 30 minutes, or until the top of a muffin bounces back when pressed lightly. Let stand 1 to 2 minutes before removing from the pan. When cool, store in an airtight container in the refrigerator. PER MUFFIN: 138 CALORIES, 3 G PROTEIN, 26 G CARBOHYDRATE, 2 G FAT, 159 MG SODIUM

May be a trigger food for some individuals.

QUINOA
Makes 3 cups

It is no wonder that quinoa (pronounced "keen-wah") was a staple in the diet of the ancient Incas. It is nutritionally impressive, with an almost-ideal balance of essential amino acids. Its light and fluffy texture makes it excellent for side dishes and salads. Also, you'll love the fact that it cooks in just 15 minutes. Quinoa is sold in natural food stores and specialty shops. It is important to wash it thoroughly before cooking.

> 1 cup quinoa
> 2 cups boiling water
> ¼ teaspoon salt

In a large bowl place quinoa and a generous amount of cold water. Rub the grains between your hands until the water is cloudy, then pour quinoa into a sieve. Repeat this process until the water stays clear, about 3 rinsings. Transfer quinoa to a medium-size pan and add the boiling water and salt. Bring to a slow simmer, then cover and cook for about 15 minutes, or until all water is absorbed. PER ½ CUP: 101 CALORIES, 4 G PROTEIN, 18 G CARBOHYDRATE, 1 G FAT, 91 MG SODIUM

SEASONED RICE
Makes 2 cups

Serve this tasty rice with steamed or grilled vegetables, or add it to soups to provide extra texture and flavor.

>2 cups hot Always Great Brown Rice (page 238) or Wild Brown
>   Rice (page 239)
>2 tablespoons Sesame Seasoning (page 299)

In a medium-size bowl combine rice and Sesame Seasoning. Toss gently to mix. PER ½ CUP: 144 CALORIES, 4 G PROTEIN, 27 G CARBOHYDRATE, 3 G FAT, 119 MG SODIUM

BUCKWHEAT
Makes 2¹/₂ cups

Despite its name, buckwheat is no relation to wheat. It is highly nutritious and has a distinct flavor that you will be familiar with if you have ever eaten buckwheat pancakes. Whole buckwheat may be sold raw (as buckwheat groats) or toasted (as kasha). Buckwheat groats are light greenish tan and have a milder flavor than the reddish tan kasha. Try both to see which you prefer. Whole buckwheat cooks quickly and makes a tasty hot breakfast cereal or side dish. Look for it in natural food and specialty stores.

>2 cups boiling water
>¼ teaspoon salt
>1 cup buckwheat groats or kasha

To the water in a medium-size pan add salt and buckwheat. Bring to a slow simmer, then cover and cook for about 10 minutes, or until all the liquid has been absorbed. PER ½ CUP: 97 CALORIES, 3 G PROTEIN, 22 G CARBOHYDRATE, 0 G FAT, 91 MG SODIUM

BARLEY

Makes 3 cups

Barley is easy to cook and is most familiar as a delicious addition to soups and stews. It may also be eaten as a breakfast cereal or used as a basis for salads and side dishes. Barley is an excellent source of protein and fiber, and scientists have also discovered that certain substances in barley, in addition to soluble fiber, inhibit cholesterol production. Hulled barley is sold in natural food stores and is significantly more nutritious than the more familiar pearled barley.

> 1 cup hulled or pearled barley*
> 3 cups water
> ¼ teaspoon salt

In a medium-size saucepan, combine all ingredients. Cover and bring to a simmer over medium heat. Continue cooking, stirring occasionally, for about 30 minutes, until the barley is tender (it will still be slightly chewy).

PER ½ CUP: 84 CALORIES, 3 G PROTEIN, 18 G CARBOHYDRATE, 0 G FAT, 91 MG SODIUM

Contains gluten, which may be a trigger food for some individuals

BARLEY TORTILLAS

Makes six 5-inch tortillas

Use these for tacos, burritos, and tostadas.

> 1 cup barley flour*
> 2 tablespoons Sesame Salt (page 298)
> 3–4 tablespoons water
> Additional Sesame Salt, for coating

Mix barley flour and Sesame Salt, then stir in just enough of the water to allow you to form a dough ball. Let stand 1 minute, then knead the dough between your hands for a few seconds.

Divide the dough into 6 equal pieces and roll each into a ball. Roll one of the balls in Sesame Salt, then place it between 2 sheets of plastic wrap. Use a rolling pin to flatten it into a ⅛-inch-thick round, starting at the

(Continued next page)

middle of the dough and rolling toward the outside edges. Carefully peel off the plastic wrap.

Heat an ungreased heavy skillet (such as cast iron). Cook rolled dough for about 2 minutes each side, or until the cooked surface appears dry with small brown flecks. Repeat with the remaining dough. To soften the tortillas, stack them while they are still warm and cover them with a dish towel or lid. Let stand about 5 minutes. PER PIECE: 85 CALORIES, 2 G PRO-TEIN, 15 G CARBOHYDRATE, 2 G FAT, 45 MG SODIUM

May be a trigger food for some individuals.

GARBANZO FLATBREAD
Makes six 5-inch flatbreads

This is quick to make, once you get the knack.

>1 cup garbanzo flour
>3 tablespoons Sesame Salt (page 298)
>3–4 tablespoons water
>Additional Sesame Salt, for coating

Mix garbanzo flour and Sesame Salt, then stir in just enough of the water to allow you to form a dough ball. Let stand 1 minute, then knead the dough between your hands for a few seconds.

Divide the dough into 6 equal pieces and roll each into a ball. Roll one of the balls in Sesame Salt, then place it between 2 sheets of plastic wrap. Use a rolling pin to flatten it into a ⅛-inch-thick round, starting at the middle of the dough and rolling toward the outside edges. Carefully peel off the plastic wrap.

Heat an ungreased heavy skillet (cast iron works well). Cook rolled dough for about 2 minutes each side, or until the cooked surface appears dry with small brown flecks. Repeat with the remaining dough. PER PIECE: 81 CALORIES, 7 G PROTEIN, 6 G CARBOHYDRATE, 3 G FAT, 70 MG SODIUM

ENSALADA DE FRIJOLES
Serves 4 as a complete meal

This salad has it all: rice, beans, corn, and greens. It is quick to prepare, especially if you use prewashed salad mix, and makes a perfect meal on a hot day. Jicama (pronounced "hick-ama") is a delicious root vegetable that is delightfully crisp and slightly sweet. It is usually sold in the unrefrigerated area of a supermarket produce section.

> 3 cups (approximately) Always Great Brown Rice (page 238)
> 8 cups prewashed salad mix
> 2 medium-size carrots, grated or cut into julienne strips
> 1 15-ounce can black beans, drained and rinsed
> 1 cup peeled and grated jicama
> 2 medium-size tomatoes, diced or cut into wedges*
> 1 15-ounce can corn, drained (or 2 cups fresh or frozen)*
> ½ cup cilantro leaves, chopped coarse (optional)
> ¼ cup salsa*
> ¼ cup seasoned rice vinegar
> 1 medium-size clove garlic, crushed or pressed
> Additional salsa, for topping*

Make a bed of warm Always Great Brown Rice on each of 4 medium-size plates. Top each with layers of salad mix; carrot strips; beans; jicama; and tomato wedges, corn, and cilantro (if used).

In a small bowl mix salsa (if used), vinegar, and garlic. Sprinkle over each of the salads, then top with generous spoonfuls of salsa.

PER SERVING: 302 CALORIES, 10 G PROTEIN, 60 G CARBOHYDRATE, 2 G FAT, 355 MG SODIUM

May be a trigger food for some individuals.

ROOTIN' TOOTIN' SALAD
Serves 6

Three root vegetables—beets, jicama, and carrots—combine to make this crunchy, nutritious salad.

> 1 15-ounce can diced beets, drained
> 1 small jicama, peeled and cut into thin strips or diced
> 2 medium-size carrots, peeled and cut into thin strips or diced
> 3 tablespoons lemon juice*
> 2 tablespoons seasoned rice vinegar
> 2 teaspoons stone-ground mustard
> ½ teaspoon dried dill weed

Place beet cubes into a large salad bowl, along with jicama and carrot pieces. In a small bowl mix lemon juice (if used), vinegar, mustard, and dill; pour over the salad. Toss to mix. Serve warm or chilled. PER SERVING: 38 CALORIES, 1 G PROTEIN, 8 G CARBOHYDRATE, 0 G FAT, 151 MG SODIUM

May be a trigger food for some individuals.

MEXICAN CORN SALAD
Serves 6

> 1 15-ounce can corn, drained*
> 1 large cucumber, peeled and diced
> ½ cup fine-chopped red onion*
> 1 medium-size red bell pepper, diced fine*
> 1 medium-size tomato, seeded and diced*
> ½ cup chopped fresh cilantro (optional)
> 2 tablespoons seasoned rice vinegar
> 2 tablespoons apple cider or distilled vinegar
> 1 tablespoon lemon juice or lime juice*
> 1 clove garlic, minced
> 1 teaspoon ground cumin
> 1 teaspoon ground coriander
> ⅛ teaspoon cayenne pepper

In a large salad bowl combine corn, cucumber, onion, pepper, tomato, and cilantro (if used). In a small bowl combine vinegars, lemon or lime juice (if used), garlic, cumin, coriander seed, and cayenne. Pour over the salad and toss gently to mix. PER SERVING: 100 CALORIES, 2 G PROTEIN, 20 G CARBOHY-DRATE, 1 G FAT, 112 MG SODIUM

May be a trigger food for some individuals.

CRISPY GREEN SALAD
Serves 6

This cool, crisp salad is a welcome addition to any meal.

>4 cups torn or chopped romaine lettuce
>1 cup fine-shredded green or red cabbage
>1 cup thin-sliced celery
>1 15-ounce can garbanzo beans, including some liquid
>¼ cup thin-sliced red onion*
>2 tablespoons seasoned rice vinegar
>1 tablespoon apple cider vinegar
>½ teaspoon sugar
>¼ teaspoon dried basil
>¼ teaspoon mixed Italian seasoning
>¼ teaspoon garlic granules or powder
>⅛ teaspoon salt
>⅛ teaspoon black pepper

In a large salad bowl combine lettuce, cabbage, and celery. Drain beans, reserving the liquid, and add them to the salad along with onion (if used).

In a small bowl stir vinegars, sugar, basil, Italian seasoning, garlic, salt, and pepper. Stir in 2 tablespoons of the reserved bean liquid. Just before serving, pour the dressing over the salad and toss to mix. PER SERV-ING: 106 CALORIES, 4 G PROTEIN, 21 G CARBOHYDRATE, 1 G FAT, 334 MG SODIUM

May be a trigger food for some individuals.

CREAMY DILL DRESSING
Makes about 1¹/₂ cups

This rich-tasting, creamy dressing has no added oil. It is made with silken tofu, which is available in most markets. Mori-Nu is one popular brand.

    1 10½-ounce package firm silken tofu*
    1½ teaspoons garlic powder or granules
    ½ teaspoon dried dill weed
    ½ teaspoon salt
    2 tablespoons water
    1½ tablespoons lemon juice*
    1 tablespoon seasoned rice vinegar

In a food processor or blender combine all ingredients. Blend until completely smooth. Store any extra dressing in an airtight container in the refrigerator. PER 1 TABLESPOON: 23 CALORIES, 3 G PROTEIN, 2 G CARBOHYDRATE, 0.5 G FAT, 115 MG SODIUM

May be a trigger food for some individuals

RED CABBAGE SALAD
Serves 8

This salad may be served warm or cold. I like to serve it with buckwheat groats or kasha.

    1 small red cabbage
    1 medium-size red onion*
    1 clove garlic, minced
    2 teaspoons toasted sesame oil*
    ¼ cup balsamic vinegar
    ¼ cup raspberry vinegar or additional balsamic vinegar
    3 tablespoons apple juice concentrate
    1 teaspoon dried thyme
    ½ teaspoon salt
    1 medium-size apple, grated*
    2 tablespoons Sesame Salt (page 298)

Cut cabbage in half, then into very thin slices (you should have about 6 cups). Peel onion (if used) and cut it in half from top to bottom. Slice each half into thin crescents. In a large skillet, heat oil (if used), then add onion and garlic. Cook 3 minutes until the onion is soft. Add sliced cabbage along with vinegars, apple juice concentrate, thyme, and salt. Stirring fairly constantly, continue cooking over high heat for 3 to 5 minutes, or until cabbage begins to soften and turns bright pink. Stir in apple (if used) and Sesame Salt. Serve warm or cold. PER SERVING: 76 CALORIES, 1 G PROTEIN, 12 G CARBOHYDRATE, 2 G FAT, 177 MG SODIUM

May be a trigger food for some individuals.

NOTE: *If sesame oil is omitted, onion and garlic may be cooked in a small amount of water (about ½ cup).*

HUMMUS (CHICKPEA PÂTÉ)
Makes about 2 cups

This Middle Eastern pâté can be used as a sandwich spread or as a dip with crackers, wedges of pita bread, or fresh vegetable slices. It is easily prepared with a food processor.

> 2 medium-size cloves garlic
> 1 tablespoon fresh parsley
> 1 15-ounce can garbanzo beans, including some liquid
> 2 tablespoons lemon juice*
> ¼ teaspoon salt
> ¼ teaspoon ground cumin
> ¼ teaspoon paprika*

In a food processor chop garlic and parsley, scraping down sides of bowl to make sure everything is chopped fine.

Drain beans, reserving the liquid. Add beans to the food processor, along with lemon juice (if used), salt, cumin, and paprika (if used). Process until smooth and spreadable, adding about ½ cup of the reserved bean liquid to achieve a spreadable consistency. PER ¼-CUP SERVING: 70 CALORIES, 3 G PROTEIN, 12 G CARBOHYDRATE, 1 G FAT, 203 MG SODIUM

May be a trigger food for some individuals.

GARBANZO SPREAD
Makes 2 cups

Use as a dip with pita bread, tortillas, or fresh vegetable slices.

> 1 15-ounce can garbanzo beans, drained
> ½ cup roasted red peppers*
> 2 tablespoons tahini
> 3 tablespoons lemon juice*

In a food processor or blender, combine all ingredients. Puree until smooth. PER ¼-CUP SERVING: 79 CALORIES, 3 G PROTEIN, 11 G CARBOHYDRATE, 2 G FAT, 112 MG SODIUM

May be a trigger food for some individuals.

CREAMY CUCUMBER DIP
Serves 6

Serve this cool, creamy dip with wedges of pita bread or pita chips with fresh vegetable slices.

> 1 medium-size cucumber
> ½ pound firm tofu*
> 2 tablespoons lemon juice*
> 1 medium-size clove garlic, minced
> ¼ teaspoon salt
> ⅛ teaspoon ground coriander
> ⅛ teaspoon ground cumin
> Pinch cayenne pepper*
> ¼ cup fine-sliced red onion*

Peel, seed, and grate cucumber. Let stand 10 minutes. In a blender, combine tofu and lemon juice (if used), garlic, salt, coriander, cumin, and pepper. Blend until completely smooth. Squeeze cucumber to remove excess moisture, then place into a medium-size serving bowl with onion (if used). Stir in the blended mixture. Chill 2 to 3 hours. PER ¼-CUP SERVING: 32 CALORIES, 3 G PROTEIN, 3 G CARBOHYDRATE, 1 G FAT, 70 MG SODIUM

May be a trigger food for some individuals.

QUICK BEAN DIP
Makes about 2 cups

Try this dip with baked tortilla chips or as a burrito filling. Instant bean flakes are sold in natural food stores and some supermarkets. (Fantastic Foods makes a widely distributed brand.)

> 1 cup water
> 1 cup instant bean flakes
> ½–1 cup salsa (you choose the heat)*

In a medium saucepan boil the water. Add bean flakes and stir. Turn off heat and let stand for 5 minutes. Stir in salsa. PER ¼-CUP SERVING: 49 CALORIES, 3 G PROTEIN, 9 G CARBOHYDRATE, 0 G FAT, 150 MG SODIUM

May be a trigger food for some individuals.

ZUCCHINI PESTO
Makes about ¹/₂ cup

Pesto is a delicious topping for steamed vegetables.

> 2 small zucchini or other summer squash
> 1 medium-size clove garlic
> 2 cups fresh basil leaves, packed
> 2 teaspoons olive oil
> ¼ teaspoon salt

Cut zucchini into 1-inch chunks (you should have about 2 cups). Steam chunks over boiling water for about 5 minutes, or until it is just tender when pierced with a sharp knife.

Place garlic and basil into a food processor fitted with a metal blade and chop until fine. Add zucchini, oil, and salt. Process in short on-off bursts until everything is chopped fine. PER 1-TABLESPOON SERVING: 15 CALORIES, 0 G PROTEIN, 1 G CARBOHYDRATE, 1 G FAT, 70 MG OF SODIUM

BLACK-BEAN SAUCE
Serves 6

This sauce is quick to prepare and delicious on broccoli, potatoes, or pasta.

> 1 15-ounce can black beans, including liquid
> ½ cup roasted red pepper*
> 2 tablespoons lemon juice*
> 2 tablespoons tahini
> ½ teaspoon chili powder*
> ¼ teaspoon ground cumin
> ¼ teaspoon ground coriander
> ¼ cup chopped fresh cilantro

In a food processor or blender, combine all ingredients. Puree until smooth. PER ¼-CUP SERVING: 94 CALORIES, 5 G PROTEIN, 14 G CARBOHYDRATE, 2 G FAT, 110 MG SODIUM

May be a trigger food for some individuals.

QUICK GARBANZO GRAVY
Makes about 2½ cups

Serve this gravy with potatoes, or as a topping for cooked green vegetables. If you omit the onion, reduce the amount of water to approximately ½ cup.

> 1 teaspoon toasted sesame oil*
> 1 medium-size onion, chopped*
> 1¼ cups water, added in increments
> 1 15-ounce can garbanzo beans, undrained
> ¼ teaspoon poultry seasoning
> 2 teaspoons soy sauce*, or to taste

In a medium-size skillet heat oil (if used). Add onion (if used), and ¼ cup of the water. Cook over high heat, stirring frequently, until all liquid has evaporated. Add another ¼ cup of the water and continue cooking until it too has evaporated and onion is lightly browned. Add another ¼ cup of the water, stirring to remove any pieces of onion that are stuck to the pan.

Transfer onion to a blender. Add beans with their liquid, poultry seasoning, and ½ cup of the water. Blend until completely smooth. Add more water for a thinner gravy. Return blended mixture to the skillet; add soy sauce (if used); heat gently, stirring occasionally until hot. PER ¼-CUP SERVING: 82 CALORIES, 4 G PROTEIN, 14 G CARBOHYDRATE, 1 G FAT, 109 MG SODIUM

May be a trigger food for some individuals.

CREAMY BROCCOLI SOUP
Makes about 8 cups

2 medium-size potatoes, scrubbed and diced
2 medium-size stalks celery, sliced
6 cups broccoli florets
2 cups water
3 cups plain rice milk
1½ teaspoons dried basil
½ teaspoon dried tarragon
¾ teaspoon salt
¼ teaspoon black pepper
3–4 tablespoons Sesame Seasoning (page 299)

Into a large pot place potato, celery, and broccoli pieces and the water. Bring to a simmer. Cover and cook over medium heat for about 10 minutes, or until potato chunks are tender when pierced with a sharp knife (do not overcook).

Transfer about 3 cups of the vegetables to a blender. Add 2 cups of rice milk, basil, tarragon, salt, and pepper. Blend for about 60 seconds, or until completely smooth. Pour blended mixture into a clean pot.

Into the blender place remaining vegetables along with the cooking liquid and remaining rice milk. Blend them until they are completely smooth or leave them slightly chunky, depending on your taste. Add them to the first batch, then stir in Sesame Seasoning. Heat gently, stirring frequently, until steamy. PER 1-CUP SERVING: 142 CALORIES, 3 G PROTEIN, 27 G CARBOHYDRATE, 2 G FAT, 316 MG SODIUM

MUSHROOM BARLEY SOUP
Makes about 3 cups

This soup takes just minutes to make if you have cooked barley on hand.

    2 cups plain rice milk
    2 tablespoons barley flour*
    1 cup cooked barley (see page 263)*
    1 4-ounce can mushrooms, including liquid
    ¼ teaspoon each: garlic powder and salt
    Pinch each: dried marjoram, sage, thyme, dill weed

Place rice milk and barley flour into a blender. Blend on high speed for a few seconds. Add barley and blend on high for about 10 seconds, or until barley is chopped coarse.

Add mushrooms with their liquid. Blend just enough to coarse-chop mushrooms.

Transfer the blended mixture to a medium-size saucepan and add all the remaining ingredients. Cook over medium heat—stirring often—for about 5 minutes, or until the soup is hot and somewhat thickened. PER 1-CUP SERVING: 159 CALORIES, 3 G PROTEIN, 34 G CARBOHYDRATE, 1 G FAT, 299 MG SODIUM

May be a trigger food for some individuals.

SUMMER VEGETABLE STEW
Makes about 8 cups

    2 teaspoons olive oil*
    2 medium-size onions, chopped*
    3 medium-size Japanese eggplants, cut into ¼-inch thick slices*
    1 medium-size green bell pepper, diced*
    5 large medium-size cloves garlic, minced
    1 12-ounce jar water-packed roasted red peppers, including liquid*
    3 small zucchini, sliced
    2 cups chopped fresh basil
    1 15-ounce can navy beans or cannelini beans, including liquid
    ½ teaspoon salt
    ¼ teaspoon black pepper

In a large skillet or pot, heat oil. Add chopped onions (if used). Cook over medium-high heat—stirring often—for about 5 minutes, or until onions are lightly browned. (Add a small amount of water if onion begins to stick.) Add eggplant and bell pepper (if used), and garlic; cover and cook—stirring occasionally—for about 5 minutes, or until eggplant begins to soften. Coarse-chop the red peppers (if used); add them, with their liquid, to the skillet. Add zucchini and basil. Cover and cook over medium heat—stirring occasionally—for about 3 minutes, or until vegetables are tender. Stir in beans with their liquid, salt, and black pepper. Cover and cook for about 3 more minutes, or until zucchini is just tender. PER 1-CUP SERVING: 121 CALORIES, 4 G PROTEIN, 22 G CARBOHYDRATE, 1 G FAT, 254 MG SODIUM

May be a trigger food for some individuals.

NOTE: *If oil is omitted, use ½ cup of water or vegetable stock to saute vegetables.*

KASHA WITH CABBAGE
Makes about 2 ½ cups

1 teaspoon olive oil*
½ cup kasha or buckwheat groats
2 cups fine-chopped cabbage
1 cup water
¼ teaspoon salt

In a large saucepan, heat oil, tilting the pan so oil completely covers the bottom. Add kasha and cabbage. Cook over medium-high heat—stirring frequently—for about 1 minute. Add the water and salt; stir to mix. When water boils, lower heat and bring liquid to a simmer. Cover and cook for about 10 minutes, or until all liquid is absorbed. PER ½-CUP SERVING: 72 CALORIES, 1 G PROTEIN, 13 G CARBOHYDRATE, 1 G FAT, 89 MG SODIUM

May be a trigger food for some individuals.

NOTE: *If oil is omitted, toast kasha in a dry skillet for 2 to 3 minutes before adding remaining ingredients.*

WONDERFUL WINTER SQUASH
Makes 4 cups

In spite of its name, winter squash is available year-round in most places. If you've never tried butternut, kabocha, or other winter squash, you're in for a real treat. For starters, be sure to try this easy recipe.

> 1 medium-size winter squash (butternut or kabocha, for example)
> ½ cup water
> 2 teaspoons soy sauce*
> 2 tablespoons maple syrup

Cut squash in half, then peel it and remove the seeds. Cut squash into 1-inch cubes (you should have about 4 cups).

Place cubes into a large pot with the water. Add soy sauce (if used) and syrup. Cover and simmer over medium heat for 15 to 20 minutes, or until squash is tender when pierced with a fork. PER ½-CUP SERVING: 52 CALORIES, 1 G PROTEIN, 11 G CARBOHYDRATE, 0 G FAT, 78 MG SODIUM

May be a trigger food for some individuals.

BROCCOLI WITH TAHINI SAUCE
Serves 2

> 2 large stalks broccoli
> 1 tablespoon tahini
> 1 tablespoon balsamic vinegar
> Pinch salt

Cut off broccoli stem. Cut or break the top into bite-size florets. Peel the stem with a sharp knife, then slice it into ½-inch-thick rounds. Transfer broccoli to a vegetable steamer. Steam over boiling water for about 5 minutes, or until broccoli is bright green and tender.

While broccoli cooks: In a small bowl mix tahini, vinegar, and salt. Add just enough water to make a thick sauce. When broccoli is cooked, place it into a medium-size serving bowl and drizzle it with the sauce.

PER SERVING: 86 CALORIES, 4 G PROTEIN, 9 G CARBOHYDRATE, 4 G FAT, 60 MG SODIUM

CREAMY YAMS
Makes about 4 cups

2 large jewel or garnet yams
1 tablespoon tahini

Scrub yams and cut them into 2-inch chunks. Steam them for about 25 minutes, or until tender when pierced with a fork. Set aside until cool enough to handle.

Peel yams, if desired, then puree them in a food processor. Add tahini and blend until completely smooth. Transfer pureed mixture to a microwavable dish. Heat 2 to 3 minutes until warm throughout; serve. PER ½-CUP SERVING: 105 CALORIES, 1 G PROTEIN, 20 G CARBOHYDRATE, 1 G FAT, 8 MG SODIUM

OVEN-ROASTED VEGETABLES
Makes 8 to 10 cups

What a happy coincidence that one of the easiest way to cook vegetables is also one of the tastiest. Serve as a vegetable side dish, or add pasta, rice, or polenta for a satisfying meal.

3 medium-size zucchini or crookneck squash
1 large red onion*
1 large red bell pepper, seeded*
2 cups small, firm mushrooms
1 teaspoon garlic granules
1 teaspoon mixed Italian seasoning
1 teaspoon chili powder*
¼ teaspoon salt
¼ teaspoon black pepper

Preheat the oven to 500° F.

Cut squash into 1-inch chunks. Do the same with onion and bell pepper (if used). Place chunks into a large bowl. Clean mushrooms and add them to the bowl. Sprinkle with the remaining ingredients; toss gently to mix.

Spread vegetable mixture in a single layer in 1 or 2 baking dishes. Bake for about 10 minutes, or until tender when pierced with a fork. PER ½-CUP SERVING: 32 CALORIES, 1 G PROTEIN, 6 G CARBOHYDRATE, 0 G FAT, 93 MG SODIUM

May be a trigger food for some individuals.

HOMESTYLE MILLET
WITH GARBANZO GRAVY

Makes about 8 cups

When you're in the mood for a comfort food reminiscent of mashed pota-toes, try this delicious millet dish with Quick Garbanzo Gravy (page 272).

    2 teaspoons toasted sesame oil*
    8 large cloves garlic, minced
    4 cups boiling water
    1 cup millet
    ½ teaspoon salt
    3 cups chopped cauliflower
    1 medium-size onion, chopped*
    1 15-ounce can garbanzo beans, including liquid
    2 teaspoons soy sauce*
    ¼ teaspoon poultry seasoning

Heat 1 teaspoon of the oil (if used) in a large pot, then add garlic and ¼ cup of the water. Cook for about 30 seconds.

Add millet and continue cooking for about 2 minutes. Then stir in 2½ cups of the boiling water; add salt. Bring to a simmer, then cover and cook for 10 minutes.

Stir in cauliflower, then cover and cook for another 15 minutes, or until millet is tender and all the water has been absorbed. (Stir occasionally during this time; add a bit more water, if necessary, to prevent the mixture from sticking.)

To prepare the gravy: Heat remaining oil (if used) in a medium-size skillet, then add onion (if used) and ¼ cup of the water. Cook over high heat about 5 minutes, stirring frequently, until all the liquid has evaporated. Add another ¼ cup of the water; continue cooking about 5 minutes until it too has evaporated and onion is lightly browned. Add ¼ cup of the water, stirring to remove any stuck pieces of onion from the pan. Transfer onion and cooking liquid to a blender.

To the blender add beans with their liquid, soy sauce (if used), poultry seasoning, and ½ cup of the water. Blend until completely smooth. Add additional water for a thinner gravy. Return blended mixture to the skillet; heat gently, stirring occasionally, until hot.

When millet is tender, place it onto serving plates and top with a generous amount of gravy.

Variation. Quinoa is also delicious prepared in this manner. Simply substitute 1 cup of well-rinsed quinoa for the millet and proceed as described, reducing the total cooking time to about 15 minutes. PER 1-CUP SERVING: 249 CALORIES, 7 G PROTEIN, 47 G CARBOHYDRATE, 3 G FAT, 351 MG SODIUM

May be a trigger food for some individuals.

RED POTATOES WITH KALE

Makes about 8 cups

4 medium-size red potatoes*
1 medium-size bunch kale
1 teaspoon toasted sesame oil* or ½ cup water
1 medium-size onion, sliced thin*
2 medium-size cloves garlic, minced
½ teaspoon black pepper
½ teaspoon paprika*
2 tablespoons water
5 teaspoons soy sauce*

Scrub potatoes and cut into ½-inch cubes. Steam over boiling water for about 10 minutes, or until just tender when pierced with a fork. Rinse with cold water, then drain and set aside.

Rinse kale, then remove the tough stems. Cut or tear the leaves into small pieces.

Heat oil or water in a large nonstick skillet. Add onion (if used) and garlic. Saute for 5 minutes, or until soft.

Add potato cubes, pepper, and paprika (if used); continue cooking for about 5 minutes, or until potatoes begin to brown. (Use a spatula to turn the mixture gently as it cooks.)

Spread kale over the top of the potato mixture. Sprinkle with the 2 tablespoons of water and soy sauce (if used). Cover and cook, turning occasionally, for about 7 minutes, or until kale is tender. PER 1-CUP SERVING: 116 CALORIES, 3 G PROTEIN, 25 G CARBOHYDRATE, 1 G FAT, 147 MG SODIUM

May be a trigger food for some individuals.

BROCCOLI WITH KASHA
AND BLACK-BEAN SAUCE

Makes about 8 cups

What a happy marriage of flavors!

1 large bunch broccoli
4 cups boiling water
2 cups kasha (use buckwheat groats for a milder flavor)
½ teaspoon salt
1 15-ounce can black beans, drained
½ cup roasted red pepper*
2 tablespoons lemon juice*
2 tablespoons tahini
½ teaspoon chili powder*
¼ teaspoon ground cumin
¼ teaspoon ground coriander
¼ cup chopped fresh cilantro

Cut off broccoli stems. Cut or break the tops into bite-size florets. Peel the stem with a sharp knife, then slice it into ½-inch-thick rounds. Set aside.

Into the water in a large saucepan, place kasha and salt. Cover and simmer for about 10 minutes, or until all the liquid has been absorbed.

While kasha is cooking, combine and puree all the remaining ingredients in a food processor or blender.

Just before you are ready to eat, steam broccoli over boiling water for about 5 minutes, or until it is bright green and just tender.

Place a generous amount of kasha on each serving plate, then top with steamed broccoli and black-bean sauce. PER 1-CUP SERVING: 133 CALORIES, 6 G PROTEIN, 21 G CARBOHYDRATE, 2 G FAT, 373 MG SODIUM

May be a trigger food for some individuals.

ZUCCHINI SKILLET HASH

Serves 8

This hearty hash is made with Boca Burger patties, delicious, fat-free vegetarian burgers that are sold in natural food stores and some super-markets.

    8 ounces gluten-free pasta (quinoa, rice, etc.)
    ½ cup water
    1 medium-size onion, chopped*
    2 medium-size cloves garlic, minced
    1½ cups sliced mushrooms
    1 medium-size stalk celery, sliced thin
    2 medium-size zucchini, diced
    3 Boca Burgers patties, chopped*
    1 15-ounce can garbanzo beans, including liquid
    ½ teaspoon salt

Cook pasta according to package directions. Drain and rinse, then set aside.

In a large skillet heat the water; add onion (if used) and garlic. Cook over high heat for about 3 minutes, or until onion is soft. Add mushrooms and celery and continue cooking—stirring frequently—for about 5 minutes, or until the mushrooms begin to brown. Add a small amount of water if the vegetables begin to stick. Add zucchini and chopped Boca Burger patties (if used); then cook, stirring often, for about 3 minutes, or until zucchini is just tender when pierced with a fork.

Puree beans, with their liquid, in a blender or food processor. Add to the vegetable mixture, along with pasta and salt. Heat gently, stirring frequently, until hot and steamy. PER SERVING: 206 CALORIES, 10 G PROTEIN, 39 G CARBOHYDRATE, 1 G FAT, 385 MG SODIUM

May be a trigger food for some individuals.

SPINACH BARLEYCAKES
Makes 10 barleycakes

Serve these tender patties with Quick Garbanzo Gravy (page 272) and a green salad.

>2 tablespoons shelled sunflower seeds
>1 small onion*
>2 medium-size cloves garlic
>1 small carrot
>2 cups fresh mushrooms
>1 10-ounce package frozen spinach
>2 cups cooked barley (page 263)
>2 tablespoons tahini
>½–1 teaspoon salt
>Vegetable-oil spray, for skillet

Grind sunflower seeds in a food processor, then add onion (if used), garlic, carrot, and mushrooms. Grind thoroughly, then add the remaining ingredients and process for about 1 minute, or until well mixed.

Preheat a large nonstick skillet and lightly coat it with vegetable-oil spray. Form the barley mixture into patties (they will be quite soft). Cook each side over medium-high heat for about 3 minutes, or until golden brown. PER BARLEYCAKE: 71 CALORIES, 3 G PROTEIN, 13 G CARBOHYDRATE, 2 G FAT, 245 MG SODIUM

May be a trigger food for some individuals.

NEAT LOAF
Makes 10 slices

½ cup pumpkin seeds or sunflower seeds
1 medium-size onion, quartered*
1 medium-size carrot, cut into 1-inch chunks
1 medium-size green bell pepper, cut into large chunks*
1 cup sliced mushrooms
2 cups Always Great Brown Rice (page 244)
1 cup oat bran*
2 tablespoons arrowroot powder
1 teaspoon agar powder (optional, serves as a binder)
1½ tablespoons stone-ground mustard
1 tablespoon nutritional yeast (optional)
¼ teaspoon dried thyme
⅛ teaspoon each: dried sage and marjoram
⅛ teaspoon black pepper
½ teaspoon salt
Vegetable-oil spray, for pan
Barbecue sauce or ketchup, for topping*

Preheat oven to 350° F.

Grind pumpkin seeds in a food processor, then add onion (if used), carrot, bell pepper, and mushrooms. Process until chopped fine.

Transfer processed mixture to a large mixing bowl. Add all the remaining ingredients except barbecue sauce. Stir to mix. Lightly coat a 5- × 9-inch loaf pan with vegetable-oil spray. Place mixture into pan, patting into place. Top with barbecue sauce. Bake for 50 minutes. Let stand for 10 minutes before serving.

Variation. To make Neat Burgers instead of Neat Loaf, form individual patties about 3 inches in diameter and ½ inch thick. Cook in a large vegetable oil–sprayed or nonstick skillet for about 4 minutes per side, or until lightly browned. PER SLICE: 141 CALORIES, 4 G PROTEIN, 20 G CARBOHYDRATE, 5 G FAT, 141 MG SODIUM

May be a trigger food for some individuals.

LENTIL BURGERS

Makes eight 3-inch burgers

1 small onion, chopped*
½ cup short-grain brown rice
½ cup lentils
¾ teaspoon salt
2 cups water
1 small carrot
1 medium-size stalk celery
2 teaspoons stone-ground mustard
1 teaspoon garlic powder
Vegetable-oil spray, for skillet

In a medium-size saucepan combine onion (if used), rice, lentils, salt, and the water. Bring to a slow simmer, then cover and cook for about 50 minutes, or until rice and lentils are tender and all the water has been absorbed.

Chop carrot and celery until fine (a food processor makes this easy). Add them to the hot lentil mixture, along with the remaining ingredients. Stir to mix, then chill completely. (You can make the patties while the mixture is still warm, but forming is much easier once it is chilled.)

Form mixture into 2- to 3-inch patties. Lightly coat a large nonstick skillet with vegetable-oil spray. Cook patties over medium heat for about 4 minutes per side, or until lightly browned. PER BURGER: 85 CALORIES, 3 G PROTEIN, 17 G CARBOHYDRATE, 0 G FAT, 223 MG SODIUM

*May be a trigger food for some individuals.

POTATO BOATS
Serves 4

These are delicious as is, or top them with Black-Bean Sauce (page 272) or Quick Garbanzo Gravy (page 272).

> 4 medium-size russet potatoes*
> 2 medium-size stalks broccoli (about 1 pound)
> 1 tablespoon tahini
> 1 tablespoon lemon juice*
> ½ teaspoon garlic powder
> ¼ teaspoon salt
> ⅛ teaspoon black pepper
> Black-Bean Sauce or Quick Garbanzo Gravy (optional)

Scrub potatoes, then steam them for about 30 minutes, or until tender when pierced with a fork.

Cut or break broccoli tops into florets. Peel the stems with a sharp knife and slice them into ½-inch-thick rounds. Steam florets and rounds over boiling water for about 5 minutes, or until bright green and just tender when pierced with a fork. Place in a food processor fitted with a metal blade; chop fine.

When potatoes are cool enough to handle, carefully cut them in half and scoop out the flesh, leaving a ¼-inch-thick shell. Add the flesh to the food processor along with tahini, lemon juice (if used), garlic, salt, and pepper. Process until smooth.

Use a large spoon to distribute the filling evenly among the shells. Top with Black-Bean Sauce, if used. PER POTATO: 273 CALORIES, 6 G PROTEIN, 57 G CARBOHYDRATE, 2 G FAT, 183 MG SODIUM

*May be a trigger food for some individuals.

BLACK-BEAN TAMALE PIE
Serves 8

¾ cup water
1 medium-size onion, chopped*
2 medium-size cloves garlic, minced
1 small bell pepper, diced fine*
½ cup crushed tomato or tomato sauce*
2 15-ounce cans black beans, including liquid
1 4-ounce can diced chiles*
½ teaspoon ground cumin
½ cup soymilk or rice milk (use rice milk if soy is a trigger for you)
2 teaspoons vinegar
1 tablespoon olive oil*
1 cup cornmeal*
¼ teaspoon salt
½ teaspoon baking soda

In a large skillet or pot, heat ½ cup of the water. Add onion (if used), garlic, and pepper (if used). Cook over high heat—stirring often—for about 5 minutes, or until all the water has evaporated. Stir in the remaining water, scraping the pan to remove any stuck bits of onion. Add tomato (if used), beans with their liquid, chiles (if used), and cumin. Stir to mix. Simmer—stirring occasionally—for 15 minutes.

Preheat the oven to 350° F.

In a medium-size bowl combine the milk, vinegar, and oil (if used). In a small bowl, mix cornmeal, salt, and baking soda. Add cornmeal mixture to milk mixture. Stir to mix completely (it will be quite stiff and crumbly).

Transfer bean mixture to a 9- × 9-inch baking dish, then spread cornmeal mixture evenly over the top. Bake for about 25 minutes, or until the crust is set and the bean mixture is hot and bubbly. PER SERVING: 147 CALORIES, 6 G PROTEIN, 25 G CARBOHYDRATE, 3 G FAT, 256 MG SODIUM

May be a trigger food for some individuals.

SIMPLE BLACK-EYED STEW
Makes 6 cups

This easy-to-prepare stew is real comfort food.

> 1½ cups dried black-eyed peas
> 6 cups cold water
> 2 teaspoons olive oil*
> 2 medium-size onions, chopped*
> 4 medium-size cloves garlic, minced
> 2 medium-size stalks celery, sliced
> ½ cup uncooked short-grain brown rice
> 1 medium-size bunch cilantro, chopped
> ¼–½ teaspoon red pepper flakes*
> 4 cups water
> 1 teaspoon salt (or less, to taste)
> Sesame Salt, for serving (page 298)

Rinse peas. In a large bowl soak them overnight in the 6 cups water.

In a large pot gently heat oil, if used. Add onion (if used), garlic, and celery. Cook over high heat—stirring often—for about 3 minutes, or until onion is soft. Add a tablespoon or two of water if the mixture begins to stick.

Drain peas and add them to the pot, along with rice, cilantro, pepper flakes (if used), and the 4 cups water. Bring to a simmer. Cover and cook for about 45 minutes, or until beans and rice are tender. Add the 1 teaspoon salt.

To serve: Ladle some stew into a small bowl and sprinkle with Sesame Salt.

Variation. For a one-dish meal, top the stew with a generous serving of Braised Kale or Collard Greens (page 245). PER 1-CUP SERVING: 192 CALORIES, 8 G PROTEIN, 34 G CARBOHYDRATE, 2 G FAT, 374 MG SODIUM

*May be a trigger food for some individuals.

NOTE: *If oil is a trigger for you, saute the onion, garlic, and celery in ½ cup water for 5 minutes.*

ALMOST-INSTANT
BLACK-BEAN CHILI

Makes 6 cups

This is a perfect make-ahead recipe, since this chili is even better the second day.

½ cup water
1 medium-size onion, chopped*
2 medium-size cloves garlic, minced
1 small bell pepper, diced fine*
½ cup crushed tomatoes or tomato sauce*
2 15-ounce cans black beans, including liquid
1 4-ounce can diced chiles*
1 teaspoon ground cumin

In a large skillet or pot, heat the water. Add onion (if used), garlic, and pepper (if used). Cook over high heat—stirring often—for about 5 minutes or until onion is translucent. Add remaining ingredients and simmer—stirring occasionally—for about 15 minutes or until flavors are blended. PER 1-CUP SERVING: 94 CALORIES, 6 G PROTEIN, 17 G CARBOHYDRATE, 0 G FAT, 188 MG SODIUM

May be a trigger food for some individuals.

PAN-GRILLED
PORTOBELLO MUSHROOMS

Serves 4

Serve with Wild Brown Rice (page 239) and Braised Kale or Collard Greens (page 245).

4 large portobello mushrooms
2 teaspoons olive oil*
2 tablespoons red wine*
2 tablespoons soy sauce*
1 tablespoon balsamic vinegar
2 medium-size cloves garlic, minced

Clean mushrooms and trim the stems flush with the bottoms of the caps. In a large skillet mix the remaining ingredients. Heat until the mixture begins to bubble; add mushrooms, tops down. Reduce to medium heat. Cover and cook for about 3 minutes, or until tops are browned. (If the pan becomes dry, add 2 to 3 tablespoons of water.) Turn the mushrooms and cook for about 5 minutes more, or until tender when pierced with a sharp knife. Serve hot. PER MUSHROOM: 75 CALORIES, 4.5 G PROTEIN, 12 G CARBOHYDRATE, 1 G FAT, 310 MG SODIUM

May be a trigger food for some individuals.

QUICK BEAN BURRITOS
Makes 4 burritos

Burritos make a quick, tasty, and very portable meal that can be eaten hot or cold. Fat-free refried beans are available in most markets. A growing number of markets also carry fat-free flour tortillas.

> 4 flour tortillas (preferably fat-free)*
> 1 15-ounce can fat-free refried beans, heated
> 1 cup shredded romaine lettuce
> 1 medium-size tomato, sliced*
> 2 medium-size green onions, sliced*
> ¼ medium-size avocado, sliced (optional)
> ½ cup salsa*

In a large, ungreased skillet heat a tortilla until it is warm and soft. Spread about ½ cup of beans down the center of the tortilla, then top with lettuce. Add tomato and onions (if used), avocado, and salsa (if used). Fold the bottom end toward the center, then roll the tortilla around the filling. Repeat with remaining tortillas. PER BURRITO: 234 CALORIES, 10 G PROTEIN, 40 G CARBOHYDRATE, 3 G FAT, 280 MG SODIUM

May be a trigger food for some individuals.

NOTE: *For even heartier burritos, add ½ cup of Always Great Brown Rice (page 244) per burrito.*

RICE AND BEANS WITH GREENS
Serves 8

If you enjoy simple, down-home food, you'll love this combination of seasoned pinto beans served with brown rice and lightly steamed kale.

BEANS
1½ cups dry pinto beans
6 cups cold water
4 cups water
4 large cloves garlic, minced
1½ teaspoons cumin seed (or 1 teaspoon ground cumin)
¾ teaspoon salt

Rinse beans. In a large pot soak beans overnight in the 6 cups water. Drain and rinse beans, then place them in a large pot with the 4 cups water, garlic, and cumin seed. Simmer for about 1 hour, or until tender. Add salt.

RICE
4 cups water
1 cup brown rice
½ teaspoon salt

In a large pot bring the water to a boil. Add rice and salt. Cover loosely and simmer for about 40 minutes, or until tender. Pour off excess water.

GREENS
1 medium-size bunch kale or collard greens (6–8 cups chopped)
½ cup water
2 teaspoons balsamic vinegar
¼ teaspoon salt
2–3 medium-size cloves garlic, minced

Wash greens, remove the stems, and chop the leaves into ½-inch-wide strips. In a large pot heat the water. Add vinegar, salt, and garlic. Cook 1 minute. Stir in greens. Cover and cook over medium heat for 3 to 5 minutes, or until tender.

To serve: Place a generous portion of rice on each plate, then top with some beans with their liquid. Serve kale on top of beans or to the side. PER 1½ CUP SERVING: 233 CALORIES, 9 G PROTEIN, 46 G CARBOHYDRATE, 1 G FAT, 432 MG SODIUM

May be a trigger food for some individuals.

BROCCOLI BURRITOS
Makes 6 burritos

The king of vegetables gets royal treatment in this recipe!

    1 medium-size bunch broccoli (about 2 cups)
    1 15-ounce can garbanzo beans, drained
    ½ cup roasted red peppers*
    2 tablespoons tahini
    3 tablespoons lemon juice*
    6 flour tortillas*
    6 tablespoons salsa (more or less, to taste)*

Cut or break broccoli into bite-size florets. Peel the stalks and cut them into ½-inch-thick rounds. Steam broccoli over boiling water for about 5 minutes, or until just barely tender when pierced with a fork.

Place beans in a food processor with peppers (if used), tahini, and lemon juice (if used). Process until smooth.

Preheat a large skillet. Spread about ¼ cup of bean mixture on a tortilla and place it face up in the skillet. Heat tortilla for about 2 minutes, or until it is warm and soft.

Spread a line of broccoli down the center of the tortilla and sprinkle it with salsa (if used). Fold the bottom of the tortilla up. Then, starting on one side, roll the tortilla around the broccoli. Repeat with remaining tortillas. PER BURRITO: 244 CALORIES, 9 G PROTEIN, 39 G CARBOHYDRATE, 5 G FAT, 130 MG SODIUM

May be a trigger food for some individuals.

NORI ROLLS

Makes 3 rolls

Vegetarian sushi, or nori rolls, make a delicious, portable meal or snack.

> 3 cups water
> 1 cup short-grain brown rice
> ¼ teaspoon salt
> ¼ cup seasoned rice vinegar
> 4 sheets nori
> 1 cup grated carrot
> 1 cup grated cucumber
> 1 cup grated baked tofu (optional)*
> ¼ medium-size avocado, sliced thin (optional)
> ¼ cup (approximately) pickled ginger

In a medium-size saucepan place the water, rice, and salt. Cover and bring to a simmer, then cook for about 1 hour, or until rice is very tender and all the water has been absorbed. Cool.

Stir in vinegar.

Set aside.

To assemble the rolls: Place a sheet of nori on a bamboo sushi mat. Spread about 1 cup of rice in a thin, even layer on the sheet, leaving uncovered a 1-inch band along the top of the sheet.

Arrange about ¼ cup each of carrot, cucumber, and tofu (if used) across the center of the rice, from edge to edge of the roll. Top with slices of avocado (if used) and pickled ginger.

To form the roll: Holding the filling ingredients in place with your fingertips, use your thumbs to lift the bottom edge of the mat so that the nori edge nearest you is lifted over to meet the top edge of the rice. Use the uncovered portion of the nori as a flap to seal the roll. Use your hands to gently shape the roll, then let it sit on its seam to seal.

If bite-size pieces are desired, use a sharp, wet knife to cut the roll crosswise; clean the knife between cuts. PER ROLL (WITH TOFU AND AVOCADO): 318 CALORIES, 13 G PROTEIN, 49 G CARBOHYDRATE, 7 G FAT, 452 MG SODIUM PER ROLL (WITHOUT TOFU AND AVOCADO): 207 CALORIES, 4 G PROTEIN, 46 G CARBOHYDRATE, 1 G FAT, 324 MG SODIUM

May be a trigger food for some individuals.

QUICK VEGETABLE CURRY
Serves 4

You can whip this tasty, colorful curry together in a flash. It is especially good served with brown basmati rice.

    ½ cup water
    1 tablespoon soy sauce*
    1 medium-size onion, chopped*
    3 medium-size cloves garlic, minced
    2 cups sliced mushrooms
    2 medium-size carrots, sliced on the diagonal
    2 medium-size stalks celery, sliced on the diagonal
    ½ pound firm tofu, cut in ½-inch cubes*
    1 medium-size red bell pepper, diced*
    2 cups kale, chopped fine
    2 teaspoons curry powder
    1 tablespoon peanut butter*
    1 tablespoon seasoned rice vinegar

In a large skillet heat the water and soy sauce (if used) to a simmer. Add onion (if used) and garlic. Cook for about 5 minutes, or until onion is soft.

Add mushrooms, carrots, and celery; cook for about 5 minutes—stirring occasionally—or until carrots just begin to soften.

Gently stir in tofu, pepper, and kale. Add curry powder. Cover and cook—stirring occasionally—for about 5 minutes, or until kale is tender.

In a small bowl combine peanut butter (if used) and vinegar. Stir into the vegetable mixture. PER SERVING: 168 CALORIES, 10 G PROTEIN, 22 G CARBOHYDRATE, 4 G FAT, 292 MG SODIUM

May be a trigger food for some individuals.

STRAWBERRY SMOOTHIE
Makes about 2 cups

Try this cold, thick smoothie with whole grain cereal or muffins for a delicious and satisfying breakfast. Buy frozen strawberries or freeze fresh ones. To freeze bananas, peel and break into pieces, pack loosely in an airtight container, and freeze.

> 1 cup frozen strawberries
> 1 frozen medium-size banana, cut into 1-inch pieces*
> ½–1 cup vanilla rice milk

Place all ingredients in a blender. Blend at high speed until smooth. (You'll have to stop the blender occasionally and move the unblended fruit to the center with a spatula to get your smoothie smooth.) PER 1-CUP SERV-ING: 105 CALORIES, 1 G PROTEIN, 23 G CARBOHYDRATE, 1 G FAT, 24 MG SODIUM

May be a trigger food for some individuals.

BANANA CAKE
Serves 9

> 2 cups whole wheat pastry flour*
> 2 teaspoons baking soda
> ½ teaspoon salt
> 1 cup wheat germ*
> 4 ripe medium-size bananas, mashed (about 2½ cups)*
> ½ cup sugar
> ¾ cup soymilk or rice milk (use rice milk if soy is a trigger food for
>   you)
> 1 teaspoon vanilla extract
> ⅛ cup raisins or dates
> Vegetable-oil spray, for pan

Preheat the oven to 350° F.

In a medium-size bowl mix whole wheat pastry flour, baking soda, salt, and wheat germ. In a large bowl, mash bananas and mix in sugar. Mix in soymilk and vanilla. Add the flour mixture, along with raisins; stir to mix. Lightly coat a 9- × 9-inch pan with vegetable-oil spray; spread batter in the pan. Bake for about 55 minutes, or until a toothpick inserted in the center comes out clean. PER SERVING: 220 CALORIES, 5 G PROTEIN, 47 G CARBOHYDRATE, 1 G FAT, 301 MG SODIUM

May be a trigger food for some individuals.

OATMEAL COOKIES
Makes about twelve 4-inch cookies

⅛ cup plain or vanilla rice milk
⅛ cup maple syrup
4 teaspoons apple cider vinegar
2 teaspoons vanilla extract
1 cup rolled oats*
1 cup barley flour*
1 teaspoon cinnamon
1 teaspoon baking powder
¼ teaspoon baking soda
¼ teaspoon salt
½ cup raisins, chopped coarse
½ cup chopped walnuts*
Vegetable-oil spray, for cookie sheet

Preheat oven to 350° F.

In a small bowl or measuring cup, mix rice milk, syrup, vinegar, and vanilla.

In a large bowl, mix rolled oats, barley flour, cinnamon, baking powder, baking soda, and salt. Add rice milk mixture, along with raisins and walnuts; mix completely.

Lightly coat a cookie sheet with vegetable-oil spray. Drop tablespoons of dough onto the sheet and flatten dough slightly with the back of the spoon. Bake 15 to 20 minutes, or until the bottoms are lightly browned. PER COOKIE: 240 CALORIES, 5 G PROTEIN, 47 G CARBOHYDRATE, 4 G FAT, 354 MG SODIUM

May be a trigger food for some individuals.

FRESH PEACH SHORTCAKE
Makes 6 servings

1 batch Barley Scones (page 258)*
3 medium-size fresh peaches or nectarines, sliced

Cut scones in half. Top with peach slices. PER SERVING: 240 CALORIES, 5 G PRO-
TEIN, 47 G CARBOHYDRATE, 4 G FAT, 354 MG SODIUM

May be a trigger food for some individuals.

FRESH STRAWBERRY SHORTCAKE
Makes 6 servings

1 batch Barley Scones (page 258)*
3 cups fresh strawberries, sliced

Cut scones in half. Top with strawberry slices. PER SERVING: 244 CALORIES,
5 G PROTEIN, 44 G CARBOHYDRATE, 4 G FAT, 355 MG SODIUM

May be a trigger food for some individuals.

FRUIT CREME
Serves 4

2 cups boysenberry-apple juice
10½ ounces firm or extra-firm silken tofu*
¼ cup plus 1 tablespoon maple syrup
1½ teaspoons agar
1 tablespoon arrowroot powder
2 tablespoons lemon juice*
2 tablespoons white grape juice concentrate
1½ teaspoons vanilla extract
¼ teaspoon salt

Place juice and tofu in a blender. Blend until completely smooth. Transfer blended mixture to a medium-size pan and stir in syrup, agar, and
arrowroot. Bring to a simmer; then cook—stirring frequently—for about

5 minutes, or until slightly thickened. Remove from heat and stir in the remaining ingredients. Pour into 4 serving dishes and chill completely.

PER SERVING: 179 CALORIES, 5 G PROTEIN, 35 G CARBOHYDRATE, 2 G FAT, 175 MG SODIUM

May be a trigger food for some individuals.

SUMMER FRUIT COBBLER
Serves 9

3 cups fresh peach slices (if desired, peel before slicing)
3 cups fresh strawberries
¾ cup white grape juice concentrate or apple juice concentrate
1 teaspoon arrowroot powder
¼ cup plain or vanilla rice milk
2 tablespoons maple syrup
1 tablespoon sunflower or canola oil
2 teaspoons vinegar
1 cup plus 3 tablespoons barley flour*
¼ teaspoon baking soda
1 teaspoon baking powder
¼ teaspoon salt
Barley flour, for dusting

Preheat oven to 350° F.

In a large saucepan combine peaches, strawberries, white grape juice concentrate, and arrowroot. Bring to a simmer and cook for about 5 minutes, or until the fruits just become soft and the liquid thickens slightly. Transfer mixture to a 9- × 9-inch baking dish.

In a small bowl mix rice milk, syrup, oil, and vinegar. Set aside.

In a medium-size bowl combine barley flour, baking soda, baking powder, and salt. Add the rice milk mixture; stir until a ball of dough forms. Transfer dough to a flat surface that has been dusted with barley flour. With your hands or a rolling pin, flatten the dough to a thickness of about ¼ inch. Cover the top of the fruit with the dough (doing this is easy if you cut the dough into a few pieces). Bake for about 30 minutes, or until the top is slightly browned and firm. PER SERVING: 213 CALORIES, 4 G PROTEIN, 41 G CARBOHYDRATE, 3 G FAT, 241 MG SODIUM

May be a trigger food for some individuals.

INDIAN PUDDING
Makes 3 cups

½ cup corn meal or masa harina*
2 cups water
1 15-ounce can corn, including liquid*
⅛ cup maple syrup
¼ teaspoon salt
¼ teaspoon cinnamon
¼ teaspoon ginger

In a medium saucepan combine cornmeal and the water. Stir until smooth.
     Puree corn, with its liquid, in a blender. Add puree to the cornmeal; stir. Bring to a simmer, then cook—stirring almost constantly—for about 10 minutes, or until thickened. Stir in the remaining ingredients, then transfer pudding to serving bowls. Serve warm or chilled. PER ½-CUP SERVING: 164 CALORIES, 3 G PROTEIN, 36 G CARBOHYDRATE, 1 G FAT, 104 MG SODIUM

May be a trigger food for some individuals.

SESAME SALT
Makes ¹/₂ cup

Sesame salt is delicious sprinkled on cooked vegetables, salads, soups, and baked potatoes. Unhulled sesame seeds (sometimes called brown sesame seeds) are sold in natural food stores and specialty shops.

½ cup unhulled sesame seeds
½ teaspoon salt

In a small dry skillet over medium heat, toast sesame seeds; stir constantly for about 5 minutes, or until seeds begin to pop and brown slightly. Transfer seeds to a blender, add salt, and grind for about 30 seconds into a uniform powder. PER 1 TABLESPOON: 54 CALORIES, 1.5 G PROTEIN, 2.5 G CARBOHYDRATE, 4 G FAT, 134 MG SODIUM

SESAME SEASONING
Makes ¼ cup

Nutritional yeast adds a cheeselike flavor to Sesame Salt.

> ¼ cup Sesame Salt (see preceding recipe)
> 1 tablespoon nutritional yeast flakes

In a small container stir Sesame Salt and nutritional yeast flakes. Store in an airtight container. PER TABLESPOON: 58 CALORIES, 2 G PROTEIN, 3 G CARBOHYDRATE, 4 G FAT, 137 MG SODIUM

ABOUT BAKING POWDER

Most commercial baking powder is made with cornstarch. A few brands are made with potato starch. Below are two recipes: One is corn-free and one is corn-free as well as potato-free. Both work equally well.

To be effective, baking powder must be kept absolutely free of moisture, so store it in an airtight container. If you have kept it for some time, test to make sure it is still active by mixing a teaspoon or two with a small amount of water. Vigorous bubbles will appear if the baking powder is still viable.

CORN-FREE BAKING POWDER
Makes 1 cup

> ½ cup cream of tartar
> ¼ cup baking soda
> ¼ cup potato starch or potato flour

In a small bowl combine all ingredients, then sift the mixture 3 times. Store in an airtight container. PER TEASPOON: 3 CALORIES, 0 G PROTEIN, 1 G CARBOHYDRATE, 0 G FAT, 205 MG SODIUM

CORN-FREE, POTATO-FREE BAKING POWDER

Makes about 1 cup

½ cup cream of tartar
¼ cup baking soda
¼ cup arrowroot powder

In a small bowl combine all ingredients, then sift the mixture 3 times. Store in an airtight container. PER TEASPOON: 3 CALORIES, 0 G PROTEIN, 1 G CARBOHYDRATE, 0 G FAT, 205 MG SODIUM

INGREDIENTS THAT MAY
BE NEW TO YOU

Most ingredients in the recipes are widely available in grocery stores. A few that may be unfamiliar are described below.

Agar powder—a sea vegetable used as a thickener and gelling agent instead of gelatin, which is a slaughterhouse by-product. Available in natural food stores and Asian markets. May also be called *agar agar*.

Apple juice concentrate—frozen apple juice concentrate works well as a sweetener in many dishes. Thaw slightly to measure. The remainder may be refrozen.

Arrowroot powder—a natural thickener that looks like cornstarch and may be substituted for it in many recipes. Sold in natural food stores.

Baking powder—may contain cornstarch or potato starch. Check the label. For corn- and potato-free baking powder, see recipe on page 300.

Balsamic vinegar—mellow-flavored wine vinegar that is delicious in salad dressings and marinades. Available in most food stores.

Barley flour—a light-textured flour that may be used in place of wheat in many baked goods. Contains gluten.

Basmati rice—an especially flavorful long-grain rice, delicious plain or in pilafs. Look for brown basmati rice in natural food stores.

Boca Burgers—a fat-free vegetarian burger with a meaty taste and texture, available in natural food stores, usually in the freezer case.

Brown rice—fuller flavored and more nutritionally complete than white rice. Long-grain varieties tend to be somewhat lighter textured than short-grain varieties.

Buckwheat groats—untoasted buckwheat kernels, which cook quickly and have a fairly mild flavor. Use as a breakfast cereal or as a side dish. Since buckwheat is not actually a wheat, it contains no gluten.

Carob powder (flour)—looks somewhat like cocoa and is often promoted as a substitute for chocolate, but its flavor, which is delicious in its own right, is

301

very different. Carob does not have the bitterness of chocolate and thus requires less sweetening.

Diced green chiles—refers to diced Anaheim chiles, which are mildly hot. These are available canned (Ortega is a common brand) or fresh. When using fresh chiles, remove skin by charring it under a broiler and rubbing it off.

Ener-G Rice Mix—a wheat-free, gluten-free baking mix made from rice. It is useful for making gluten-free pancakes, muffins, and other baked goods. Available in natural food stores, or check the resource list on pages 335–336.

Garbanzo flour—has a pleasant, slightly sweet flavor, excellent for flatbread or tortillas. Sold in natural food stores.

Garlic granules—granulated form of garlic powder. Granules remain free-flowing.

Gluten-free pasta—made from rice, corn, buckwheat, Jerusalem artichokes, or other nonglutinous grains. Usually sold in natural food stores.

Instant bean flakes—precooked black or pinto beans. Can be reconstituted quickly with boiling water and used as a side dish, dip, sauce, or burrito filling. Fantastic Foods and Taste Adventure are two brands that are available in natural food stores and some supermarkets.

Italian seasoning—a commercially prepared mixture of commonly used Italian herbs.

Jicama—"hick-ama." Jicama is a delicious root vegetable that is a crisp, slightly sweet addition to salads. Usually sold in the unrefrigerated area of the supermarket produce section.

Kasha—buckwheat groats that have been toasted to bring out the full buckwheat flavor.

Masa harina—cornmeal processed with lime and water to enhance its flavor and calcium content. Commonly used for making corn tortillas. Sold in most supermarkets.

Mochi—a dense cake of sweet brown rice sold in natural food stores.

Natural fruit preserves—preserves, jams, and jellies made with just fruit and fruit juice—no granulated sugar.

Nori—a sea vegetable used for wrapping sushi. Sold in natural food stores and Asian markets.

Nutritional yeast—yeast produced specifically to provide nutrition, including protein and some B vitamins. Certain brands are a source of vitamin B_{12}. Sold in natural food stores. Do not confuse with baking yeast.

Poultry seasoning—a commercial blend of marjoram, sage, and thyme. Sold in supermarkets.

Prune puree—can be used in place of fat (eggs and some or all oil) in baked goods. Commercial brands are WonderSlim and Lekvar. Prune baby food or pureed stewed prunes may also be used. Also called prune butter.

Quinoa—looks and cooks like a grain, though it is actually a member of the beet family. Its light, fluffy texture makes it an excellent choice for side dishes and salads.

Red pepper flakes—dried, crushed chile peppers. At the supermarket, available in the spice section or with the Mexican foods.

Reduced-sodium soy sauce—see Soy sauce.

Rice bread—yeast-raised bread made with rice flour. Sold in natural food stores. Be sure to read the label to see what other ingredients are used.

Rice milk—beverage made from partially fermented rice. Can be used in place of dairy milk on cereal and in most recipes. Comes in a variety of flavors, including plain (also called original), vanilla, and chocolate. Some brands are fortified with calcium and vitamin D. Available in natural food stores and some supermarkets. One widely distributed brand is Rice Dream.

Roasted red peppers—roasted red bell peppers. Add great flavor and color to a variety of dishes. Roast your own or purchase them already roasted and packed in water. Available in most grocery stores, usually near the pickles.

Salad mix—mixture of lettuce, spinach, and other salad ingredients. All ingredients have been cleaned and dried. They store well and make salad preparation a snap. Several different mixes are available in the produce department of most foodstores. Spring mix is particularly flavorful.

Seasoned rice vinegar—mild vinegar seasoned with sugar and salt. Great for salad dressings and on cooked vegetables. Available in most grocery stores, with other vinegars or in the Asian foods section.

Silken tofu—smooth, delicate tofu excellent for sauces, cream soups, and dips. Often available in special packaging that allows storage without refrigeration for up to a year. Refrigerate after opening. One popular brand, Mori-Nu, is available in most grocery stores. Ask for the reduced-fat, "lite" variety.

Soymilk—made from soybeans. Use as a beverage, on cereal, or as a substitute for dairy milk and cream in most recipes. Available in regular, low-fat, fat-free, and calcium-fortified varieties. Sold in natural food stores and many supermarkets.

Soy sauce—made from soybeans, salt, water, and sometimes wheat. Adds saltiness as well as flavor to foods. **Tamari,** a naturally fermented variety sold in natural food stores, is usually made without wheat, but be sure to check the label if wheat is something you want to avoid. Commercial varieties sold in supermarkets often contain caramel color, derived from corn, and they may also contain corn syrup. **Lite soy sauce:** Soy sauce with a lower than usual amount of sodium. Compare labels to find the brand with the smallest amount. Also called reduced-sodium soy sauce.

Tahini—sesame seed butter, often used in Middle Eastern cooking. Available raw and toasted; toasted varieties have a slightly nuttier flavor.

Tamari—naturally fermented, usually wheat-free soy sauce. Check the label to be sure a specific product is wheat-free.

Tofu—see Silken tofu.

White grape concentrate—frozen white grape juice concentrate. May be used as a sweetener in many dishes. Keep frozen; thaw slightly to measure. The remainder may be refrozen.

Whole wheat pastry flour—milled from soft spring wheat. Contains wheat bran and wheat germ and produces lighter textured baked goods than does regular whole wheat flour. Available in natural food stores.

Notes

PREFACE

1. Wipf JE, Deyo RA. Low back pain. *Med Clin N Am* 1995;79:231–46.
2. Long DM, BenDebba M, Torgerson WS, et al. Persistent back pain and sciatica in the United States: patient characteristics. *J Spinal Disorders* 1996; 9:40–58.

1. OH, MY ACHING BACK!

1. Long DM, BenDebba M, Torgerson WS, et al. Persistent back pain and sciatica in the United States: patient characteristics. *J Spinal Disorders* 1996;9:40–58.
2. Borenstein D. Epidemiology, etiology, diagnostic evaluation, and treatment of low back pain. *Curr Op Rheumatol* 1995;7:141–46.
3. Indahl A, Velund L, Reikeraas O. Good prognosis for low back pain when left untampered: a randomized clinical trial. *Spine* 1995;20:473–77.
4. Kirkaldy-Willis WH, Wedge JH, Yong-Hing K, Reilly J. Pathology and pathogenesis of lumbar spondylosis and stenosis. Spine 1978;3:319–28.
5. Garfin SR. A 50-year-old woman with disabling spinal stenosis. *JAMA* 1995;274:1949–54.
6. Freemont AJ, Peacock TE, Goupille P, Hoyland JA, O'Brien J, Jayson MIV. Nerve ingrowth into diseased intervertebral disc in chronic back pain. *Lancet* 1997;350:178–81.
7. Hollingworth P. Back pain in children. *Br J Rheumatol* 1996;35:1022–28.
8. Silman AJ, Ferry S, Papageorgiou AC, Jayson MIV, Croft PR. Number of children as a risk factor for low back pain in men and women. *Arth Rheum* 1995;38:1232–35.
9. Finkelstein MM. Back pain and parenthood. *Occup Environ Med* 1995;52:51–53.
10. Wipf JE, Deyo RA. Low back pain. *Med Clin N Am* 1995;79:231–46.
11. Dreisinger TE, Nelson B. Management of back pain in athletes. *Sports Med* 1996;21:313–20.

12. Wilkinson MJB. Does 48 hours' bed rest influence the outcome of acute low back pain. *Br J Gen Pract* 1995;45:481–84.

13. Kauppila LI. Can low-back pain be due to lumbar-artery disease? *Lancet* 1995;346:888–89.

14. Vihert AM. Atherosclerosis of the aorta in five towns. Chapter 2. *Bull Wld Health Org* 1976;53:501–8.

15. Kauppila LI, Penttilä A, Karhunen PJ, Lalu K, Hannikainen P. Lumbar disc degeneration and atherosclerosis of the abdominal aorta. *Spine* 1994; 19:923–29.

16. Svensson HO, Vedin A, Wilhelmsson C, Andersson GBJ. Low-back pain in relation to other diseases and cardiovascular risk factors. *Spine* 1983; 8:277–85.

17. Deyo RA, Bass JE. Lifestyle and low-back pain: the influence of smoking and obesity. *Spine* 1989;14:501–6.

18. Ernst E. Smoking, a cause of back trouble? *Br J Rheumatol* 1993;32:239–42.

19. Huang C, Ross PD, Wasnich RD. Vertebral fractures and other predictors of back pain among older women. *J Bone Miner Res* 1996;11:1026–32.

20. Kelsey JL, Githens PB, O'Connor T, et al. Acute prolapsed lumbar intervertebral disc: an epidemiologic study with special reference to driving automobiles and cigarette smoking. *Spine* 1984;9:608–13.

21. Zimmermann M, Bartoszyk GD, Bonke D, Jurna I, Wild A. Antinociceptive properties of pyridoxine: neurophysiological and behavioral findings. *Ann MY Acad Sci* 1990;585:219–30.

22. Schwieger G, Karl H, Schonhaber E. Relapse prevention of painful vertebral syndromes in follow-up treatment with a combination of vitamins B_1, B_6, and B_{12}. *Ann NY Acad Sci* 1990;585:540–42.

23. Sternbach RA, Janowsky DS, Huey LY, Segal DS. Effects of altering brain serotonin activity on human chronic pain. *Adv in Pain Res Ther* 1996;1:601–6.

24. Seltzer S, Stoch R, Marcus R, Jackson E. Alteration of human pain thresholds by nutritional manipulation and L-tryptophan supplementation. *Pain* 1982;13:35–93.

25. Srivastava KC, Mustafa T. Ginger *(Zingiber officinale)* in rheumatism and musculoskeletal disorders. *Med Hypoth* 1992;39:342–48.

26. Remer T, Manz F. Estimation of the renal net acid excretion by adults consuming diets containing variable amounts of protein. *Am Clin Nutr* 1994;59:1356–61.

27. Nordin BEC, Need AG, Morris HA, Horowitz M. The nature and significance of the relationship between urinary sodium and urinary calcium in women. *J Nutr* 1993;123:1615–22.

28. Massey LK, Whiting SJ. Caffeine, urinary calcium, calcium metabolism and bone. *J Nutr* 1993;123:1611–14.
29. Hopper JL, Seeman E. The bone density of female twins discordant for tobacco use. *N Engl J Med* 1994;330:387–92.
30. Curhan GC, Willett WC, Speizer FE, Spiegelman D, Stampfer MJ. Comparison of dietary calcium with supplemental calcium and other nutrients as factors affecting the risk for kidney stones in women. *Ann Int Med* 1997;126:497–504.
31. Feskanich D, Willett WC, Stampfer MJ, Colditz GA. Milk, dietary calcium, and bone fractures in women: a 12-year prospective study. *Am J Publ Health* 1997;87:992–97.
32. Colditz GA, Stampfer MJ, Willett WC, et al. Type of postmenopausal hormone use and risk of breast cancer: 12-year follow-up from the Nurses' Health Study. *Cancer Causes and Control* 1992;3:433–39.
33. Lee JR. Osteoporosis reversal; the role of progesterone. *Int Clin Nutr Rev* 1990;10:384–91.
34. Peris P, Guanabens N, Monegal A, et al. Aetiology and presenting symptoms in male osteoporosis. *Br J Rheumatol* 1995;34:936–41.
35. Shekelle PG, Adams AH, Chassin MR, Hurwitz EL, Brook RH. Spinal manipulation for low-back pain. *Ann Int Med* 1992;117:590–98.
36. Meade TW, Dyer S, Browne W, Frank AO. Randomized comparison of chiropractic and hospital outpatient management for low back pain: results from extended follow up. *BMJ* 1995;311:349–51.

2. DISSOLVING CHEST PAIN, CLEANING YOUR ARTERIES

1. Roach GW, Kanchuger M, Mora Mangano C, et al. Adverse cerebral outcomes after coronary bypass surgery. *N Engl J Med* 1996;335:1857–63.
2. Ornish D, Brown SE, Scherwitz LW, et al. Can lifestyle changes reverse coronary heart disease? *Lancet* 1990;336:129–33.
3. Gould KL, Ornish D, Scherwitz L, et al. Changes in myocardial perfusion abnormalities by positron emission tomography after long-term intense risk factor modification. *JAMA* 1995;274:894–901.
4. Barnard ND, Scherwitz LW, Ornish D. Adherence and acceptability of a low-fat, vegetarian diet among patients with cardiac disease. *J Cardiopulmary Rehabil* 1992;12:423–31.
5. Lichtenstein AH, Ausman LM, Carrasco W, Jenner JL, Ordovas JM, Schae-

fer EJ. Hypercholesterolemic effect of dietary cholesterol in diets enriched in polyunsaturated and saturated fat. *Arterioscler Thromb* 1994;14:168–75.

6. Vuoristo M, Miettinen TA. Absorption, metabolism, and serum concentrations of cholesterol in vegetarians: effects of cholesterol feeding. *Am J Clin Nutr* 1994;59:1325–31.

7. Shekelle RB, Stamler J. Dietary cholesterol and ischemic heart disease. *Lancet* 1989;1:1177–79.

8. Hunninghake DB, Stein EA, Dujovne Ca. The efficacy of intensive dietary therapy alone or combined with lovastatin in outpatients with hypercholesterolemia. *N Engl J Med* 1993;328:1213–19.

9. Anderson JW, Gustafson NJ, Spencer DB, Tietyen J, Bryant CA. Serum lipid response of hypercholesterolemic men to single and divided doses of canned beans. *Am J Clin Nutr* 1990;51:1013–19.

10. Messina M, Messina V. The simple soybean and your health. Garden City Park, New York, Avery Publishing Group, 1994.

11. Bordia A. Effect of garlic on blood lipids in patients with coronary heart disease. *Am J Clin Nutr* 1981;34:2100–2103.

12. Sabate J, Fraser GE, Burke K, Knutsen SF, Bennett H, Lindsted KD. Effects of walnuts on serum lipid levels and blood pressure in normal men. *N Engl J Med* 1993;328:603–7.

13. Belcher JD, Balla J, Balla G, et al. Vitamin E, LDL, and endothelium. Brief oral vitamin supplementation prevents oxidized LDL-mediated vascular injury in vitro. *Arterioscler Thromb* 1993;13:1779–89.

14. Salonen JT, Salonen R, Nyyssonen K, Korpela H. Iron sufficiency is associated with hypertension and excess risk of myocardial infarction: the Kuopio Ischaemic Heart Disease Risk Factor Study (KIHD). *Circulation* 1992; 85:864.

15. Ascherio A, Willett WC, Rimm EB, Giovannucci EL, Stampfer MJ. Dietary iron intake and risk of coronary disease among men. *Circulation* 1994;89:969–74.

16. Stampfer MJ, Malinow MR, Willett WC, et al. A prospective study of plasma homocyst[e]ine and risk of myocardial infarction in U.S. physicians. *JAMA* 1992;268:877–81.

17. Selhub J, Jacques PF, Wilson PWF, Rush D, Rosenberg IH. Vitamin status and intake as primary determinants of homocysteinemia in an elderly population. *JAMA* 1993;270:2693–98.

18. Trout DL. Vitamin C and cardiovascular risk factors. *Am J Clin Nutr* 1991;53:322S–25S.

19. Wood PD, Stefanick ML, Dreon DM, et al. Changes in plasma lipids and lipoproteins in overweight men during weight loss through dieting as compared with exercise. *N Engl J Med* 1988;319:1173–79.

20. Castelli WP. Epidemiology of coronary heart disease. *Am J Medicine* 1984;76:4–12.
21. Hunninghake DB. Drug treatment of dyslipoprotenemia. *Endocrin Metab Clin N Am* 1990;19:345–60.
22. Stone NJ. Lipid management: current diet and drug treatment options. *Am J Med* 1996;101(suppl 4A):40S–49S.
23. Rouse IL, Beilin LJ. Editorial review: vegetarian diet and blood pressure. *J Hypertension* 1984;2:231–40.
24. Lindahl O, Lindwall L, Spangberg A, Stenram A, Ockerman PA. A vegan regimen with reduced medication in the treatment of hypertension. *Br J Nutr* 1984;52:11–20.
25. Ernst E, Pietsch L, Matrai A, Eisenberg J. Blood rheology in vegetarians. *Br J Nutr* 1986;56:555–60.

3. MIGRAINE KNOCKOUTS

1. Diener HC. A review of current treatments for migraine. *Eur Neurol* 1994;34(suppl 2):18–25.
2. Trotsky MB. Neurogenic vascular headaches, food and chemical triggers. *ENT Journal* 1994;73:228–36.
3. Hanington E. Migraine. London, Priory Press, 1974, pp. 10–11.
4. Egger J, Carter CM, Wilson J, Turner MW. Is migraine food allergy? A double-blind controlled trial of oligoantigenic diet treatment. *Lancet* 1983; 2:865–69.
5. Mansfield LE, Vaughan TR, Waller SF, Haverly RW, Ting S. Food allergy and adult migraine: double-blind and mediator confirmation of an allergic etiology. *Ann Allergy* 1985;55:126–29.
6. Vaughan TR. The role of food in the pathogenesis of migraine headache. *Clin Rev Allergy* 1994;12:167–80.
7. Vaughan TR, Mansfield LE, Haverly RW, Chamberlin WM, Waller SF. The value of cutaneous testing for food allergy in the diagnostic evaluation of migraine headache. *Ann Allergy* 1983;50:363.
8. Solomon S. Migraine diagnosis and clinical symptomatology. *Headache* 1994;34:S8–S12.
9. Littlewood JT, Gibb C, Glover V, Sandler M, Davies PTG, Rose FC. Red wine as a cause of migraine. *Lancet* 1988;1:558–59.
10. Wantke F, Gotz M, Jarisch R. The red wine provocation test: intolerance to histamine as a model for food intolerance. *Allergy Proc* 1994;15:27–32.
11. Chaytor JP, Crathorne B, Saxby MJ. The identification and significance of 2-phenylethylamine in foods. *J Sci Fd Agric* 1975;26:593–98.

12. Heatley RV, Denburg JA, Bayer N, Bienenstock J. Increased plasma histamine levels in migraine patients. *Clin Allergy* 1982;12:145–49.

13. McGee H. On food and cooking: the science and lore of the kitchen. New York, Macmillan, 1984, pp. 400–404.

14. Mansfield LE. The role of food allergy in migraine: a review. *Ann Allergy* 1987;58:313–17.

15. Steinberg M, Page R, Wolfson S, Friday G, Fireman P. Food induced late phase headache. *J Allergy Clin Immunol* 1988;81:185.

16. Hampl KF, Schneider MC, Ruttimann U, Ummenhofer W, Drewe J. Perioperative administration of caffeine tablets for prevention of postoperative headaches. *Can J Anaesth* 1995;42:789–92.

17. Silverman K, Evans SM, Strain EC, Griffiths RR. Withdrawal syndrome after the double-blind cessation of caffeine consumption. *N Engl J Med* 1992; 327:1109–14.

18. Sawynok J. Pharmacological rationale for the clinical use of caffeine. *Drugs* 1995;49:37–50.

19. Johnson ES, Kadam NP, Hylands DM, Hylands PJ. Efficacy of feverfew as prophylactic treatment of migraine. *Br Med J* 1985;291:569–73.

20. Murphy JJ, Heptinstall S, Mitchell JRA. Randomised double-blind placebo-controlled trial of feverfew in migraine prevention. *Lancet* 1988;2:189–92.

21. Groenewegen WA, Knight DW, Heptinstall S. Progress in the medicinal chemistry of the herb feverfew. *Prog Med Chem* 1992;29:217–38.

22. Mowrey DB, Clayson DE. Motion sickness, ginger, and psychophysics. *Lancet* 1982;1:655–57.

23. Grontved A, Brask T, Kambskard J, Hentzer E. Ginger root against seasickness. *Acta Otolaryngol* (Stockh) 1988;105:45–49.

24. Mustafa T, Srivastava KC. Ginger *(Zingiber officinale)* in migraine headache. *J Ethnopharmacol* 1990;29:267–73.

25. Swanson DR. Migraine and magnesium: eleven neglected connections. *Perspect Biol Med* 1988;31:526–57.

26. Weaver K. Migraine and magnesium (letter). *Perspect Biol Med* 1989; 33:150–51.

27. Seelig MS. The requirement of magnesium by the normal adult. *Am J Clin Nutr* 1964;14:342–90.

28. Abraham GE, Hargrove JT. Effect of vitamin B_6 on premenstrual symptomatology in women with premenstrual tension syndromes: a double-blind cross-over study. *Infertility* 1980;3:155–65.

29. Brush MG. Vitamin B_6 treatment of premenstrual syndrome. In Leklum JE, Reynolds RD, eds. Clinical and physiological applications of vitamin B_6. Current topics in nutrition and disease, vol. 19. New York, Alan R. Liss, 1988, pp. 363–79.

30. Somerville BW. The role of estradiol withdrawal in the etiology of menstrual migraine. *Neurology* 1972;22:355–65.

31. Dalton K. Migraine and oral contraceptives. *Headache* 1976;15:247–51.

32. Scheife RT, Hills JR. Migraine headache: signs and symptoms, biochemistry, and current therapy. *Am J Hosp Pharm* 1980;37:365–74.

33. Chen TC, Leviton A. Headache recurrence in pregnant women with migraine. *Headache* 1994;34:107–10.

34. Stewart WF, Lipton RB, Celentano DD, Reed ML. Prevalence of migraine headache in the United States. *JAMA* 1992;267:64–69.

35. Cheng XM, Ziegler DK, Li SC, Dai QS, Chandra V, Schoenberg BS. A prevalence survey of "incapacitating headache" in the People's Republic of China. *Neurology* 1986;36:831–34.

36. Wong TW, Wong KS, Yu TS, Kay R. Prevalence of migraine and other headaches in Hong Kong. *Neuroepidemiol* 1995;14:82–91.

37. Sachs H, Sevilla F, Barberis P, Bolis L, Schoenberg B, Cruz M. Headache in the rural village of Quiroga, Ecuador. *Headache* 1985;25:190–93.

38. Mitsikostas DD, Thomas A, Gatzonis S, Ilias A, Papageorgiou C. An epidemiological study of headache among the monks of Athos. *Headache* 1994; 34:539–41.

39. Singh I, Singh I, Singh D. Progesterone in the treatment of migraine. *Lancet* 1947;1:745–47.

40. Green R, Dalton K. The premenstrual syndrome. *Brit Med J* 1953; 1:1007–14.

41. Lundberg PO. Prophylactic treatment of migraine with flumedroxone. *Acta Neurol Scandinav* 1969;45:309–26.

42. Bradley WG, Hudgson P, Foster JB, Newell DJ. Double-blind controlled trial of a micronized preparation of flumedroxone (Demigran) in the prophylaxis of migraine. *Brit Med J* 1968;3:531–33.

43. Blau JN, Diamond S. Dietary factors in migraine precipitation: the physicians' view. *Headache* 1985;25:184–87.

44. Thys-Jacobs S. Vitamin D and calcium in menstrual migraine. *Headache* 1994;34:544–46.

45. Thys-Jacobs S. Alleviation of migraines with therapeutic vitamin D and calcium. *Headache* 1994;34:590–92.

46. McGrady A, Wauquier A, McNeil A, Gerard G. Effect of biofeedback-assisted relaxation on migraine headache and changes in cerebral blood flow velocity in the middle cerebral artery. *Headache* 1994;34:424–28.

47. Wilkinson M. Migraine treatment: the British perspective. *Headache* 1994;34:S13–S16.

48. Edmeads J. The diagnosis and treatment of migraine: a clinician's view. *Eur Neurol* 1994;34(suppl 2):2–5.

49. Pilgrim AJ. The clinical profile of sumatriptan: efficacy in migraine. *Eur Neurol* 1994;34(suppl 2):26–34.
50. Wilkinson M, Pfaffenrath V, Schoenen J, Diener HC, Steiner TJ. Migraine and cluster headache—their management with sumatriptan: a critical review of the current clinical experience. *Cephalalgia* 1995;15:337–57.
51. Maizels M, Scott B, Cohen W, Chen W. Intranasal lidocaine for treatment of migraine. *JAMA* 1996;276:319–21.
52. Silberstein SD. Headaches and women: treatment of the pregnant and lactating migraineur. *Headache* 1993;33:533–40.
53. Bernstein AL. Vitamin B_6 in clinical neurology. *Ann NY Acad Sci* 1990; 585:250–60.
54. Silberstein SD. Tension-type headache. *Headache* 1994;34:S2–S7.

4. FOODS FOR OTHER KINDS OF HEADACHES

1. Raskin NH. Chemical headaches. *Ann Rev Med* 1981;32:63–71.
2. Cerrato PS. Headaches? Change your diet. RN 1993;May:69–72.
3. Anonymous. Nitrates and nitrites in food. *Medical Letter* 1974;16(18):75–76.
4. Wantke F, Gotz M, Jarisch R. The red wine provocation test: intolerance to histamine as a model for food intolerance. *Allergy Proc* 1994;15:27–32.
5. Martin RW, Becker C. Headaches from chemical exposures. *Headache* 1993;33:555–59.
6. Connors MJ. Cluster headache: a review. *J Amer Osteopathic Assoc* 1995; 95:533–39.
7. Marks DR, Rapoport AM. Cluster headache syndrome. *Postgraduate Med* 1992;91:96–104.
8. Hardebo JE. How cluster headache is explained as an intracavernous inflammatory process lesioning sympathetic fibers. *Headache* 1994;34:125–31.
9. Peatfield RC. Relationships between food, wine, and beer-precipitated migrainous headaches. *Headache* 1995;35:355–57.
10. Heatley RV, Denburg JA, Bayer N, Bienenstock J. Increased plasma histamine levels in migraine patients. *Clin Allergy* 1982;12:145–49.
11. Goadsby PJ. The clinical profile of sumatriptan: cluster headache. *Eur Neurol* 1994;34(suppl 2):35–39.
12. Sicuteri F, Fusco BM, Marabini S, et al. Beneficial effect of capsaicin application to the nasal mucosa in cluster headache. *Clin J Pain* 1989;5:49–53.
13. Mansfield LE. Food allergy and headache: whom to evaluate and how to treat. *Postgraduate Med* 1988;83:46–55.
14. Silberstein SD. Tension-type headache. *Headache* 1994;34:S2–S7.

15. Castillo J, Martinez F, Leira R, Lema M, Noya M. Plasma monoamines in tension-type headache. *Headache* 1994;34:531–35.

5. COOLING YOUR JOINTS

1. Williams R. Rheumatoid arthritis and food: a case study. *BMJ* 1981;283:563.
2. Kjeldsen-Kragh J, Haugen M, Borchgrevink CF, et al. Controlled trial of fasting and one-year vegetarian diet in rheumatoid arthritis. *Lancet* 1991; 338:899–902.
3. Hicklin JA, McEwen LM, Morgan JE. The effect of diet in rheumatoid arthritis. *Clin Allergy* 1980;10:463.
4. Panush RS, Carter RL, Katz P, Kowsari B, Longley S, Finnie S. Diet therapy for rheumatoid arthritis. *Arth Rheum* 1983;26:462–71.
5. Skoldstam L. Fasting and vegan diet in rheumatoid arthritis. *Scand J Rheumatol* 1986;15:219–23.
6. Kjeldsen-Kragh J, Haugen M, Borchgrevink CF, Forre O. Vegetarian diet for patients with rheumatoid arthritis—status: two years after introduction of the diet. *Clin Rheum* 1994;13:475–82.
7. Ratner D, Eshel E, Vigder K. Juvenile rheumatoid arthritis and milk allergy. *J Royal Soc Med* 1985;78:410–13.
8. Leventhal LJ, Boyce EG, Zurier RB. Treatment of rheumatoid arthritis with gamma-linolenic acid. *Ann Int Med* 1993;119:867–73.
9. Pullman-Moor S, Laposata M, Lem D, et al. Alteration of the cellular fatty acid profile and the production of eicosanoids in human monocytes by gamma linolenic acid. *Arthritis Rheum* 1990;33:1526–33.
10. Belch JJF, Ansell D, Madho KAR, O'Dowd A, Sturrock RD. Effects of altering dietary essential fatty acids on requirements for non-steroidal anti-inflammatory drugs in patients with rheumatoid arthritis: a double blind placebo controlled study. *Ann Rheum Dis* 1988;47:96–104.
11. Watson J, Madhok R, Wijelath E, et al. Mechanism of action of polyunsaturated fatty acids in rheumatoid arthritis. *Biochem Soc Trans* 1990;18:284–85.
12. Hunter JE. n-3 Fatty acids from vegetable oils. *Am J Clin Nutr* 1990; 51:809–14.
13. Mantzioris E, James MJ, Gibson RA, Cleland LG. Dietary substitution with an alpha-linolenic acid-rich vegetable oil increases eicosapentaenoic acid concentrations in tissues. *Am J Clin Nutr* 1994;59:1304–9.
14. Phinney SD, Odin RS, Johnson SB, Holman RT. Reduced arachidonate in serum phospholipids and cholesteryl esters associated with vegetarian diets in humans. *Am J Clin Nutr* 1990;51:385–92.

15. Siguel EN, Maclure M. Relative activity of unsaturated fatty acid metabolic pathways in humans. *Metabolism* 1987;36:664–69.
16. Okuyama H. Minimum requirements of n-3 and n-6 essential fatty acids for the function of the central nervous system and for the prevention of chronic disease. *Proc Exp Biol Med* 1992;200:174–76.
17. Chan JK, McDonald BE, Gerrard JM, Bruce VM, Weaver BJ, Holub BJ. Effect of dietary alpha-linolenic acid and its ratio to linoleic acid on platelet and plasma fatty acids and thrombogenesis. *Lipids* 1993;28:811–17.
18. Field CJ, Clandinin MT. Modulation of adipose tissue fat composition by diet: a review. *Nutr Research* 1984;4:743–55.
19. Dayton S, Hashimoto S, Dixon W, Pearce ML. Composition of lipids in human serum and adipose tissue during prolonged feeding of a diet high in unsaturated fat. *J Lipid Res* 1966;76:103–11.
20. Holman RT, Johnson SB, Hatch TF. A case of human linolenic acid deficiency involving neurological abnormalities. *Am J Clin Nutr* 1982;35:617–23.
21. Crary EJ, McCarthy MF. Potential clinical applications for high-dose nutritional antioxidants. *Med Hypotheses* 1984;13:77–98.
22. Woodruff I, Blake DR, Freeman J, Andrews FJ, Salt P, Lunec J. Is chronic synovitis an example of reperfusion injury? *Ann Rheum Dis* 1986;45:608–11.
23. Henning B, Chow CK. Lipid peroxidation and endothelial cell injury: implications in atherosclerosis. *Free Radic Biol Med* 1988;4:99–106.
24. Srivastava KC, Mustafa T. Ginger *(Zingiber officinale)* in rheumatism and musculoskeletal disorders. *Med Hypoth* 1992;39:342–48.
25. Srivastava KC. Effect of onion and ginger consumption on platelet thromboxane production in humans. *Prostaglandins Leukot Essent Fatty Acids* 1989;35:183–85.
26. Srivastava KC. Antiplatelet principles from a food spice clove *(Syzygium aromaticum L)*. *Prostaglandins Leukot Essent Fatty Acids* 1993;48:363–72.
27. Srivastava KC, Tyagi OD. Effects of a garlic-derived principle (ajoene) on aggregation and arachidonic acid metabolism in human blood platelets. *Prostaglandins Leukot Essent Fatty Acids* 1993;49:587–95.
28. Lipsky PE, Tao XL. A potential new treatment for rheumatoid arthritis: thunder god vine. *Semin Arth Rheum* 1997;26:713–23.
29. Xue-Lian T, Ying S, Yi D, et al. A prospective, controlled, double-blind, crossover study of tripterygium wilfodii hook F in the treatment of rheumatoid arthritis. *Chin Med J* 1989;102:327–32.
30. Merry P, Grootveld M, Lunec J, Blake DR. Oxidative damage to lipids within the inflamed human joint provides evidence of radical-medicated hypoxic-reperfusion injury. *Am J Clin Nutr* 1991;53:362S–69S.

31. Inman RD. Antigens, the gastrointestinal tract, and arthritis. *Rheum Dis Clin N Am* 1991;17:309–21.

32. Aoki S, Yoshikawa K, Yokoyama T, et al. Role of enteric bacteria in the pathogenesis of rheumatoid arthritis: evidence for antibodies to enterobacterial common antigens in rheumatoid sera and synovial fluids. *Ann Rheum Dis* 1996;55:363–69.

33. Hochberg MC. Epidemiologic considerations in the primary prevention of osteoarthritis. *J Rheumatol* 1991;18:1438–40.

34. Peyron JG. Is osteoarthritis a preventable disease? *J Rheumatol* 1991;18 (suppl 27):2–3.

35. Felson DT, Hannan MT, Naimark A, et al. Occupational physical demands, knee bending, and knee osteoarthritis, results from the Framingham study. *J Rheumatol* 1991;18:1587–92.

36. Cooper C, McAlindon T, Coggon D, Egger P, Dieppe P. Occupational activity and osteoarthritis of the knee. *Ann Rheum Dis* 1994;53:90–93.

37. Lane NE, Michel B, Bjorkengren A, et al. The risk of osteoarthritis with running and aging: a 5-year longitudinal study. *J Rheumatol* 1993;20:461–68.

38. Hart DJ, Spector TD. The relationship of obesity, fat distribution and osteoarthritis in women in the general population: the Chingford Study. *J Rheumatol* 1993;20:331–35.

39. Carman WJ, Sowers MF, Hawthorne VM, Weissfeld LA. Obesity as a risk factor for osteoarthritis of the hand and wrist: a prospective study. *Am J Epidemiol* 1994;139:119–29.

40. Cauley JA, Kwoh CK, Egeland G, et al. Serum sex hormones and severity of osteoarthritis of the hand. *J Rheumatol* 1993;20:1170–75.

41. Spector TD, Hart DJ, Brown P, et al. Frequency of osteoarthritis in hysterectomized women. *J Rheumatol* 1991;18:1877–83.

42. Packer L. Interactions among antioxidants in health and disease: vitamin E and its redox cycle. *Proc Soc Exp Biol Med* 1992;200:271–76.

43. Watson CPN, Evans RJ, Watt VR. Post-herpetic neuralgia and topical capsaicin. *Pain* 1988;33:333–40.

44. Schnitzer TJ, Posner M, Lawrence ID. High strength capsaicin cream for osteoarthritis pain: rapid onset of action and improved efficacy with twice daily dosing. *J Clin Rheumatol* 1995;268–73.

45. Gibson T, Rodgers AV, Simmonds HA, Court-Brown F, Todd E, Meilton V. A controlled study of diet in patients with gout. *Ann Rheum Dis* 1983;42:123–27.

46. Cleland LG, Hill CL, James MJ. Diet and arthritis. *Ballière's Clinical Rheumatology* 1995;9:771–85.

47. Stack BC Jr, Stack BC Sr. Temporomandibular joint disorder. *Am Fam Phys* 1992;46:143–50.
48. Bernstein AL. Vitamin B$_6$ in clinical neurology. *Ann NY Acad Sci* 1990;585:250–60.
49. Milam SB, Schmitz JP. Molecular biology of temporomandibular joint disorders: proposed mechanisms of disease. *J Oral Maxillofac Surg* 1995;53:1448–54.

6. CURING STOMACHACHES AND DIGESTIVE PROBLEMS

1. Marshall BJ, Warren JR. Unidentified curved bacilli in the stomach of patients with gastritis and peptic ulceration. *Lancet* 1984;1:1311–15.
2. Mégraud F. Epidemiology of *Helicobacter pylori* infection. *Gastroenterol Clin N Am* 1993;22:73–88.
3. Goodwin CS, Mendall MM, Northfield TC. *Helicobacter pylori* infection. *Lancet* 1997;349:265–69.
4. Marshall BJ. Treatment strategies for *Helicobacter pylori* infection. *Gastroenterol Clin N Am* 1993;22:183–98.
5. Wotherspoon AC, Doglioni C, Diss TC, et al. Regression of primary low-grade B-cell gastric lymphoma of mucosa-associated lymphoid tissue type after eradication of *Helicobacter pylori*. *Lancet* 1993;342:575–77.
6. Friedman G. Diet and the irritable bowel syndrome. *Gastroenterol Clin N Am* 1991;20:313–24.
7. Chin D, Milhorn HT, Robbins JG. Irritable bowel syndrome. *J Fam Prac* 1985;20:125–38.
8. Levinson S, Bhasker M, Gibson TR, Morin R, Snape WJ Jr. Comparison of intraluminal and intravenous mediators of colonic response to eating. *Dig Dis Sci* 1985;30:33–39.
9. Olesen M, Gudmand-Hoyer E. Maldigestion and colonic fermentation of wheat bread in humans and the influence of dietary fat. *Am J Clin Nutr* 1997;66:62–66.
10. Alun Jones V, McLaughlan P, Shorthouse M, Workman E, Hunter JO. Food intolerance: a major factor in the pathogenesis of irritable bowel syndrome. *Lancet* 1982;2:1115–18.
11. Petitpierre M, Gumowski P, Girard JP. Irritable bowel syndrome and hypersensitivity to food. *Ann Allergy* 1985;54:538–40.
12. Cuatrecasas P, Lockwood DH, Caldwell JR. Lactase deficiency in the adult: a common occurrence. *Lancet* 1965;1:14–18.
13. Bayless TM, Rosensweig NS. A racial difference in incidence of lactase defi-

ciency: a survey of milk intolerance and lactase deficiency in healthy adult males. *JAMA* 1966;197:968–72.

14. Hertzler SR, Huynh BCL, Savaiano DA. How much lactose is low lactose? *J Am Dietetic Asso* 1996;96:243–46.

15. Mishkin S. Dairy sensitivity, lactose malabsorption, and elimination diets in inflammatory bowel disease. *Am J Clin Nutr* 1997;65:564–67.

16. Scrimshaw NS, Murray EB. The acceptability of milk and milk products in populations with a high prevalence of lactose intolerance. *Am J Clin Nutr* 1988;48:1083–85.

17. Outwater JL, Nicholson A, Barnard N. Dairy products and breast cancer: the IGF-1, estrogen, and bGH hypothesis. *Med Hypoth* 1997;48:453–61.

18. McGee H. On food and cooking: the science and lore of the kitchen. New York, Macmillan, 1984.

19. Rees WDW, Evans BK, Rhodes J. Treating irritable bowel syndrome with peppermint oil. *Brit Med J* 1979;2:835–36.

20. Leicester RJ, Hunt RH. Peppermint oil to reduce colonic spasm during endoscopy. *Lancet* 1982;2:989.

21. Somerville KW, Richmond CR, Bell GD. Delayed release peppermint oil capsules (Colpermin) for the spastic colon syndrome: a pharmacokinetic study. *Br J Clin Pharmac* 1984;18:638–40.

22. Grontved A, Brask T, Kambskard J, Hentzer E. Ginger root against seasickness: a controlled trial on the open sea. *Acta Otolaryngol* (Stockh) 1988; 105:45–49.

23. Mowrey DB, Clayson DE. Motion sickness, ginger, and psychophysics. *Lancet* 1982;1:655–57.

24. Srivastava KC, Mustafa T. Ginger *(Zingiber officinale)* in rheumatism and musculoskeletal disorders. *Med Hypoth* 1992;39:342–48.

25. Narducci F, Snape WJ Jr, Battle WM, London RL, Cohen S. Increased colonic motility during exposure to a stressful situation. *Dig Dis Sci* 1985; 30:40–44.

26. Clyne PS, Kulczycki A. Human breast milk contains bovine IgG. Relationship to infant colic? *Pediatrics* 1991;87:439–44.

27. Lust KD, Brown JE, Thomas W. Maternal intake of cruciferous vegetables and other foods and colic symptoms in exclusively breast-fed infants. *J Am Dietetic Asso* 1996;96:46–48.

28. Sartor RB. Current concepts of the etiology and pathogenesis of ulcerative colitis and Crohn's disease. *Gastroenterol Clin N Am* 1995;24:475–507.

29. Yang VW. Eicosanoids and inflammatory bowel disease. *Gastroenterol Clin N Am* 1995;25:317–32.

30. Sanderson JD, Moss MT, Tizard MLV, Hermon-Taylor J. *Mycobacterium paratuberculosis* DNA in Crohn's disease tissue. *Gut* 1992;33:890–96.

31. Lashner BA. Epidemiology of inflammatory bowel disease. *Gastroenterol Clin N Am* 1995;24:467–74.

32. Thornton JR, Emmett PM, Heaton KW. Diet and Crohn's disease: characteristics of the pre-illness diet. *Br Med J* 1979;2:762–64.

33. Heaton KW, Thornton JR, Emmett PM. Treatment of Crohn's disease with an unrefined-carbohydrate, fibre-rich diet. *Br Med J* 1979;2:764–66.

34. Alun Jones V. Comparison of total parenteral nutrition and elemental diet in induction of remission of Crohn's disease: long-term maintenance of remission by personalized food exclusion diets. *Dig Dis Sci* 1987;32 (suppl): 100S–107S.

35. Pearson M, Teahon K, Jonathan Levi A, Bjarnason I. Food intolerance and Crohn's disease. *Gut* 1993;34:783–87.

36. Gudmand-Hoyer E, Jarnum S. Incidence and clinical significance of lactose malabsorption in ulcerative colitis and Crohn's disease. *Gut* 1970;11:338–43.

37. Kelly DG, Fleming CR. Nutritional considerations in inflammatory bowel diseases. *Gastroenterol Clin N Am* 1995;24:597–611.

38. Biancone L, Paganelli R, Fais S, Squarcia O, D'Offizi G, Pallone F. Peripheral and intestinal lymphocyte activation after in vitro exposure to cow's milk antigens in normal subjects and in patients with Crohn's disease. *Clin Immunol Immunopathol* 1987;45:491–98.

39. Alun Jones V, Dickinson RJ, Workman E, Wilson AJ, Freeman AH, Hunter JO. Crohn's disease: maintenance of remission by diet. *Lancet* 1985;2:177–80.

40. Aslan A, Triadafilopoulos G. Fish oil fatty acid supplementation in active ulcerative colitis: a double-blind, placebo-controlled, crossover study. *Am J Gastroenterol* 1992;87:432–37.

41. Hawthorne AB, Daneshmend TK, Hawkey CJ, et al. Treatment of ulcerative colitis with fish oil supplementation: a prospective 12 month randomised controlled trial. *Gut* 1992;33:922–28.

42. Stenson WF, Cort D, Rodgers J, et al. Dietary supplementation with fish oil in ulcerative colitis. *Ann Intern Med* 1992;116:609–14.

7. FIBROMYALGIA

1. Wolfe F, Smythe HA, Yunus MB, et al. The American College of Rheumatology 1990 criteria for the classification of fibromyalgia. Report of the Multicenter Criteria Committee. *Arthritis Rheum* 1990;33:160–72.

2. Wolfe F, Ross K, Anderson J, Russell IJ, Hebert L. The prevalence and char-

acteristics of fibromyalgia in the general population. *Arthritis Rheum* 1995; 38:19–28.

3. Buskila D, Press J, Gedalia A, et al. Assessment of nonarticular tenderness and prevalence of fibromyalgia in children. *J Rheumatol* 1993;20:368–70.

4. Clauw DJ. The pathogenesis of chronic pain and fatigue syndromes, with special reference to fibromyalgia. *Med Hypoth* 1995;44:369–78.

5. Behan PO, Haniffah BAG, Doogan DP, Loudon M. A pilot study of sertraline for the treatment of chronic fatigue syndrome. *Clin Inf Dis* 1994; 18(suppl):S111.

6. Wiebe E. N of 1 trials. Managing patients with chronic fatigue syndrome: two case reports. *Can Fam Phys* 1996;42:2214–17.

7. Granges G, Littlejohn GO. A comparative study of clinical signs in fibromyalgia/fibrositis syndrome, healthy and exercising subjects. *J Rheumatol* 1993; 20:344–51.

8. McCain GA, Bell DA, Mai FM, Halliday PD. A controlled study of the effects of a supervised cardiovascular fitness training program on the manifestations of primary fibromyalgia. *Arthritis Rheum* 1988;31:1135–41.

9. Moldofsky H, Scarisbrick P, England R, Smythe H. Musculoskeletal symptoms and non-REM sleep disturbance in patients with "fibrositis syndrome" and healthy subjects. *Psychosom Med* 1975;37:341–51.

10. Klug GA, McAuley E, Clark S. Factors influencing the development and maintenance of aerobic fitness: lessons applicable to the fibrositis syndrome. *J Rheumatol* 1989;16:30–39.

11. Martin L, Nutting A, Macintosh BR, Edworthy SM, Butterwick D, Cook J. An exercise program in the treatment of fibromyalgia. *J Rheumatol* 1996; 23:1050–53.

12. McCully KK, Sisto SA, Natelson BH. Use of exercise for treatment of chronic fatigue syndrome. *Sports Med* 1996;21:35–48.

13. Fulcher KY, White PD. Randomised controlled trial of graded exercise in patients with the chronic fatigue syndrome. *BMJ* 1997;314:1647–52.

14. Russell IJ, Michalek JE, Flechas JD, Abraham GE. Treatment of fibromyalgia syndrome with Super Malic: a randomized, double blind, placebo controlled, crossover study. *J Rheumatol* 1995;22:953–58.

15. Cox IM, Campbell MJ, Dowson D. Red blood cell magnesium and chronic fatigue syndrome. *Lancet* 1991;337:757–60.

16. Jaffe RM, Deuster PA. A novel treatment for fibromyalgia improves clinical outcomes in a community-based study. Presented to the Annual Conference of the Clinical Immunology Society, New Orleans, May 31–June 3, 1996.

17. Jennum P, Drewes AM, Andreasen A, Nielsen KD. Sleep and other symp-

toms in primary fibromyalgia and in healthy controls. *J Rheumatol* 1993; 20:1756–59.

18. Seltzer S, Stoch R, Marcus R, Jackson E. Alteration of human pain thresholds by nutritional manipulation and L-tryptophan supplementation. *Pain* 1982;13:35–93.

19. Rowe PC, Bou-Holaigah I, Kan JS, Calkins H. Is neurally mediated hypotension an unrecognised cause of chronic fatigue? *Lancet* 1995;345:623–24.

20. Kennedy M, Felson DT. A prospective long-term study of fibromyalgia syndrome. *Arthritis Rheum* 1996;39:682–85.

8. USING FOODS AGAINST MENSTRUAL PAIN

1. Chan WY. Prostaglandins and nonsteroidal antiinflammatory drugs in dysmenorrhea. *Ann Rev Pharmacol Toxicol* 1983;23:131–49.

2. Ylikorkala O, Dawood MY. New concepts in dysmenorrhea. *Am J Obstet Gynecol* 1978;130:833–47.

3. Prentice R, Thompson D, Clifford C, Gorbach S, Goldin B, Byar D. Dietary fat reduction and plasma estradiol concentration in healthy postmenopausal women. *J Natl Cancer Inst* 1990;82:129–34.

4. Thys-Jacobs S, Ceccarelli S, Bierman A, Weisman H, Cohen M, Alvir A. Calcium supplementation in premenstrual syndrome. *J Gen Intern Med* 1989; 4:183–89.

5. Penland JG, Johnson PE. Dietary calcium and manganese effects on menstrual cycle symptoms. *Am J Obstet Gynecol* 1993;168:1417–23.

6. Remer T, Manz F. Estimation of the renal net acid excretion by adults consuming diets containing variable amounts of protein. *Am J Clin Nutr* 1994; 59:1356–61.

7. Bernstein AL. Vitamin B_6 in clinical neurology. *Ann NY Acad Sci* 1990; 585:250–60.

8. Biskin MS. Nutritional deficiency in the etiology of menorrhagia, metrorrhagia, cystic mastitis and premenstrual tension: treatment with vitamin B complex. *J Clin Endocr Metab* 1943;3:227.

9. Abraham GE, Rumley RE. The role of nutrition in managing the premenstrual tension syndromes. *J Reprod Med* 1987;32:405–22.

10. Kleijnen J, Ter Riet G, Knipschild P. Vitamin B_6 in the treatment of premenstrual syndrome—a review. *Br J Obstet Gynaecol* 1990;97:847–52.

11. Abraham GE, Hargrove JT. Effect of vitamin B_6 on premenstrual symptomatology in women with premenstrual tension syndromes: a double-blind crossover study. *Infertility* 1980;3:155–65.

12. Brush MG. Vitamin B_6 treatment of premenstrual syndrome. *Curr Topics in Nutr Dis* 1988;19:363–79.

13. Deutch B. Menstrual pain in Danish women correlated with low n-3 polyunsaturated fatty acid intake. *Eur J Clin Nutr* 1995;49:508–16.

14. Ahlborg UG, Lipworth L, Titus-Ernstoff L, et al. Organochlorine compounds in relation to breast cancer, endometrial cancer, and endometriosis: an assessment of the biological and epidemiological evidence. *Crit Rev Toxicol* 1995;25:463–531.

15. Moen MH, Magnus P. The familial risk of endometriosis. *Acta Obstet Gynecol Scand* 1993;72:560–64.

16. Mangtani P, Booth M. Epidemiology of endometriosis. *J Epidem Comm Health* 1993;47:84–88.

17. Dmowski WP. Immunological aspects of endometriosis. *Int J Gynecol Obstet* 1995;50(suppl 1):S3–S10.

18. Balasch J, Creus M, Fabregues F, et al. Visible and nonvisible endometriosis at laparoscopy in fertile and infertile women and in patients with chronic pelvic pain: a prospective study. *Human Repro* 1996;11:387–91.

19. Grodstein F, Goldman MB, Ryan L, Cramer DW. Relation of female infertility to consumption of caffeinated beverages. *Am J Epidemiol* 1993; 37:1353–60.

20. Holloway M. An epidemic ignored: endometriosis linked to dioxin and immunologic dysfunction. *Sci Am* 1994;270:24–26.

21. Koninckx PK, Braet P, Kennedy SH, Barlow DH. Dioxin pollution and endometriosis in Belgium. *Human Reproduction* 1994;9:1001–2.

22. Hergenrather J, Hlady G, Wallace B, Savage E. Pollutants in breast milk of vegetarians. *N Engl J Med* 1981;304:792.

23. Dawood MY. Considerations in selecting appropriate medical therapy for endometriosis. *Int J Gynecol Obstet* 1993;40(suppl):S29–S42.

24. Revelli A, Modotti M, Ansaldi C, Massobrio M. Recurrent endometriosis: a review of biological and clinical aspects. *Obstet Gynecol Survey* 1995; 50:747–54.

25. Barone J, Hebert JR, Reddy MM. Dietary fat and natural-killer-cell activity. *Am J Clin Nutr* 1989;50:861–67.

26. Cuthbert JA, Lipsky PE. Immunoregulation by low density lipoproteins in man. *J Clin Invest* 1984;73:992–1003.

27. Pepe MG, Curtiss LK. Apolipoprotein E is a biologically active constituent of the normal immunoregulatory lipoprotein, LDL-In. *J Immunol* 1986; 136:3716–23.

28. Traill KN, Huber LA, Wick G, Jurgens G. Lipoprotein interactions with T cells: an update. *Immunol Today* 1990;11:411–17.

29. Malter M, Schriever G, Eilber U. Natural killer cells, vitamins, and other blood components of vegetarian and omnivorous men. *Nutr Cancer* 1989; 12:271–78.

30. Yamamoto T, Noguchi T, Tamura T, Kitawaki J, Okada H. Evidence of estrogen synthesis in adenomyotic tissues. *Am J Obstet Gynecol* 1993;169:734–38.
31. Srivastava KC. Antiplatelet principles from a food spice clove *(Syzygium aromaticum L)*. *Prostglandins Leukot Essent Fatty Acids* 1993;48:363–72.

9. BREAST PAIN

1. Sitruk-Ware R, Sterkers N, Mauvais-Jarvis P. Benign breast disease I: hormonal investigation. *Obstet Gynecol* 1979;53:457–60.
2. Watt-Boolsen S, Eskildsen PC, Blaehr H. Release of prolactin, thyrotropin, and growth hormone in women with cyclical mastalgia and fibrocystic disease of the breast. *Cancer* 1985;56:500–502.
3. Rose DP, Boyar AP, Cohen C, Strong LE. Effect of a low-fat diet on hormone levels in women with cystic breast disease. I. Serum steroids and gonadotropins. *J Natl Cancer Inst* 1987;78:623–26.
4. Rose DP, Cohen LA, Berke B, Boyar AP. Effect of a low-fat diet on hormone levels in women with cystic breast disease. II. Serum radioimmunoassayable prolactin and growth hormone and bioactive lactogenic hormones. *J Natl Cancer Inst* 1987;78:627–31.
5. Minton JP, Foecking MK, Webster DJT, Matthews RH. Caffeine, cyclic nucleotides, and breast disease. *Surgery* 1979;86:105–9.
6. Ferrini RL, Barrett-Connor E. Caffeine intake and endogenous sex steroid levels in postmenopausal women. *Am J Epidemiol* 1996;144:642–44.
7. Pye JK, Mansel RE, Hughes LE. Clinical experience of drug treatments for mastalgia. *Lancet* 1985;2:373–76.
8. Brush MG. Vitamin B$_6$ treatment of premenstrual syndrome. *Curr Topics in Nutr Dis* 1988;19:363–79.

10. CANCER PAIN

1. Armstrong B, Doll R. Environmental factors and cancer incidence and mortality in different countries, with special reference to dietary practices. *Int J Cancer* 1975;15:617–31.
2. Howell MA. Factor analysis of international cancer mortality data and per capita food consumption. *Br J Cancer* 1974;29:328–36.
3. Blair A, Fraumeni JF Jr. Geographic patterns of prostate cancer in the United States. *J Natl Cancer Inst* 1978;61:1379–84.
4. Kolonel LN, Hankin JH, Lee J, Chu SY, Nomura AMY, Hinds MW. Nutrient intakes in relation to cancer incidence in Hawaii. *Br J Cancer* 1981;44:332–39.

5. Rotkin ID. Studies in the epidemiology of prostatic cancer: expanded sampling. *Cancer Treat Rep* 1977;61:173–80.
6. Schuman LM, Mandel JS, Radke A, Seal U, Halberg F. Some selected features of the epidemiology of prostatic cancer: Minneapolis–St. Paul, Minnesota, case control study, 1976–1979. In Magnus K, ed. Trends in cancer incidence: causes and practical implications. Washington, D.C., Hemisphere Publishing Corp., 1982.
7. Graham S, et al. Diet in the epidemiology of carcinoma of the prostate gland. *J Natl Cancer Inst* 1983;70:687–92.
8. Ross RK, Shimizu H, Paganini-Hill A, Honda G, Henderson BE. Case-control studies of prostate cancer in blacks and whites in Southern California. *J Natl Cancer Inst* 1987;78:869–74.
9. Severson RK, Nomura AM, Grove JS, Stemmermann GN. A prospective study of demographics, diet, and prostate cancer among men of Japanese ancestry in Hawaii. *Cancer Research* 1989;49:1857–60.
10. Oishi K, Okada K, Yoshida O, et al. A case-control study of prostatic cancer with reference to dietary habits. *Prostate* 1988;12:179–90.
11. Mettlin C, Selenskas S, Natarajan N, Huben R. Beta-carotene and animal fats and their relationship to prostate cancer risk: a case-control study. *Cancer* 1989;64:605–12.
12. National Research Council. Diet, nutrition, and cancer. Washington, D.C., National Academy Press, 1982.
13. Hirayama T. Changing patterns of cancer in Japan with special reference to the decrease in stomach cancer mortality. In Hiatt HH, Watson JD, Winsten JA, eds. Origins of human cancer. Book A, incidence of cancer in humans. Cold Spring Harbor, N.Y., Cold Spring Harbor Laboratory, 1977, pp. 55–75.
14. Hirayama T. Epidemiology of prostate cancer with special reference to the role of diet. *Natl Cancer Inst Monogr* 1979;53:149–54.
15. Phillips RL. Role of life-style and dietary habits in risk of cancer among Seventh-Day Adventists. *Cancer Research* 1975;35:3513–22.
16. Mills P, Beeson WL, Phillips RL, Fraser GE. Cohort study of diet, lifestyle, and prostate cancer in Adventist men. *Cancer* 1989;64:598–604.
17. Gray A, Jackson DN, McKinlay JB. The relation between dominance, anger, and hormones in normally aging men: results from the Massachusetts Male Aging Study. *Psychosom Med* 1991;53:375–85.
18. Giovannucci E, Ascherio A, Rimm EB, Stampfer MJ, Colditz GA, Willett WA. Intake of carotenoids and retinol in relation to risk of prostate cancer. *J Natl Cancer Inst* 1995;87:1767–76.
19. Wynder EL, Fujita Y, Harris RE, Hirayama T, Hiyama T. Comparative

epidemiology of cancer between the United States and Japan. *Cancer* 1991;67:746–63.

20. Hirayama T. Epidemiology of breast cancer with special reference to the role of diet. *Prev Med* 1978;7:173–95.

21. Rose DP, Boyar AP, Cohen C, Strong LE. Effect of a low-fat diet on hormone levels in women with cystic breast disease. 1. Serum steroids and gonadotropins. *J Natl Cancer Inst* 1987;78:6223–26.

22. Ingram DM, Bennett FC, Willcox D, de Klerk N. Effect of low-fat diet on female sex hormone levels. *J Natl Cancer Inst* 1987;79:1225–29.

23. Goldin BR, Gorbach SL. Effect of diet on the plasma levels, metabolism and excretion of estrogens. *Am J Clin Nutr* 1988;48:787–90.

24. Toniolo P, Riboli E, Protta F, Charrel M, Cappa AP. Calorie-providing nutrients and risk of breast cancer. *J Natl Cancer Inst* 1989;81:278.

25. Messina MJ, Barnes S. The role of soy products in reducing risk of cancer. *J Natl Cancer Inst* 1991;83:541–46.

26. Outwater JL, Nicholson A, Barnard ND. Dairy products and breast cancer: the IGF-1, estrogen, and bGH hypothesis. *Med Hypoth* 1997;48:453–61.

27. Willett WC, Stampfer MJ, Colditz FA, et al. Moderate alcohol consumption and the risk of breast cancer. *N Engl J Med* 1987;316:1174–80.

28. Miller DR, Rosenberg L, Kaufman DW, et al. Breast cancer before age 45 and oral contraceptive use: new findings. *Am J Epidemiol* 1989;129:269.

29. Bergkvist L, Adami AO, Persson I., et al. The risk of breast cancer after estrogen and estrogen-progestin replacement. *New Engl J Med* 1989; 321:293.

30. Lubin F, Ruder AM, Wax Y, Modan B. Overweight and changes in weight throughout adult life in breast cancer etiology. *Am J Epidemiol* 1985; 122:579–88.

31. Miller FA, Hempelmann LH, Dutton AM, Pifer JW, Toyooka ET, Ames WR. Breast neoplasms in women treated with X rays for acute postpartum mastitis. A pilot study. *J Natl Cancer Inst* 1969;43:803–11.

32. Lynch HT, Albano WA, Heieck JJ, et al. Genetics, biomarkers, and control of breast cancer: a review. *Cancer, Genetics, and Cytogenetics* 1984; 13:43–92.

33. Goldman BA. The truth about where you live. New York, Random House, 1991.

34. Wynder EL, Kajitani T, Kuno J, Lucas JC Jr, DePalo A, Farrow J. A comparison of survival rates between American and Japanese patients with breast cancer. *Surg Gynec Obstet* 1963;117:196–200.

35. Gregorio DI, Emrich LJ, Graham S, Marshall JR, Nemoto T. Dietary fat

consumption and survival among women with breast cancer. *J Natl Cancer Inst* 1985;75:37–41.

36. Verreault R, Brisson J, Deschenes L, Naud F, Meyer F, Belanger L. Dietary fat in relation to prognostic indicators in breast cancer. *J Natl Cancer Inst* 1988;80:819–25.

37. Zhang S, Folsom AR, Sellers TA, Kushi LH, Potter JD. Better breast cancer survival for postmenopausal women who are less overweight and eat less fat. *Cancer* 1995;76:275–83.

38. Newman SC, Miller AB, Howe GR. A study of the effect of weight and dietary fat on breast cancer survival time. *Am J Epidemiol* 1986;123:767–74.

39. Holm LE, Callmer E, Hjalmar ML, Lidbrink E, Nilsson B, Skoog L. Dietary habits and prognostic factors in breast cancer. *J Natl Cancer Inst* 1989; 81:1218–23.

40. Donegan WL, Hartz AJ, Rimm AA. The association of body weight with recurrent cancer of the breast. *Cancer* 1978;41:1590–94.

41. Schapira DV, Kumar NB, Lyman GH, Cox CE. Obesity and body fat distribution and breast cancer prognosis. *Cancer* 1991;67:523–28.

42. Watson CPN. Topical capsaicin as an adjuvant analgesic. *J Pain Symptom Management* 1994;9:425–33.

43. Lingeman CH. Etiology of cancer of the human ovary: a review. *J Natl Cancer Inst* 1974;53:1603–18.

44. Helzlsouer KJ, Alberg AJ, Norkus EP, Morris JS, Hoffman SC, Comstock GW. Prospective study of serum micronutrients and ovarian cancer. *J Natl Cancer Inst* 1996;88:32–37.

45. Wynder EL, Escher GC, Mantel N. An epidemiological investigation of cancer of the endometrium. *Cancer* 1966;19:489–520.

46. Elwood JM, Cole P, Rothman KJ, Kaplan SD. Epidemiology of endometrial cancer. *J Natl Cancer Inst* 1977;59:1055–60.

47. Cramer DW, Willett WC, Bell DA, et al. Galactose consumption and metabolism in relation to the risk of ovarian cancer. *Lancet* 1989;2:66–71.

48. Sinha R, Rothman N, Brown ED, et al. High concentrations of the carcinogen 2-amino-1-methyl-6-phenylimidazo-[4,5]pyridine (PhIP) occur in chicken but are dependent on the cooking method. *Cancer Research* 1995;55:4516–19.

49. Knekt P, Steineck G, Jarvinen R, Hakulinen T, Aromaa A. Intake of fried meat and risk of cancer: a follow-up study in Finland. *Int J Cancer* 1994; 59:756–60.

50. Willett WC, Stampfer MJ, Colditz GA, Rosner BA, Speizer FE. Relation of meat, fat, and fiber intake to the risk of colon cancer in a prospective study among women. *N Engl J Med* 1990;323:1664–72.

51. Giovannucci E, Rimm EB, Stampfer MJ, Colditz GA, Ascherio A, Willett WC. Intake of fat, meat, and fiber in relation to risk of colon cancer in men. *Cancer Res* 1994;54:2390–97.
52. Gerhardsson de Verdier M, Hagman U, Peters RK, Steineck G, Overvik E. Meat, cooking methods and colorectal cancer: a case-referrent study in Stockholm. *Int J Cancer* 1991;49:520–25.
53. DeCosse JJ, Miller HH, Lesser ML. Effect of wheat fiber and vitamins C and E on rectal polyps in patients with familial adenomatous polyposis. *J Natl Cancer Inst* 1989;81:1290–97.
54. Block F. Epidemiologic evidence regarding vitamin C and cancer. *Am J Clin Nutr* 1991;54:1310S–14S.
55. Kromhout D. Essential micronutrients in relation to carcinogenesis. *Am J Clin Nutr* 1987;45:1361–67.
56. Barone J, Hebert JR, Reddy MM. Dietary fat and natural-killer-cell activity. *Am J Clin Nutr* 1989;50:861–67.
57. Nordenstrom J, Jarstrand C, Wiernik A. Decreased chemotactic and random migration of leukocytes during intralipid infusion. *Am J Clin Nutr* 1979;32:2416–22.
58. Hawley HP, Gordon GB. The effects of long chain free fatty acids on human neutrophil function and structure. *Lab Invest* 1976;34:216–22.
59. Beisel WR. Single nutrients and immunity. *Am J Clin Nutr* 1982;35 (February suppl):417–68.
60. Watson RR. Immunological enhancement by fat-soluble vitamins, minerals, and trace metals: a factor in cancer prevention. *Cancer and Prevention* 1986; 9:67–77.
61. Chandra S, Chandra RK. Nutrition, immune response, and outcome. *Progress in Food and Nutrition Science* 1986;10:1–65.
62. Watson RR, Prabhala RH, Plezia PM, Alberts DS. Effect of beta-carotene on lymphocyte subpopulations in elderly humans: evidence for a dose-response relationship. *Am J Clin Nutr* 1991;53:90–94.
63. Malter M, Schriever G, Eilber U. Natural killer cells, vitamins, and other blood components of vegetarian and omnivorous men. *Nutr Cancer* 1989; 12:271–78.

11. CARPAL TUNNEL SYNDROME

1. Kerwin G, Williams CS, Seiler JG. The pathophysiology of carpal tunnel syndrome. *Hand Clinics* 1996;12:243–51.
2. Osorio AM, Ames RG, Jones J, et al. Carpal tunnel syndome among grocery store workers. *Am J Industrial Med* 1994;25:229–45.

3. Putnam JJ. A series of cases of paresthesiae, mainly of the hands, of periodic occurrence and possibly of vasomotor origin. *Arch Med* 1880;4:147–51.

4. Bernstein AL. Vitamin B$_6$ in clinical neurology. *Ann NY Acad Sci* 1990; 585:250–60.

5. Copeland DA, Stoukides CA. Pyridoxine in carpal tunnel syndrome. *Ann Pharmacother* 1994;28:1042–44.

6. Jacobsen MD, Plancher KD, Kleinman WB. Vitamin B$_6$ (pyridoxine) therapy for carpal tunnel syndrome. *Hand Clinics* 1996;12:253–57.

7. Spooner GR, Desai HB, Angel JF, Reeder BA, Donat JR. Using pyridoxine to treat carpal tunnel syndrome. *Can Fam Phys* 1993;39:2122–27.

8. Ellis JM, Folkers K, Levy M, et al. Therapy with vitamin B$_6$ with and without surgery for treatment of patients having the idiopathic carpal tunnel syndrome. *Res Commun Chem Pathol Pharmacol* 1981;33:331–44.

9. Ellis JM, Folkers K, Levy M, et al. Response of vitamin B$_6$ deficiency and the carpal tunnel syndrome to pyridoxine. *Proc Natl Acad Sci* 1982;79:7494–98.

10. Hamfelt A. Carpal tunnel syndrome and vitamin B$_6$ deficiency. *Clin Chem* 1982;28:721.

11. Kasdan ML, Janes C. Carpal tunnel syndrome and vitamin B$_6$. *Plast Reconstr Surg* 1987;79:456–62.

12. Fuhr JE, Farrow A, Nelson HS Jr. Vitamin B$_6$ levels in patients with carpal tunnel syndrome. *Arch Surg* 1989;124:1329–30.

13. Laso Guzman FJ, Gonzalez-Buitrago JM, de Arriba F, Mateos F, Moyano JC, Lopez-Alburquerque T. Carpal tunnel syndrome and vitamin B$_6$. *Klin Wochenschr* 1989;67:38–41.

14. Lewis PJ. Pyridoxine supplements may help patients with carpal tunnel syndrome. *BMJ* 1995;310:1534.

15. Ellis JM, Kishi T, Azuma J, et al. Vitamin B$_6$ deficiency in patients with a clinical syndrome including the carpal tunnel defect. Biochemical and clinical response to therapy with pyridoxine. *Res Commun Chem Pathol Pharmacol* 1976;13:743–57.

16. Ellis JM, Azuma J, Watanabe T, et al. Survey and new data on treatment with pyridoxine of patients having a clinical syndrome including carpal tunnel and other defects. *Res Commun Chem Pathol Pharmacol* 1977; 17:165–77.

17. Zimmermann M, Bartoszyk GD, Bonke D, Jurna I, Wild A. Antinociceptive properties of pyridoxine: neurophysiological and behavioral findings. *Ann NY Acad Sci* 1990;585:219–30.

18. Dakshinamurti K, Paulose CS, Viswanathan M, Siow YL, Sharma SK. Neurobiology of pyridoxine. *Ann NY Acad Sci* 1990;585:128–44.

19. Stransky M, Rubin A, Lava NS, Lazoro RP. Treatment of carpal tunnel syndrome with vitamin B$_6$: a double-blind study. *South Med J* 1989;82:841–42.

20. Ellis JM. Treatment of carpal tunnel syndrome with vitamin B₆. *South Med J* 1987;80:882–84.

21. Nathan PA, Keniston RC, Lockwood RS, Meadows KD. Tobacco, caffeine, alcohol, and carpal tunnel syndrome in American industry. *J Occup Environ Med* 1996;38:593–601.

22. Stahl S, Blumenfeld Z, Yarnitsky D. Carpal tunnel syndrome in pregnancy: indications for early surgery. *J Neuro Sci* 1996;136:182–84.

23. Wand JS. Carpal tunnel syndrome in pregnancy and lactation. *J Hand Surg* (British volume 1990)15-B:93–95.

24. Sabour MS, Fadel HE. The carpal tunnel syndrome—a new complication ascribed to the "pill." *Am J Obstet Gynecol* 1970;107:1265–67.

25. Danforth DN. Obstetrics and gynecology, 3rd ed. New York, Harper and Row, 1977, p. 224.

26. Linder MC. Nutritional biochemistry and metabolism with clinical applications, 2nd ed. New York, Elsevier Science Publishing, 1991, pp. 127–37.

27. Courts RB. Splinting for symptoms of carpal tunnel syndrome during pregnancy. *J Hand Ther* 1995;8:31–34.

12. DIABETES

1. Max MB, Lynch SA, Muir J, Shoaf SE, Smoller B, Dubner R. Effects of desipramine, amitriptyline, and fluoxetine on pain in diabetic neuropathy. *N Eng J Med* 1992;326:1250–56.

2. Crane MG, Sample C. Regression of diabetic neuropathy with total vegetarian (vegan) diet. *J Nutr Med* 1994;4:431–39.

3. Barnard RJ, Lattimore L, Holly RA, Cherny S, Pritikin N. Response of non-insulin-dependent diabetic patients to an intensive program of diet and exercise. *Diabetes Care* 1982;5:370–74.

4. Barnard RJ, Massey MR, Cherny S, O'Brien LT, Pritikin N. Long-term use of a high-complex-carbohydrate, high-fiber, low-fat diet and exercise in the treatment of NIDDM patients. *Diabetes Care* 1983;6:268–73.

5. Anderson JW. Plant fiber and blood pressure. *Ann Intern Med* 1983;98(pt 2):842.

6. Dodson PM, Pacey PJ, Bal P, Kubicki AJ, Fletcher RF, Taylor KG. A controlled trial of a high-fiber, low fat, and low sodium diet for mild hypertension in type 2 (non-insulin-dependent) diabetic patients. *Diabetologia* 1984;27:522.

7. Roy MS, Stables G, Collier B, Roy A, Bou E. Nutritional factors in diabetics with and without retinopathy. *Am J Clin Nutr* 1989;50:728–30.

8. Morley GK, Mooradian AD, Levine AS, Morley JE. Mechanism of pain in diabetic peripheral neuropathy. *Am J Med* 1984;77:79–82.

9. Nicholson AS, Sklar M, Gore S, Sullivan R, Browning S. The very-low-fat, high-fiber diet in treatment of NIDDM: a randomized, controlled, intervention study. 1997, in press.

10. Bernstein AL. Vitamin B$_6$ in clinical neurology. *Ann NY Acad Sci* 1990; 585:250–60.

11. Capsaicin Study Group. Effect of treatment with capsaicin on daily activities of patients with painful diabetic neuropathy. *Diabetes Care* 1992; 15:159–65.

12. Karjalainen J, Martin JM, Knop M, et al. A bovine albumin peptide as a possible trigger of insulin-dependent diabetes mellitus. *N Engl J Med* 1992; 327:302–7.

13. American Academy of Pediatrics Work Group on Cow's Milk Protein and Diabetes Mellitus. Infant feeding practices and their possible relationship to the etiology of diabetes mellitus. *Pediatrics* 1994;94:752–54.

14. Cavallo MG, Fava D, Monetini L, Barone F, Pozzilli P. Cell-mediated immune response to beta-casein in recent-onset insulin-dependent diabetes: implications for disease pathogenesis. *Lancet* 1996;348:926–28.

13. HERPES AND SHINGLES

1. Tankersley RW. Amino acid requirements of herpes simplex virus in human cells. *J Bacteriology* 1964;87:609–13.

2. Griffith RS, DeLong DC, Nelson JD. Relation of arginine-lysine antagonism to herpes simplex growth in tissue culture. *Chemotherapy* 1981;27:209–13.

3. Griffith RS, Walsh DE, Myrmel KH, Thompson RW, Behforooz A. Success of L-lysine therapy in frequently recurrent herpes simplex infection. *Dermatologica* 1987;175:183–90.

4. Milman N, Scheibel J, Jessen O. Lysine prophylaxis in recurrent herpes simplex labialis: a double-blind, controlled crossover study. *Acta Dermato Venereologica* 1980;60:85–87.

5. DiGiovanna JJ, Blank H. Failure of lysine in frequently recurrent herpes simplex infection. *Arch Dermatol* 1984;102:48–51.

6. Griffith RS, Norins AL, Kagan C. A multicentered study of lysine therapy in herpes simplex infection. *Dermatologica* 1978;156:257–67.

7. Flodin NW. The metabolic roles, pharmacology, and toxicology of lysine. *J Am Coll Nutr* 1997;16:7–21.

8. Walsh DE, Griffith RS, Behforooz A. Subjective response to lysine in the therapy of herpes simplex. *J Antimicrobial Chemother* 1983;12:489–96.

9. Wright EF. Clinical effectiveness of lysine in treating recurrent aphthous ulcers and herpes labialis. *Gen Dent* 1994;42:40–42.

10. Bowsher D. Pathophysiology of postherpetic neuralgia. *Neurology* 1995; 45(suppl 8):S56–S57.

11. Nikkels AF, Pierard GE. Recognition and treatment of shingles. *Drugs* 1994;48:529–48.

12. Straus SE. Shingles: sorrows, salves, and solutions. *JAMA* 1993; 269:1836–39.

13. Watson CPN, Tyler KL, Bickers DR, Millikan LE, Smith S, Coleman E. A randomized vehicle-controlled trial of topical capsaicin in the treatment of post-herpetic neuralgia. *Clin Therapeutics* 1993;15:510–26.

14. Oxman MN. Immunization to reduce the frequency and severity of herpes zoster and its complications. *Neurology* 1995;45(suppl 8):S41–S46.

15. Bogden JD, Oleske JM, Lavenhar MA, et al. Effects of one year of supplementation with zinc and other micronutrients on cellular immunity in the elderly. *J Am Coll Nutr* 1990; 9: 214–215.

14. SICKLE-CELL ANEMIA

1. Nagel RL, Fleming AF. Genetic epidemiology of the ß^s gene. *Baillière's Clinical Haematology* 1992;5:331–65.

2. Burdick E. Sickle cell disease: still a management challenge. *Postgrad Med* 1994;107–15.

3. Reed JD, Redding-Lallinger R, Orringer EP. Nutrition and sickle cell disease. *Am J Hematol* 1987;24:441–55.

4. Enwonwu CO. Nutritional support in sickle cell anemia: theoretical considerations. *J Nat Med Asso* 1988;80:139–44.

5. Gillette PN, Peterson CM, Lu YS, Cerami A. Sodium cyanate as a potential treatment for sickle-cell disease. *N Engl J Med* 1974;290:654–60.

6. Harkness DR, Roth S. Clinical evaluation of cyanate in sickle cell anemia. *Progr Hematol* 1975;9:157–84.

7. Houston RG. Sickle cell anemia and dietary precursors of cyanate. *Am J Clin Nutr* 1973;26:1261–64.

8. Sergeant GR. Observations on the epidemiology of sickle cell disease. *Trans Roy Soc Trop Med Hygiene* 1981;75:228–33.

9. Lambotte C. Sickle cell anemia and dietary precursors of cyanate. *Am J Clin Nutr* 1974;27:765–73.

10. Kark JA, Ward FT. Exercise and hemoglobin S. *Seminars in Hematology* 1994;31:181–225.

15. KIDNEY STONES AND URINARY INFECTIONS

1. Curhan GC, Willett WC, Rimm EB, Stamper MJ. A prospective study of dietary calcium and other nutrients and the risk of symptomatic kidney stones. *N Engl J Med* 1993;328:833–38.
2. Curhan GC, Willett WC, Rimm EB, Spiegelman D, Stampfer MJ. Prospective study of beverage use and the risk of kidney stones. *Am J Epidemiol* 1996; 143:240–47.
3. Curhan GC, Willett WC, Speizer FE, Spiegelman D, Stampfer MJ. Comparison of dietary calcium with supplemental calcium and other nutrients as factors affecting the risk for kidney stones in women. *Ann Int Med* 1997; 126:497–504.
4. Soucie JM, Thun MJ, Coates RJ, McClellan W, Austin H. Demographic and geographic variability of kidney stones in the United States. *Kidney Int* 1994;46:893–99.
5. Nordin BEC, Need AG, Morris HA, Horowitz M. The nature and significance of the relationship between urinary sodium and urinary calcium in women. *J Nutr* 1993;123:1615–22.
6. Lemann J. Composition of the diet and calcium kidney stones. *N Engl J Med* 1993;328:880–82.
7. Remer T, Manz F. Estimation of the renal net acid excretion by adults consuming diets containing variable amounts of protein. *Am J Clin Nutr* 1994; 59:1356–61.
8. Breslau NA, Brinkley L, Hill KD, Pak CYC. Relationship of animal protein-rich diet to kidney stone formation and calcium metabolism. *J Clin Endocrinol* 1988;66:140–46.
9. Robertson WG, Peacock M, Hodgkinson A. Dietary changes and the incidence of urinary calculi in the U.K. between 1958 and 1976. *J Chron Dis* 1979; 32:469–76.
10. Lemann J Jr, Adams ND, Gray RW. Urinary calcium excretion in human beings. *N Engl J Med* 1979;301:535–41.
11. Soucie JM, Coates RJ, McClellan W, Austin H, Thun MJ. Relation between geographic variability in kidney stones prevalence and risk factors for stones. *Am J Epidemiol* 1996;143:487–95.
12. Avorn J, Monane M, Gurwitz JH, Glynn RJ, Choodnovskiy I, Lipsitz LA. Reduction of bacteriuria and pyuria after ingestion of cranberry juice. *JAMA* 1994;271:751–54.
13. Haverkorn MJ, Mandigers J. Reduction of bacteriuria and pyuria after using cranberry juice. *JAMA* 1994;272:590.

14. Smith SD, Wheeler MA, Foster HE Jr., Weiss RM. Improvement in interstitial cystitis symptom scores during treatment with oral L-arginine. *J Urol* 1997;158:703–8.

16. EXERCISE AND ENDORPHINS

1. Granges G, Littlejohn GO. A comparative study of clinical signs in fibromyalgia/fibrositis syndrome, healthy and exercising subjects. *J Rheumatol* 1993; 20:344–51.
2. Janal MN, Colt EWD, Clark WC, Glusman M. Pain sensitivity, mood and plasma endocrine levels in man following long-distance running: effects of naloxone. *Pain* 1984;19:13–25.

17. REST AND SLEEP

1. Moldofsky H, Scarisbrick P. Induction of neurasthenic musculoskeletal pain syndrome by selective sleep stage deprivation. *Psychosomatic Med* 1976; 38:35–44.
2. McCain GA, Bell DA, Mai FM, Halliday PD. A controlled study of the effects of a supervised cardiovascular fitness training program on the manifestations of primary fibromyalgia. *Arthritis Rheum* 1988;31:1135–41.
3. von Wartburg JP, Buhler R. Alcoholism and aldehydism. *New Biomedical Concepts* 1984;50:5–15.

18. YOGURT AND CORN DOGS: WHY OUR BODIES REBEL AGAINST CERTAIN FOODS

1. Alun Jones V. Comparison of total parenteral nutrition and elemental diet in induction of remission of Crohn's disease: long-term maintenance of remission by personalized food exclusion diets. *Dig Dis Sci* 1987;32(suppl):100S–107S.
2. Blau JN, Diamond S. Dietary factors in migraine precipitation: the physicians' view. *Headache* 1985;25:184–87.
3. Curtis-Brown R. A protein poison theory: its application to the treatment of headache and especially migraine. *Br Med J* 1925;1:155–56.
4. Darlington LG, Ramsey NW. Review of dietary therapy for rheumatoid arthritis. *Br J Rheum* 1993;32:507–14.
5. Egger J, Carter CM, Wilson J, Turner MW. Is migraine food allergy? A double-blind controlled trial of oligoantigenic diet treatment. *Lancet* 1983; 2:865–69.

6. Eyermann CH. Allergic headache. *J Allergy* 1930;2:106–12.

7. McClure CW, Huntsinger ME. Observations on migraine. *Boston Med Surg J* 1927;196:270–73.

8. Glover V, Littlewood J, Sandler M, Peatfield R, Petty R, Rose FC. Biochemical predisposition to dietary migraine: the role of phenolsulphotransferase. *Headache* 1983;23:53–58.

9. Guariso G, Bertoli S, Cernetti R, Battistella PA, Setari M, Zacchello F. Emicrania e intolleranza alimentare: studio controllato in età evolutiva. *Ped Med Chir* 1993;15:57–61.

10. Hicklin JA, McEwen LM, Morgan JE. The effect of diet in rheumatoid arthritis. *Clin Allergy* 1980;10:463.

11. Jaffe RM, Deuster PA. A novel treatment for fibromyalgia improves clinical outcomes in a community-based study. Presented to the Annual Conference of the Clinical Immunology Society, New Orleans, May 31–June 3, 1996.

12. Mansfield LE, Vaughan TR, Waller SF, Haverly RW, Ting S. Food allergy and adult migraine: double-blind and mediator confirmation of an allergic etiology. *Ann Allergy* 1985;55:126–29.

13. McClure CW, Huntsinger ME. Observations on migraine. *Boston Med Surg J* 1927;196:270–73.

14. Panush RS, Carter RL, Katz P, Kowsari B, Longley S, Finnie S. Diet therapy for rheumatoid arthritis. *Arth Rheum* 1983;26:462–71.

15. Parke AC, Hughes GRV. Rheumatoid arthritis and food. A case study. *BMJ* 1981;282:2027–29.

16. Pearson M, Teahon K, Jonathan Levi A, Bjarnason I. Food intolerance and Crohn's disease. *Gut* 1993;34:783–87.

17. Peatfield RC. Relationships between food, wine, and beer-precipitated migrainous headaches. *Headache* 1995;35:355–57.

18. Solomon S. Migraine diagnosis and clinical symptomatology. *Headache* 1994;34:S8–S12.

19. van de Laar MAFJ, van der Korst JK. Food intolerance in rheumatoid arthritis. I. A double blind, controlled trial of the clinical effects of elimination of milk allergens and azo dyes. *Ann Rheum Dis* 1992;51:298–302.

20. van de Laar MAFJ, Aalbers M, Bruins FG, van Dinther-Janssen ACHM, van der Korst JK, Meijer CJLM. Food intolerance in rheumatoid arthritis. I. Clinical and histological aspects. *Ann Rheum Dis* 1992;51:303–6.

21. Williams R. Rheumatoid arthritis and food: a case study. *BMJ* 1981;283:563.

22. Leakey R. The origin of humankind. New York, Basic Books, 1994, p. 21.

23. McGee H. On food and cooking: the science and lore of the kitchen. New York, Macmillan, 1984, p. 3.

24. Cramer DW, Xu H, Sahi T. Adult hypolactasia, milk consumption, and age-specific fertility. *Am J Epidemiol* 1994;139:282–89.
25. Outwater JL, Nicholson A, Barnard ND. Dairy products and breast cancer: the IGF-1, estrogen, and bGH hypothesis. *Med Hypoth* 1997;48:453–61.
26. Trager J. The food chronology. New York, Henry Holt, 1995, p. 8.
27. McGee, op cit., 220.
28. Barnard ND. The power of your plate. Summertown, Tenn., Book Publishing, 1995, p. 172–73.

Resources

Allergy Resources, Inc.
745 Powderhorn
Monument, CO 80132
(800) USE-FLAX
Mail order source of specialty flours, cereals, pasta, and many other foods.

American Holistic Medical Association
4101 Lake Boone Trail
Suite 201
Raleigh, NC 27607
(919) 787-5146
AHMA has a referral network of holistic physicians.

Arrowhead Mills, Inc.
Box 2059
Hereford, TX 79045
Wide selection of grains and flours; available in most natural food stores and some supermarkets.

Eden Foods, Inc.
701 Tecumseh Rd.
Clinton, MI 49236
(800) 248-0301
(517) 456-7424
Gluten-free pasta products; soy and rice milks; sold in natural food stores and some supermarkets.

Ener-G Foods, Inc.
P.O. Box 24723

6901 Fox Ave. S.
Seattle, WA 98124
(206) 767-6660
Gluten-free rice bread, egg replacer; sold in many natural food stores.

Featherweight Baking Powder
Sandoz Nutrition Corporation
P.O. Box 40
405 E. Shawmut Avenue
LaGrange, IL 60525
(312) 352-6900
Featherweight Baking Powder (gluten-free); sold in many natural food stores.

Food for Life Baking Co., Inc.
P.O. Box 1434
Corona, CA 91718-1434
(800) 797-5090
Rice bread and rice pastas; sold in many natural food stores.

The Kushi Institute
P.O. Box 7
Becket, MA 01223
(800) 975-8744
(413) 623-5741
The Kushi Institute offers information on macrobiotic diets.

Physicians Committee for Responsible Medicine
5100 Wisconsin Avenue
Suite 404
Washington, DC 20016
(202) 686-2210
www.pcrm.org
PCRM publishes Good Medicine, *a quarterly magazine of emerging information on health, nutrition, and research controversies.*

Special Foods
9207 Shotgun Ct.
Springfield, VA 22153
(703) 644-0991
Large selection of gluten-free pasta products; sold in many natural food stores.

Transitions for Health
(800-648-8211) is a reliable source of natural progesterone cream, which is useful in treating osteoporosis, menstrual problems, and other conditions.

Recommended Reading

NUTRITION INFORMATION

Akers, Keith. *A Vegetarian Sourcebook*. Vegetarian Press, 1993.

Attwood, Charles. *Dr. Attwood's Low-Fat Prescription for Kids*. Viking, 1995.

Barnard, Neal. *Eat Right, Live Longer*. Harmony Books, 1995.

Barnard, Neal. *Food for Life*. Harmony Books, 1993.

Barnard, Neal. *The Power of Your Plate*. Book Publishing Company, 1994.

Fuhrmann, Joel. *Fasting—and Eating—for Health*. St. Martin's Press, 1995.

Kushi, Michio. *The Cancer Prevention Diet*. St. Martin's Press, 1993.

Ludington, Aileen, and Hans Diehl. *Lifestyle Capsules*. Woodbridge Press, 1991.

McDougall, John. *The McDougall Program*. Plume Books, 1991.

Melina, Vasanto, Brenda Davis, and Victoria Harrison. *Becoming Vegetarian*. Book Publishing Company, 1995.

Messina, Virginia, and Mark Messina. *The Vegetarian Way*. Crown Trade Paperbacks, 1996.

Moran, Victoria. *Get the Fat Out: 501 Simple Ways*. Crown Trade Paperbacks, 1994.

———. *The Love-Powered Diet*. New World Library, 1992.

Ornish, Dean. *Dr. Dean Ornish's Program for Reversing Heart Disease*. Random House, 1990.

———. *Eat More, Weigh Less*. HarperCollins, 1993.

COOKBOOKS

Diamond, Marilyn. *The American Vegetarian Cookbook*. Warner Books, 1990.

Dumke, Nicolette M. *Allergy Cooking with Ease*. Starburst Publishers, 1992.

Frazier, Claude A. *Coping with Food Allergy.* Times Books, 1985.

Havala, Suzanne. *Simple, Low-Fat, and Vegetarian.* Vegetarian Resource Group, 1994.

Jones, Marjorie Hurt. *The Allergy Self-Help Cookbook.* Rodale Books, 1984.

Ornish, Dean. *Everyday Cooking with Dr. Dean Ornish.* HarperCollins, 1996.

People for the Ethical Treatment of Animals. *The Compassionate Cook.* Warner Books, 1993.

Raymond, Jennifer. *Fat-Free & Easy.* Heart & Soul Publications, 1997.

———. *The Peaceful Palate.* Heart & Soul Publications, 1992.

Sass, Lorna. *Great Vegetarian Cooking Under Pressure.* William Morrow & Co., 1994.

———. *Recipes from an Ecological Kitchen.* William Morrow and Co., 1982.

Shattuck, Ruth R. *The Allergy Cookbook.* New American Library, 1984.

Stepaniak, Joanne, and Kathy Hecker. *Ecological Cooking.* Book Publishing Co., 1991.

———. *The Uncheese Cookbook.* Book Publishing Co., 1994.

Wasserman, Debra. *Conveniently Vegan.* Vegetarian Resource Group, 1997.

Wasserman, Debra, and Reed Mangels. *Simply Vegan.* Vegetarian Resource Group, 1991.

Yoder, Eileen Rhude. *Allergy-Free Cooking.* Addison-Wesley, 1990.

Index

Acupuncture, 4, 60
adenomyosis, 140
ALA (alpha-linolenic acid), 80–85
alcohol
  effects on bones, 21
  effects on sleep, 207
  headaches and, 65, 66
  help in preventing kidney stones, 195
  link to breast cancer, 155
  link to carpal tunnel syndrome, 170
  wine, 49–50, 65, 77–78
allergens, 51
  ELISA/ACT test, 119–20
  sinus headaches, 43, 67–68
alpha-linolenic acid. See ALA
amino acids, 183–84, 196, 199
  See also tryptophan
animal products
  as arthritis trigger, 79
  avoiding in diabetes diet, 176
  avoiding to prevent migraines, 47–48
  effect on kidneys, 190, 195–97
  eggs, 27, 216
  proteins, 16, 17, 19
  See also dairy products; meat
ankylosing spondylitis, 8
anthropologists, 212, 215
antibiotics, 92, 98, 107
antidepressants, 70, 122, 173, 177, 185
antioxidants, 86, 89–90, 94
  See also beta-carotene; vitamin E
apples
  poached, 253
  sauce, 236
apricot-pineapple gel, 249
arginine, 183, 184
arteries
  blocked, 11–13, 23, 27
  coronary, 33

lumbar, xiii, 11–14
  preventing blockages, 12–13
  reversing blockages, 13–14, 23–26,
    37–38, 204
arthritis
  food triggers, xv, 72, 74–79, 80, 225
  reducing inflammation, 80–87
  stopping joint damage, 89–91
  treatments, 73, 92–94
  See also rheumatoid arthritis
Asian diets, benefits of, 13, 57–58, 148,
  154
asparagus soup, 240–41
aspartame, 64–65

Back. See back pain; osteoporosis
back pain
  causes, xii–xiv, 7–8, 9, 11–12, 14
  in children, 9
  preventing, xiii–xiv
  surgery, 9–10
  treatments, 10–11, 14–16, 21–22
baking powder, 299–300
bananas, 132, 217
  cake, 294–95
barley, 263
  breakfast, 254
  mushroom soup, 274
  pancakes, 256–57
  scones, 258–59
  spinach barleycakes, 282
  tortillas, 263–64
  waffles, 258
Barnett, Martha, 50
basil-lover's green beans, 244
beans
  basil-lover's green beans, 244
  benefits, 106, 132
  black-bean chili, 288

black-bean sauce, 272, 280
black-bean tamale pie, 286
burritos, 289
calcium in, 18, 19
digestive problems, 106
dip, 271
ensalada de frijoles, 265
garbanzo, 264, 270, 272–73, 278–79
rice and greens with, 290–91
beef. *See* meat
beet soup, 239
beta-carotene, 32, 89–90, 140, 162
beverages
date cooler, 250
rice milk, 252
strawberry smoothie, 294
biofeedback, 60
black-bean chili, 288
black-bean sauce, 272, 280
black-bean tamale pie, 286
black currant oil, 81, 82, 83–84, 115
blood pressure, controlling, 37–38
blood vessel abnormalities, 43
bones. *See* osteoporosis
borage oil, 81, 82, 83–84, 115, 144
braised cabbage, 244
braised kale or collard greens, 245
braised summer squash, 245
breakfast barley, 254
breakfast rice pudding, 235
breast cancer, 20, 104, 153–57, 159
breastfeeding, 110, 137–38
breast pain, 142–45
breathing exercises, 207–8, 209
broccoli
burritos, 291
with kasha and black-bean sauce,
280
soup, 273
with tahini sauce, 276
brown rice, 238–39
buckwheat, 262
pancakes, 257
Burdick, Bruce, 178–79
Burmeister, Ronald, 138–39
burritos
bean, 289
broccoli, 291

Cabbage
braised, 244
kasha with, 275
red, salad, 268–69
rolls, 248
caffeine, 16, 137, 143–44, 195, 207, 215
caffeine withdrawal headaches, 43, 52
cake, banana, 294–95
calcium
amount needed, 19
dietary sources, 18, 19, 195
in kidney stones, 192–93, 196
loss of, 16–18, 131, 197
as menstrual pain aid, 130–31
migraines and, 51, 56, 60
cancer, 150
breast, 20, 104, 153–57, 159
causes, 150
colon, 159–60
diet and, 146–51, 152–53, 156, 160,
161–62
of digestive tract, 159–61
of esophagus, 160
feeling to blame for, 158–59
ovarian, 104, 157–58, 159
pain medications, 147, 162–63
pancreatic, 161
prostate, 147, 151–53
stomach, 99, 160–61
uterine, 157–58, 159
canker sores, 184
capsaicin, 3, 67, 93–94, 157, 179, 185–86
carbohydrates, 121, 175–76, 177
carpal tunnel syndrome, 167–72
carrots
pudding, 251
soup, 240
cars, vibrations, 14
cataracts, 104
cauliflower, and green-pea soup, 241
celiac disease, 101
cheese, 218
See also dairy products
chemical headaches, 64–65
chemicals, environmental, 65, 119–20, 137,
155
chest pains. *See* heart disease
chicken. *See* meat

chicken pox, 184
chickpeas, hummus, 269
children
    back pain, 9
    digestive problems, 111
    juvenile-onset diabetes, 174, 180–81
    risks of dairy products to, 180–81
chili, black-bean, 288
chili peppers. *See* capsaicin
chiropractic treatments, 4, 22
chocolate, 49, 50, 77–78, 215, 218
cholesterol, 26–27
    in foods, 27, 29
    HDL ("good"), 34, 35–36
    lowering, 14, 28–32, 36–37
    negative effects on immune system, 140
    tests, 33–34, 35
chronic fatigue syndrome, 116–18, 121–22
claudication, 24, 33
cluster headaches, 42–43, 62, 65–67
cobalamin. *See* vitamin B$_{12}$
coffee, 52, 59, 105, 215
    See also caffeine
cold sores, 182–84, 186–87
colic, 110, 217
collard greens, braised, 245
colon cancer, 159–60
condiments, 107
    See also spices
cookies, oatmeal, 295
corn, 214–15
    as arthritis trigger, 78
    ingredients derived from, 227, 299
    recipes, 265, 266–67, 298
corn oil, 30
cranberry juice, 198–99
Crane, Milton, 173–74, 177
cream of asparagus soup, 240–41
creamy broccoli soup, 273
creamy carrot soup, 240
creamy cucumber dip, 270
creamy dill dressing, 268
creamy yams, 277
crispy green salad, 267
Crohn's disease, 111–15
cucumbers, dip, 270
curry, vegetable, 293
cyanate, 190–91

cyanocobalamin. *See* vitamin B$_{12}$
cyclic mastalgia. *See* breast pain

Dairy products
    as arthritis trigger, 75–76, 77
    calcium in, 17, 19
    digestive problems, 103–5, 113–14,
        213–14
    health effects of, 213–14
    ingredients derived from, 227
    risks to children, 180–81
    sinus headaches and, 68
    See also animal products; milk
dates
    cooler, 250
    muffins, 259
    spread, 254
DeCosse, Jerome J., 160
degenerative joint disease. *See*
    osteoarthritis
deglycyrrhizinated licorice (DGL), 99
desserts. *See* fruits, *specific recipes*
diabetes, 174–75
    adult-onset, 174
    diets for, 175–79, 180
    exercise and, 176–77, 178, 180
    juvenile-onset, 174, 180–81
    pains associated with, 2–3, 173–74, 179
digestive problems, 97
    celiac disease, 101
    changing eating habits, 109–10
    in children, 111
    colic, 110, 217
    Crohn's disease, 111–15
    diverticulitis, 111
    heartburn, 99
    inflammatory bowel disease, 111–15
    irritable bowel syndrome (IBS),
        100–109
    ulcerative colitis, 111–12, 114, 115
    ulcers, 97–99
digestive tract, cancers, 159–61
dips
    creamy cucumber, 270
    garbanzo spread, 270
    quick bean, 271
directed breathing, 207–8
disks. *See* back pain

diverticulitis, 111
dried fruit compote, 237

Eating habits, 109–10
eggs, 27, 216
    See also animal products
elimination diet, 47–49, 228–30
    menus, 230–33
    recipes, 234–54
ELISA/ACT allergy test, 119–20
Ellis, John, 168
endometriosis, 136–40
endorphins, 3–4, 61, 203
enkephalins, 3
ensalada de frijoles, 265
esophagus, cancer of, 160
estrogens
    breast cells stimulated by, 142–43
    in cow's milk, 155
    effects on fibroids, 135
    effects of food on levels, 57–58, 127–30,
        143, 171
    elimination of, 57, 129, 131
    joint pain and, 93, 95–96
    levels in menstrual cycle, 127
    link to breast cancer, 154
    link to carpal tunnel syndrome, 170–71
    plant sources, 133–34, 155
    supplements, 19–20
evening primrose oil, 81, 82, 83–84, 115,
    144
evolution, 212–13
exercise
    aerobic, 10, 139, 203
    amount of, 204–5
    benefits, 16, 37, 176–77, 178, 180, 203–4,
        206–7
    effects on hormones, 139
    increased pain resistance, 3–4, 117,
        203–4
    sickle-cell anemia and, 191
    stress-reducing, 207–10
eyes, resting, 209

Fats
    balancing, 90
    effects on estrogen levels, 57, 127–30,
        143, 154

effects on immune system, 140
effects on insulin, 175
effects on testosterone levels, 152
irritable bowel syndrome and, 101–2
reducing in diet, 14, 28–31, 85, 102
saturated, 28, 31
topping substitutes, 31
triglycerides, 34–35
unsaturated, 28
    See also ALA; GLA; omega-3 fatty
        acids
feverfew, 51, 52–53
fiber
    benefits for sugar absorption, 176
    effects on estrogen levels, 57, 143
    foods high in, 111
    soluble, 31, 101
fibroids, 135
fibromyalgia, 8, 116–17, 118–22
fish oils, 83–84, 90
5-hydroxytryptophan, 15
flatbread, garbanzo, 264
flax oil, 81, 82, 83–84, 115
folic acid, 32–33, 190
Folkers, Karl, 168
food groups, 30, 221
foods
    benefits of changing diet, 219–20
    diets of early humans, 212, 215–16, 218
    fighting pain with, xiv-xvi, 2–4
    processed, 226–28
food sensitivities
    arthritis triggers, xv, 72, 74–79, 80, 225
    blood tests, 49, 119–20
    ingredients in processed foods, 226–28
    irritable bowel syndrome and, 101–7
    kidney stones and, 195–97
    migraine triggers, 41–43, 44–45, 46,
        49–50
    multi-symptom triggers, 211–16,
        217–18, 225–28
Fothergill, John, 44
four-seven-eight breathing, 209
free radicals, 89–91
French toast, 234
French vegetable salad, 243
fresh peach shortcake, 296
fruit creme, 296–97

fruited breakfast quinoa, 255
fruit gel, 249
fruits
 citrus, 77, 214
 in elimination diet, 230
 juices, 105
 raw, 86, 105
 recipes, 236–37, 249, 250, 251, 252–54,
  256, 294–97

Gamma-linolenic acid. *See* GLA
garbanzo flatbread, 264
garbanzo gravy, 272–73, 278–79
garbanzo spread, 270
garlic, 32, 87–88
gastric lymphoma, 99
gastritis, 98
genital herpes, 182–84, 186–87
ginger, 51
 anti-inflammatory effects, 86–87, 141
 as back pain aid, 15–16
 as digestive aid, 108–9
 as migraine treatment, 52, 54, 60
GLA (gamma-linolenic acid), 81–84, 86,
  115, 132, 133, 144, 145
glaucoma, headaches and, 43
gout, 94–95
grains
 digestive problems, 105
 quinoa, 255, 261
 whole, 132, 176
 See also barley; oats; rice; wheat
green-pea and cauliflower soup, 241
Griffith, Richard, 184

Headaches
 blood vessel abnormalities, 43
 caffeine withdrawal, 43, 52
 chemical, 64–65
 cluster, 42–43, 62, 65–67
 consulting physicians about, 44
 as glaucoma symptom, 43
 premenstrual, 55, 132
 sinus, 43, 67–68
 temporal arteritis, 43
 tension, 43, 60, 68–70
 See also migraines
heartburn, 99

heart disease, 23, 33, 34
 lowering cholesterol, 28–32
 reversing blockages, 23–26, 37–38
helicobacter bacteria, 98–99
hemp oil, 115
herbs. *See* feverfew
herpes simplex virus type 1 (HSV-1),
  182–84, 186–87
herpes simplex virus type 2 (HSV-2),
  182–84, 186–87
herpes zoster (shingles), 184–87
histamine, 49–51, 66
homestyle millet with garbanzo gravy,
  278–79
homocysteine, 32–33
hormone replacement therapy. *See*
  estrogens; progesterone
hormones
 breast pain and, 142–43
 carpal tunnel syndrome and, 170–71
 effects of aerobic exercise, 139
 in menstrual cycle, 49, 57–58, 127,
  142–43
 migraines and, 49
 testosterone, 21, 152, 153
hummus, 269

IBS. *See* irritable bowel syndrome
immune system, 74, 137, 140, 161–62,
  186
Indian pudding, 298
infants
 breastfeeding, 110, 137–38
 colic, 110, 217
 foods tolerated by, 216–17
inflammation, reducing, 80–87
inflammatory bowel disease, 111–15
ingredients, descriptions, 301–4
insulin, 174, 175
interstitial cystitis, 199
iron, 32, 90–91, 190
irritable bowel syndrome (IBS), 100–109

Jaffe, Russell M., 119–20
Japan. *See* Asian diets
joints. *See* arthritis; temporomandibular
  joint pain
juvenile-onset diabetes, 174, 180–81

Kale
  braised, 245
  red potatoes with, 279
kasha
  broccoli with, 280
  with cabbage, 275
kidney stones, 192–97, 198

Lactose, 103–5, 158, 213–14
L-arginine, 199
Lee, John, 58, 171
lentil burgers, 284
licorice, 99
low-fat vegetarian diet. *See* vegetarian
    diet
lumbar arteries, xiii, 11–14
lycopene, 152–53
lysine, 183–84, 185

Macrobiotic diet, 147–50, 153
magnesium, 18, 51, 55, 118, 122, 132
malaria, 189
Marshall, Barry, 98
mastectomies, pain following, 157
McGee, Harold, 106
meals
  eating habits, 109–10
  elimination diet menus, 230–33
measurements, conversion chart, 305
meat
  carcinogens in, 159
  cholesterol in, 27
  fats in, 28
  in human diet, 215–16
  ingredients derived from, 227
  iron in, 32, 91
  See also animal products
medication. *See* antidepressants;
    painkillers
men
  impotence, 12
  osteoporosis, 21
  prostate cancer, 147, 151–53
menopausal symptoms, reducing, 134
menstrual cycles, 49, 57–58, 127,
    142–43
menstrual pain
  causes, 126, 136–40

foods to help reduce, 125, 126–30, 132–34
  treatments, 130–32, 134–35, 141
menus, elimination diet, 230–33
Mexican corn salad, 266–67
migraines, 41, 42
  elimination diet, 47–49
  food triggers, 41–43, 44–45, 46, 49–50
  hormones and, 57
  pain-safe foods, 45–46, 47, 55, 58
  prevention, 42, 62–63
  treatments, 42, 51–56, 59–61
milk
  babies' intolerance of, 110, 217
  cholesterol in, 27
  digestive problems, 103–5, 213–14
  link to cancer risks, 155, 158
  link to diabetes in children, 180–81
  skim, 25
  substitutes, 105
  See also dairy products
millet, 191, 278–79
mixed fruit muffins, 260–61
monosodium glutamate (MSG), 64
Moore, Ellen, 125
motion sickness, 108–9
muffins
  date, 259
  mixed fruit, 260–61
  yam spice, 260
mushrooms
  barley soup, 274
  pan-grilled portobello, 288–89
Musickant, Claire, 119, 120

Neat loaf, 283
neck circles, 208–9
nerves, 2–3, 7
niacin, 36–37
Nicholson, Andrew, 178
noradrenaline, 177, 185
nori rolls, 292
Norman, Greg, 208
NutraSweet, 64–65
nutritional supplements, xvi
  back pain aids, 14–16
  vitamins, 33, 186, 190
  See also specific nutrients
nuts, 32, 106, 132, 216

Oats, 31, 101
  oatmeal, 255
  oatmeal Cookies, 295
oils
  botanical, 81, 82, 83–84, 115, 144
  fish, 83–84, 90
  olive, 30
  peppermint, 108
  See also vegetable oils
olive oil, 30
omega-3 fatty acids, 83–84, 86, 115,
    132–33
Ornish, Dean, xiv, 13, 24–25, 204
Oski, Frank, 181
osteoarthritis, 73, 92–94
  See also arthritis
osteoporosis, 16–18, 20–21
ovarian cancer, 104, 157–58, 159
oven fries, 246
oven-roasted vegetables, 277
oxalates, 192–93, 195, 197

Pain
  fighting with foods, xiv-xvi, 2–4
  increasing resistance to, 15
  nutrients' roles in reducing, xii
  sensitivity to, xv, 177
  as series of reactions, 1
  strategies to fight, 1–4
painkillers, 4
  for arthritis, 73, 80
  for back pain, 22
  for cancer, 147, 162–63
  for migraines, 60–61
  narcotic, 147, 162–63, 189
  overuse of, 61
  for sickle-cell crises, 189
  for tension headaches, 69
pancakes
  barley, 256–57
  buckwheat, 257
  rice, 235
pancreatic cancer, 161
pan-grilled portobello mushrooms,
    288–89
Panush, Richard S., 76
pasta, rice, 247
Pauling, Linus, 197

peaches
  shortcake, 296
  sorbet, 251
  sweet potatoes and, 238
peanuts, 216
pears, poached, 252
peas
  black-eyed, 287
  green-pea and cauliflower soup, 241
peppermint oil, 108
peppers. *See* capsaicin
pesto, zucchini, 271
physicians, xvi-xviii
Physicians Committee for Responsible
    Medicine (PCRM), 222
phytoestrogens, 133–34, 155
pineapple
  apricot gel, 249
  yams with, 246–47
poached apples, 253
poached pears, 252
portobello mushrooms, 288–89
postherpetic neuralgia, 185, 187
potassium, 194
potatoes
  boats, 285
  oven fries, 246
  red, with kale, 279
  vegetable soup, 242
potato starch, 299
pregnancy, carpal tunnel syndrome
    during, 170
premenstrual pain, 55, 130–31, 132, 135
primates, diet of, 215, 217
Pro-Gest, 20, 22, 58, 134–35, 144
progesterone, 143
  natural, 20, 58, 134–35, 139, 144,
    171–72
  supplements, 20
progesterone cream. *See* Pro-Gest
progressive relaxation, 208
prostaglandins, 82–83, 126, 132–33
prostate cancer, 147, 151–53
protein
  animal, 16, 17, 19
  dietary sources, 221
  effect on sleep, 206
  plant, 16

prunes
    puree, 253
    stewed, 237
    whip, 250
puddings
    carrot, 251
    Indian, 298
    peachy sweet potatoes, 238
    quick breakfast, 256
    rice, 235
    tapioca, 250
pyridoxine. *See* vitamin B₆

Quinoa, 255, 261

Raymond, Jennifer, 128
red cabbage salad, 268–69
relaxation techniques, 69, 70, 207–10
rheumatoid arthritis
    diet, 78–80
    food triggers, xv, 72, 74–79, 80
    pain-safe foods, 77, 79
    reducing inflammation, 80–87
    in spine, 8
    treatment with antibiotics, 92
rice, 101
    and beans with greens, 290–91
    brown, 238–39
    milk, 252
    pancakes, 235
    pasta, 247
    pudding, 235
    seasoned, 262
    wild, 239
Rootin' Tootin' salad, 266

Salad dressings, 31
    creamy dill, 268
salads
    crispy green, 267
    ensalada de frijoles, 265
    French vegetable, 243
    Mexican corn, 266–67
    red cabbage, 268–69
    Rootin' Tootin', 266
salt, sesame, 298
    See also sodium
Sandys, George, 215

Sattilaro, Anthony J., 146–50
sauces
    black-bean, 272, 280
    garbanzo gravy, 272–73, 278–79
Scherwitz, Larry, 25
Scialli, Anthony, 128
scones, barley, 258–59
selenium, 89, 162
serotonin, 4, 15, 120–21, 177, 206
sesame salt, 298
sesame seasoning, 299
sex-hormone binding globulin (SHBG),
    152, 155
shingles, 184–87
shortcake, peach and strawberry, 296
sickle-cell anemia, 188–91
simple black-eyed stew, 287
sinus headaches, 43, 67–68
sleep, 206–7
smoking, 16, 37, 156, 170
sodium
    in foods, 194–95
    high-sodium diets, 121
    increased risk of kidney stones, 194,
        197
    reducing intake, 16, 194
sorbets, peach, 251
soups
    beet, 239
    carrot, 240
    cream of asparagus, 240–41
    creamy broccoli, 273
    green-pea and cauliflower, 241
    mushroom barley, 274
    potato-vegetable, 242
    vegetable, 242–43
soy products
    cholesterol-lowering effect, 31–32
    ingredients derived from, 228
    phytoestrogens, 133–34
    progesterone in, 20
spastic colon. *See* irritable bowel
    syndrome
spices, 87–88, 107
    See also garlic; ginger
spinach barleycakes, 282
spinal stenosis, 7–8, 10
spine. *See* back pain; osteoporosis

Spock, Benjamin, 181
squash
    summer, 245
    winter, 276
    See also zucchini
starches, in elimination diet, 229
steamed yams, 247
stews
    simple black-eyed, 287
    summer vegetable, 274–75
stimulants, 207
stomach
    cancer, 99, 160–61
    See also digestive problems
strawberries
    applesauce, 236
    shortcake, 296
    smoothie, 294
stress
    reducing, 37, 122, 207–10
    as trigger for herpes viruses, 186–87
substance P. *See* capsaicin
sugar
    absorption by body, 175–76
    calcium loss increased by, 17, 197
    in foods, 197
    in milk. *See* milk
    pain tolerance reduced by, 177
    as sleep aid, 206
summer fruit cobbler, 297
summer fruit compote, 237
summer vegetable stew, 274–75
sushi, 292
sweet potatoes, peachy, 238

Tapioca pudding, 250
tea, 105, 215
    See also caffeine
temporal arteritis, 43
temporomandibular joint (TMJ) pain, 95–96
tension headaches, 43, 60, 68–70
testosterone, 21, 152, 153
thunder-god vine, 88
TMJ. *See* temporomandibular joint pain
tobacco. *See* smoking
tomatoes, 152–53, 214

triglycerides, 34–35
tryptophan, 4, 15, 121, 214–15
turmeric, 87–88

Ulcerative colitis, 111–12, 114, 115
ulcers, 97–99
uric acid, 94, 192–93, 196
urinary infections, 198–99
uterus
    adenomyosis, 140
    cancer, 157–58, 159
    endometriosis, 136–40
    fibroids, 135

Vegetable oils, 28, 30, 31, 176
vegetables
    curry, 293
    in elimination diet, 229
    fiber in, 101
    oven-roasted, 277
    raw, 86, 105–6
    salads, 243, 265–67
    soups, 242–43
    stews, 274–75, 287
vegetarian diet
    artery blockages reversed by, 24–26, 28–31
    benefits for breastfeeding, 137–38
    calcium loss reduced by, 16
    cancer risk lowered by, 156, 161
    for diabetics, 177, 180
    food groups, 30, 221
    lowering cholesterol with, 28–31
    low-fat, 14, 28–32, 36, 120, 156
    recipes, 254–99
vertebrae. *See* back pain
visualization, 210
vitamin B₃ (niacin), 36–37
vitamin B₆
    for back pain, 15
    benefits for diabetes, 179
    benefits for heart disease, 32–33
    for carpal tunnel syndrome, 168–70
    dietary sources, 132, 169, 170
    dosages, 15, 55, 169
    for menstrual pain, 131–32
    for premenstrual headaches, 55
    for TMJ pain, 95

vitamin B$_{12}$, 30, 32–33, 221–22
vitamin C, 32, 89–90, 140, 162, 197
vitamin D, 17, 21, 56, 197, 221
vitamin E
    antioxidant benefits, 89–90
    as arthritis treatment, 93
    benefits for cholesterol levels, 32
    benefits for immune system, 140, 162
    for sickle-cell anemia, 190
    taking with botanical oils, 83

Waffles, barley, 258
walnuts, 32
water, drinking, 193
weight loss, 219
Weil, Andrew, 209
wheat, 59–60
    as arthritis trigger, 78
    digestive problems, 105, 113–14, 214
    ingredients derived from, 227–28
    substitutes, 47
wild brown rice, 239
wine, 49–50, 65, 77–78

women
    breast cancer, 20, 104, 153–57, 159
    breast pain, 142–45
    cancer of uterus and ovary, 104, 157–58, 159
    endometriosis, 136–40
    pregnancy, 170
    premenstrual pain, 55, 130–31, 132, 135
    See also menstrual pain
Wynder, Ernst, 156

Yams, 20, 191
    creamy, 277
    with pineapple, 246–47
    spice muffins, 260
    steamed, 247
yogurt, 107
    See also dairy products

Zucchini
    basil-lover's green beans, 244
    pesto, 247, 271
    skillet hash, 281

Conversion Chart
EQUIVALENT IMPERIAL AND METRIC MEASUREMENTS

American cooks use standard containers, the 8-ounce cup and a tablespoon that takes exactly 16 level fillings to fill that cup level. Measuring by cup makes it very difficult to give weight equivalents, as a cup of densely packed butter will weigh considerably more than a cup of flour. The easiest way therefore to deal with cup measurements in recipes is to take the amount by volume rather than by weight. Thus the equation reads:

1 cup = 240 ml = 8 fl. oz.
½ cup = 120 ml = 4 fl. oz.

It is possible to buy a set of American cup measures in major stores around the world.

In the States, butter is often measured in sticks. One stick is the equivalent of 8 tablespoons. One tablespoon of butter is therefore the equivalent to ½ ounce/15 grams.

LIQUID MEASURES

Fluid Ounces	U.S.	Imperial	Milliliters
	1 tsp	1 tsp	5
¼	2 tsps	1 dessertspoon	10
½	1 tb	1 tbn	14
1	2 tbs	2 tbs	28
2	¼ cup	4 tbs	56
4	½ cup		110
5		¼ pt or 1 gill	140
6	¾ cup		170
8	1 cup		225
9			250, ¼ liter
10	1¼ cups	½ pt	280
12	1½ cups		340
15		¾ pt	420
16	2 cups		450
18	2¼ cups		500, ½ liter
20	2½ cups	1 pt	560
24	3 cups or 1½ pts		675
25		1¼ pts	700
27	3½ cups		750, ¾ liter
30	3¾ cups	1½ pts	840
32	4 cups or 2 pts or 1 qt		900
35		1¾ pts	980
36	4½ cups		1000, 1 liter
40	5 cups	2 pts or 1 qt	1120

SOLID MEASURES

U.S. and Imperial		Metric	
Ounces	Pounds	Grams	Kilos
1		28	
2		56	
3½		100	
4	¼	112	
5		140	
6		168	
8	½	225	
9		250	¼
12	¾	340	
16	1	450	

OVEN TEMPERATURE EQUIVALENTS

F	C	Gas Mark	Description
225	110	¼	Cool
250	130	½	
275	140	1	Very Slow
300	150	2	
325	170	3	Slow
350	180	4	Moderate
375	190	5	
400	200	6	Moderately Hot
425	220	7	Fairly Hot
450	230	8	Hot
475	240	9	Very Hot
500	250	10	Extremely Hot

Any broiling recipes can be used with the grill of the oven, but beware of high-temperature grills.

EQUIVALENTS FOR INGREDIENTS

all-purpose flour—plain flour
arugula—rocket
beet—beetroot
coarse salt—kitchen salt
cornstarch—cornflour
eggplant—aubergine
fava beans—broad beans
granulated sugar—caster sugar
lima beans—broad beans
scallion—spring onion
shortening—white fat
snow pea—mangetout
squash—courgettes or marrow
unbleached flour—strong, white flour
zest—rind
zucchini—courgettes or marrow
baking sheet—oven tray
plastic wrap—cling film